Bottom Line's

Breakthroughs in
Natural
Healing
2011

Bill Gottlieb
and the Editors of Bottom Line Publications

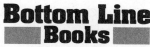
**Bottom Line
Books**
www.BottomLineSecrets.com

Bottom Line's Breakthroughs in Natural Healing 2011
Bill Gottlieb and the Editors of Bottom Line Publications

Copyright © 2010 by Boardroom® Inc.

10   9   8   7   6   5   4   3   2   1

Cover design by Aimee Zaleski and Gretchen Bruno

ISBN 0-88723-606-5

Bottom Line Books® publishes the advice of expert authorities in many fields. These opinions
may at times conflict as there are often different approaches to solving problems. The use
of a book is not a substitute for legal, accounting, investment, health or any other professional
services. Consult competent professionals for answers to your specific questions.

Offers, prices, rates, addresses, telephone numbers and Web sites
listed in this book are accurate at the time of publication,
but they are subject to frequent change.

Bottom Line Books® is a registered trademark of
Boardroom® Inc.
281 Tresser Boulevard, Stamford, CT 06901

www.bottomlinesecrets.com

Bottom Line Books® is an imprint of Boardroom® Inc., publisher of print periodicals,
e-letters and books. We are dedicated to bringing you the best information from the most
knowledgeable sources in the world. Our goal is to help you gain greater wealth,
better health, more wisdom, extra time and increased happiness.

Printed in the United States of America

CONTENTS

Contents

Contents

Chapter 9:
HEART DISEASE

Chapter 10:
MEMORY

Chapter 11:
MEN'S HEALTH

Contents

Chapter 17:
WOMEN'S HEALTH

Appendix:
NATURAL HEALING MODALITIES

PREFACE

Natural Healing That Really Works

If you're in a car accident—don't ask the ambulance driver to take you to the acupuncturist. If you have a case of pneumonia—don't rely on aromatherapy. If you're having a heart attack—don't call the nutritionist.

Conventional medicine—high-tech tests, prescription medications and surgery—is your best bet for treating medical disasters. But while conventional medicine is ideal for handling a medical *crisis*, it's often second-rate for preventing and treating routine conditions (such as headaches or heartburn) and chronic diseases (such as arthritis and diabetes).

However, everyday and chronic health problems "respond wonderfully" to *natural* therapies, says Jacob Teitelbaum, MD, a physician in Hawaii, and author of *Pain-Free 1-2-3!* (McGraw-Hill) and several other books on natural healing.

Dr. Teitelbaum and thousands of other naturally oriented health professionals favor the modalities of natural and alternative healing—nutritional therapy, herbal therapy, acupuncture, homeopathy and many others—for several reasons.

• **Natural therapies address the *cause* of the problem rather than a symptom.** "Masking a symptom with a medication is like shooting out the blinking oil light on the dashboard of your car," says Dr. Teitelbaum.

"Yes, you're no longer *aware* of the problem—but you're not *solving* the problem, either." On the other hand, he says, natural modalities work *with* nature to help the body heal. As the underlying problem is resolved, symptoms recede and disappear.

• **Natural therapies are safe.** Medication-related problems kill nearly 200,000 people a year and put nearly 9 million in hospitals, accounting for 28% of hospital admissions, says Dr. Teitelbaum. Problems caused by natural modalities are rare.

• **Natural therapies are often more effective than conventional care.** For example, a major 10-year study shows that lifestyle methods such as diet and exercise are more effective than a prescription medication in preventing and controlling type 2 diabetes. Studies also show that regular exercise clears up mild to moderate depression more effectively than antidepressant medications. And that acupuncture relieves back pain as effectively as surgery. In fact, name almost any everyday or chronic problem, and natural healing handles it as well as, or *better* than conventional medicine.

• **Compared with conventional care, natural therapies are low-cost.** "A good example is carpal tunnel syndrome, from a pinched nerve in the wrist, which causes pain and numbness in the hands," says Dr. Teitelbaum. "The usual medical approach is surgery, which costs around $3,000. But those same symptoms can be alleviated in six to 12 weeks by *inexpensive* remedies—

ix

taking vitamin B-6 and a thyroid supplement, wearing a wrist splint and reducing or stopping the activity that caused the problem."

• **Natural therapies have as much scientific evidence to support their use as conventional therapies.** This point is very much *the* point of *Bottom Line's Breakthroughs in Natural Healing, 2011*. Here you'll find fascinating news about the latest scientific research on natural therapies, from acidophilus to zinc, and acupuncture to yoga. And you'll also find expert advice on how to *apply* that science to your own life, for health and healing.

For example, in just the first chapter of this book—"Aches & Pains from Head to Toe"—you'll discover...

• A simple exercise that quickly and permanently relieves the pain of tennis elbow—without surgery or drugs.

• How to use homeopathy to beat back pain, including how to find the remedy that's exactly right for your personal pain.

• How wearing the right kind of underwear can quickly ease the pain of fibromyalgia, particularly when the condition worsens in the winter. (That's right—*underwear!*)

• How swearing when you hurt yourself can muffle pain *immediately.*

• How three, 20-minute sessions of meditation can train your brain to feel less pain.

And those are only a few of the scientifically proven benefits from *one* of the seventeen chapters in this remarkable new book.

How did I find them?

As a researcher and advocate for natural healing, I spend my time (and have spent my career) finding and learning about natural remedies to help you and millions of other readers achieve robust health. I relentlessly study the scientific literature on health and healing...I find the newest and most useful science-supported natural remedies...I interview hundreds of the top medical scientists and health-care practitioners about these findings...and I present to you the practical information that is proven and that *really works.* (And only *after* that information has also been reviewed and vetted by medical experts and the editors at Bottom Line Publications.)

My family and friends are always asking me about the latest breakthroughs in the field of natural health and healing, and I share with them this same research—so I've seen the benefits of my findings firsthand. I know you will find the same benefits in the pages of this book. Enjoy it in good (and better!) health.

Bill Gottlieb
September 2010

Chapter 1

ACHES & PAINS
FROM HEAD TO TOE

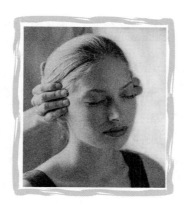

Say Goodbye To Your Chronic Headaches

Of all the medical conditions that send patients to their doctors, chronic headaches (including migraines) are among the least likely to be treated effectively.*

Problem: Most chronic headache sufferers would like to simply pop a pill to relieve their pain. Although there are many helpful medications, each can have side effects and is designed to reduce headache pain rather than prevent it.

Solution: After treating thousands of headache patients, Alexander Mauskop, MD, director of the New York Headache Center in New York City, devised a natural "triple therapy" that helps prevent migraines from developing in the first place.

What you need to know...

*To find a headache specialist or headache support group near you, contact the National Headache Foundation (888-643-5552, *www.headaches.org*).

When the Pain Won't Go Away

Approximately 15 million Americans have chronic headaches (occurring on at least 15 days a month).

The most common forms, in order of prevalence, are tension-type headaches (head pain caused by tight muscles—for example, in the neck—often due to stress)...and migraines (throbbing head pain accompanied by other symptoms, such as nausea or dizziness, and sometimes preceded by light sensitivity and visual disturbance known as an *aura*).

Natural Therapy

Doctors don't know the exact cause of migraines, but the most popular theory focuses on disturbances in the release of pain-modulating brain chemicals, including the neurotransmitter serotonin.

In reviewing the medical literature, Dr. Mauskop found several references to the mineral magnesium, which has been shown to prevent migraines by helping open up blood vessels in the brain. Studies indicate that half of all migraine sufferers are deficient in this mineral.

Within a short time, Dr. Mauskop also discovered several references that supported the use of riboflavin (vitamin B-2), which plays a role in energy production in brain cells… and the herb *feverfew*, which promotes the health of blood vessels.

Advice: Each day, take a total of 400 mg of magnesium (as magnesium oxide or in a chelated form—if one form causes diarrhea, try the other)…400 mg of riboflavin…and a total of 100 mg of feverfew, divided in two doses with meals. Many people take this therapy indefinitely. Ask your doctor about the appropriate duration of treatment for you.

Caution: Feverfew may interfere with your blood's ability to clot, so consult your doctor before taking this herb. Riboflavin may turn your urine bright yellow, but the change is harmless.

For Even More Pain Relief

Coenzyme Q10 (CoQ10) is a substance that, like riboflavin, is believed to fight migraines by boosting energy production in brain cells. Research has shown that 100 mg of CoQ10 three times a day reduces migraine frequency.

Advice: Take a total of 300 mg of CoQ10 daily, in one or two doses.

An extract from the root of the butterbur plant is another supplement that has shown promise as a remedy for migraines. In one study, 75 mg of butterbur taken twice daily for four months helped reduce the frequency of migraine attacks.

Although the exact mechanism of action is unclear, the herb might help reduce inflammatory substances in the body that can trigger headaches. Butterbur is sold in the US under the brand name Petadolex (888-301-1084, *www.petadolex.com*).

Advice: Take a total of 150 mg of butterbur daily, in one or two doses.

Other Helpful Strategies

All the natural therapies described earlier help prevent migraines, but you're likely to achieve even better results if you adopt a holistic approach that includes the following steps. These strategies also help guard against chronic tension headaches but are overlooked by many doctors. *My advice…*

● **Get regular aerobic exercise.** Exercise supplies more blood to the brain and boosts levels of feel-good hormones known as *endorphins*, which help fight migraines. Physical activity also helps release muscle tension that contributes to tension-type headaches.

Scientific evidence: In data collected from 43,770 Swedes, men and women who regularly worked out were less likely to have migraines and recurring headaches than those who did not exercise.

Helpful: Do some type of moderate-intensity aerobic activity for at least 30 minutes five times a week.

● **Use relaxation techniques.** A mind-body approach, such as *progressive muscle relaxation* (deliberately tensing then releasing muscles from toe to head)…guided imagery (in which you create calm, peaceful images in your mind)…or breathing exercises (a method of slow inhalation and exhalation), can ease muscle tension and relax blood vessels to help prevent migraines and tension headaches.

Also helpful: Biofeedback, which involves learning to control such involuntary functions as skin temperature, heart rate or muscle tension while sensors are attached to the body, helps prevent migraines and tension headaches. Biofeedback usually can be learned in about eight sessions and should be practiced daily by migraine and tension headache sufferers. To find a biofeedback practitioner near you, consult the Biofeedback Certification International Alliance (866-908-8713, *www.bcia.org*). (For more information on biofeedback, see appendix page 358.)

● **Try acupuncture.** There's good evidence that this centuries-old needling technique can reduce the severity and frequency of migraines and tension headaches.** It typically requires at least 10 sessions to see benefits.

**To find an acupuncturist near you, go to the National Certification Commission for Acupuncture and Oriental Medicine Web site (*www.nccaom.org*) and click on "Find a Practitioner."

Ask your health insurer whether acupuncture is covered. If not, each session, typically an hour long, will cost $50 to $100, depending on your location. (For more information on acupuncture, see appendix page 354.)

If you feel that you are developing a migraine or tension headache: Perform a simple *acupressure* treatment on yourself to help relieve headache pain.

What to do: Place your right thumb on the webbing at the base of your left thumb and index finger, and your right index finger on the palm side of this point. Gently squeeze and massage this area, using small circular motions, for one to two minutes. Repeat on the right hand. (See appendix page 351, for more information on acupressure.)

Alexander Mauskop, MD, director of the New York Headache Center in New York City (*www.nyheadache.com*). He is author of *What Your Doctor May Not Tell You About Migraines* (Grand Central Publishing).

Illustration by Shawn Banner.

The Vegetable That Cures Hangovers

Asparagus may help when you *feel* like a vegetable, when a night of alcohol-assisted revelry has turned into a morning of regret. An herbal extract of asparagus (*Asparagus officinalis*) is a remedy for the aching head, dry mouth, queasy stomach and the other misery-making symptoms of a hangover.

However, "little is known" about how asparagus works at the cellular level in the "alleviation of alcohol hangover," said a team of Korean researchers, who set out to discover the mechanisms behind the green spears' metabolic magic.

Here's what they found…

Asparagus Protects Your Liver

Studying human liver cells in the laboratory, researchers found that asparagus extract reduced by an estimated 70% the production of "radical oxygen species" (ROS)—the free radicals that steal electrons from other molecules, damaging cells. Drinking a lot of alcohol triggers the production of ROS, say the researchers.

And they found that adding the extract to liver cells more than doubled their production of two enzymes, *alcohol dehydrogenase* and *aldehyde dehydrogenase*. Those enzymes help get rid of *acetaldehyde*, a byproduct of alcohol that is the "main component causing the hangover symptoms," says Deok-Bae Park, PhD, the study's lead researcher.

The Pre-Party Treatment

Asparagus may help in the treatment of an alcohol hangover and also protect the liver from the toxic results of alcohol, agrees Ray Sahelian, MD, an expert in nutritional and herbal therapies.

• **Take a supplement.** "It's best to take the extract before an evening of drinking—if you take it after drinking, the liver damage is already done," he says.

Suggested intake: 200 milligrams of standardized extract.

• **Make asparagus tea.** A supplement isn't your only option. You also can use asparagus as a remedy (not a preventive) for a hangover, says Phyllis Light, a professor of herbal studies at the Clayton College of Natural Health in Alabama (*www.ccnh.edu*). "Asparagus is an Appalachian folk remedy for hangover," she says.

Her advice: Wash one bunch of asparagus, removing any wilted or bruised spears. Trim the large, whitish ends off the bottom of the spears. Cut the asparagus spears in half and place in a nonreactive pot with one quart of water. Bring to a boil and reduce the heat to simmer, for 10 to 12 minutes. Remove spears from pot (save for a future meal). Pour the light-green asparagus broth into a mug, drinking 1 cup every hour until you've consumed the entire quart.

3

"The asparagus detoxifies the alcohol and also increases levels of *glutathione*, an antioxidant that protects the liver," says Light.

Deok-Bae Park, PhD, professor of medicine, Jeju National University School of Medicine, Republic of Korea.

Ray Sahelian, MD, (*www.raysahelian.com*), expert in nutritional and herbal therapies, author of *Mind Boosting Secrets* (Bottom Line Books).

Phyllis Light, herbalist and author, and professor of herbal studies, Clayton College of Natural Health in Alabama. *www.ccnh.edu.*

Dealing with Your Fear of Dental Pain

Redhead or not (see next page) an estimated 20% of the general population say they have an extreme fear of the dentist, with another 45% reporting a moderate level of fear. What's the best way to overcome that dental anxiety?

Jaw with Your Dentist

• **Talk to your dentist about previous experiences with inadequate pain relief.** "Mention any bad experiences you've had with local anesthesia, so your dentist knows you might require more anesthesia than usual," says Daniel Sessler, MD, professor and chair, Department of Outcomes Research, Cleveland, Clinic. Studies show that people with dental anxiety are so anxious, they typically don't mention those bad experiences (or even the fact that they're afraid of going to the dentist).

• **Don't put up with pain.** "The dentist should wait and confirm that the anesthesia is actually working," says Dr. Sessler. "If it's not, the dentist should stop and give another dose."

• **Reduce your dental anxiety—with "tapping."** There's a simple way to cure your dental fear, says Roberta Temes, PhD, a psychotherapist and clinical professor in the Department of Psychiatry at SUNY Health Science Center in Brooklyn, New York and author of *The Tapping Cure: A Revolutionary System for Rapid Relief from Phobias,* *Anxiety, Post-Traumatic Stress Disorder and More* (Da Capo). *Tap on your collarbone...*

Overcoming Dental Phobia

But before you learn about tapping, it is important to understand that the terms *dental fear* and *dental anxiety* are misnomers, says Dr. Temes. The problem is more correctly called *dental phobia*—a persistent, illogical fear of a specific situation. "Modern dentistry is pain-free if done professionally. The dentist asks if you can still feel sensation during a procedure, and if you can, he administers more anesthesia. There is no reason to be afraid of the dentist."

However, if you have dental phobia—and millions do—tapping is the best way to overcome it. Tapping—also called the Emotional Freedom Technique—is a procedure to separate a specific thought from a negative feeling, she explains. *Here's how to do it...*

1. Create one sentence about your fear, making it as specific as possible. Example: "I'm afraid of going to the dentist" or "I'm afraid of sitting in the dentist's chair."

2. Put words in front of and after the sentence that change it from negative to positive. Example: "Even though I'm afraid of going to the dentist, I can do it—it's no big deal."

3. Say the original sentence over and over, so that you bring up all your feelings, upset and fears. As you say the sentence, picture the worst possible scenario associated with the fear, and become very frightened.

4. While you're frightened, use four fingers of one hand to tap fairly hard on one of your collarbones, for ten to fifteen seconds. ("You can use either hand to tap either collarbone," says Dr. Temes. "Some people say that tapping both collarbones at once works best.")

5. As you tap, say the positive version of your sentence.

"For 90% of people, tapping on the collarbone while saying the positive sentence a few times completely relieves the phobia—

Why Redheads Are Afraid of Dentists

Anesthesiologists are wary about redheads.

Redheads don't go under general anesthesia as easily as they should…redheads have more pain…redheads take longer to wake up from anesthesia…

Doctors theorize that the cause might be the *melanocortin-1 receptor gene* (MC1R), which colors hair (and skin and eyes). Redheads have a mutation of this gene, which might also raise their sensitivity to pain. (About 25% of nonredheads also have a mutation of MC1R.)

After conducting two studies that revealed redheads needed 20% more general anesthesia and that they are only about half as sensitive to local anesthesia than blondes or brunettes, the researchers received more than 100 e-mails from redheads across the US, says Daniel Sessler, MD, a study researcher, and professor and chair of the Department of Outcomes Research at the Cleveland Clinic. "They didn't complain about problems with general anesthesia," he says. "They complained about problems with local dental anesthesia—specifically, not receiving enough anesthesia to numb their dental pain."

Based on those e-mails, the researchers conducted a study to determine if redheads have more fear of dental pain and more avoidance of routine dental care. Among 144 adults—67 with red hair and 77 with dark—they found that those with a mutation of MC1R (65 of the redheads and 20 of the brunettes) had more dental anxiety than those without the mutation. They were also more likely to avoid going to the dentist. The findings were published in the *Journal of the American Dental Association*.

That's no small matter. Studies show that people with dental fear and avoidance have more cavities and pulled teeth, and other studies link unhealthy teeth with higher death rates.

they just don't feel scared anymore," says Dr. Temes.

For the other 10%, a combination of two techniques works.

1. Perform the collarbone tapping.

2. Put your right hand over the chest (in the same spot you would place your right hand while pledging allegiance to the flag).

3. Make a fist with the right hand—your knuckles are now on the pledge spot.

4. Move your fist in a circle, lightly rubbing the knuckles on that spot, saying the positive sentence.

You're done with the technique when you feel done—when you're completely relieved of your phobia. "If you feel somewhat relieved, or not so worried, or a little more calm—continue to perform the technique daily for several days," says Dr. Temes. "Once you notice the phobia stays away permanently, you're done."

Important: Nobody knows how tapping works, she explains. "The reason for why it works hasn't been discovered yet. It's sufficient to say, 'We don't know why it works, but it does work, so just do it. There's no way it can harm you—and why deprive yourself of the fantastic results?"

Daniel Sessler, MD, professor and chair, Department of Outcomes Research, Cleveland Clinic.

Roberta Temes, PhD, psychotherapist and clinical professor in the Department of Psychiatry at SUNY Health Science Center in Brooklyn, New York, and author of *The Tapping Cure* (Da Capo). *www.drroberta.com.*

Heal Carpal Tunnel Without Surgery

The wrist pain or sensations of numbness, tingling and/or weakness in the fingers that you may be experiencing stem from inflammation in the carpal tunnel, a small opening below the base of the wrist where the median nerve passes between the muscles and bones. This area is vulnerable to overuse from repetitive tasks such as playing a musical instrument, knitting or working on a computer. To facilitate healing, rest the affected wrist(s) as much as you can for several weeks minimum.

Recommendation: Take 100 mg of vitamin B-6 three times daily for two months (then reduce to 100 mg daily). Acupuncture can reduce pain, tightness and swelling—typically within three treatments. And chiropractic manipulations to the neck, elbow and wrist area can reduce nerve impingement.

Mark A. Stengler, NMD, naturopathic medical doctor in private practice, La Jolla, California, and author of the *Bottom Line/Natural Healing* newsletter. *www.drstengler.com.*

Better Back Pain Prevention

When researchers analyzed 20 studies involving nearly 30,000 people with a history of low back pain, exercise regimens designed to build muscle strength and endurance, including leg lifts and weight lifting, were effective in preventing back symptoms. Other strategies, such as shoe inserts (to reduce pressure on the spine) and lumbar supports (belts that support the back), did not reduce back pain.

If you suffer from low back pain: Discuss an exercise program with your doctor.

Stanley J. Bigos, MD, professor emeritus of orthopedics, University of Washington, Seattle.

Vitamin D Eases Back Pain

After taking vitamin D supplements for three months, 95% of patients with chronic back pain reported improve-

ment. Low levels of vitamin D may soften bone surfaces, leading to pain. Increasing vitamin D improves calcium absorption and bone health.

Best: Ask your doctor about taking 1,000 international units (IU) of vitamin D-3 daily...or 2,000 IU daily if you have back pain.

Stewart B. Leavitt, PhD, editor of the Web site Pain Treatment Topics (*www.pain-topics.org*) and leader of an analysis of 22 studies on back pain.

Stop Disc Deterioration

As we age, we all develop some degree of degenerative disc disease, in which our discs, the shock-absorbing pads between the vertebrae, begin to wear down. Symptoms can include neck or back pain, pain that radiates down the back of the shoulder or into the arms, numbness, tingling, muscle weakness, even difficulty with hand dexterity or walking.

Risk factors: Smoking, heavy lifting and a history of back injuries. To diagnose degenerative disc disease, your doctor may order an x-ray, computed tomography (CT) scan or magnetic resonance imaging (MRI) to examine your discs.

For treatment and prevention: Drink 48 ounces or more of water daily to keep discs hydrated (they are made up primarily of water)...eat an anti-inflammatory diet that is high in vegetables and fruits with moderate lean protein and carbs...take nutritional supplements to strengthen disc tissue, including collagen (500 mg twice daily), glucosamine sulfate (1,500 mg daily), and vitamin C (1,000 mg twice daily). In addition, stretch daily—to keep tight muscles from pulling on discs.

Mark A. Stengler, NMD, naturopathic medical doctor in private practice, La Jolla, California, and author of the *Bottom Line/Natural Healing* newsletter. *www.drstengler.com.*

Fast (and Cheap) Relief For Tennis Elbow

Tennis elbow—what doctors and physical therapists call lateral *epicondylitis*—is a classic overuse injury, afflicting an estimated nine million Americans.

What happens: Tendons (tissue that connects muscle to bone) on the outside of the elbow become inflamed, from repeatedly performing an activity that tightens the forearm muscles. That activity might be tennis, golfing, painting (housepainters), using a screwdriver (plumbers), hammering (carpenters), raking (gardeners) or carrying a heavy briefcase (white-collar workers).

Symptoms can include pain that shoots from the outside of the elbow to the forearm and wrist…a weak forearm…and a painful grip, while shaking hands or turning a doorknob. Over time, the pain can worsen and become debilitating, limiting activity.

Now, a recent study shows there is a simple, cheap cure for tennis elbow—at-home exercises for the wrist extensors (the muscles in the forearm), using a bendable rubber bar.

Simple Effective Exercise

Twenty-one people with severe, debilitating pain from chronic tennis elbow were divided into two groups. For several weeks, both groups received typical treatments for tennis elbow, such as stretching, ultrasound, massage and heat and ice.

But the two groups performed two different types of at-home strengthening exercises, with one group doing "eccentric" exercises using a Thera-Band FlexBar, a rubber bar about eight inches long.

What most people don't know: There are two types of strengthening exercises. In a concentric exercise, the muscle tightens and shortens. In an eccentric exercise, the muscle tightens and lengthens.

Example: In a biceps curl, raising the dumbbell shortens and tightens the muscle—a concentric exercise. Lowering the dumbbell lengthens and tightens the muscle—an eccentric exercise. Recent research shows eccentric exercises can help heal damaged tendons.

Those using the FlexBar saw remarkable improvement—81% less elbow pain, 70% less tenderness and 72% more strength. Those not using the FlexBar had 22% less pain, 4% less tenderness and 11% more strength.

In fact, the group using the FlexBar had such quick and remarkable improvement that the researchers ended the study earlier than planned so that all the patients could do the FlexBar exercise.

"Our study showed that this new exercise, using an inexpensive rubber bar, provides a practical and effective way of helping treat tennis elbow," says study leader Timothy Tyler, a physical therapist and clinical research associate at the Nicholas Institute of Sports Medicine and Athletic Trauma in New York City.

"Compared with other treatment for tennis elbow—such as cortisone injections or topical nitric oxide, both of which require direct medical supervision and may have significant side effects—this treatment is cost effective, and doesn't require the patient to come to a clinic."

Less Pain and Tenderness

Three times a day, slowly perform this exercise 15 times.

1. Hold your arms at each side of your body. With the affected arm, hold the rubber bar, with the bar upright and the wrist fully extended.

2. Grasp the bar at the top with unaffected hand, with the palm facing away from you.

3. Use the unaffected wrist to twist the bar, flexing the wrist. Keep the affected wrist extended.

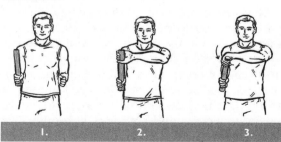

7

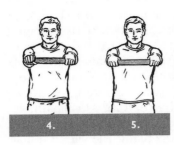

4. Maintaining the twist, extend both arms fully out in front of the body, holding the bar perpendicular to the body. Keep the affected wrist extended and the unaffected wrist flexed.

5. Slowly untwist the rubber bar with the affected arm, moving the wrist from its extended to a flexed position. This is the eccentric contraction of the wrist extensors.

"You should feel sore afterward," says Tyler. "That's how you know it's effective."

Resource: You can order the Thera-Band FlexBar—the same device used in the study—from *www.amazon.com.* You can also call the Hygenic Corporation at 800-321-2135 to find a dealer near you.

Timothy Tyler, physical therapist and clinical research associate at the Nicholas Institute of Sports Medicine and Athletic Trauma in New York City.

Illustrations by Shawn Banner.

Homeopathy for Back Pain

Imagine taking a super-small amount of a substance that would cause the health problem you're having if you took a normal quantity of it—and expecting that infinitesimal dose to heal you. Sound impossible?

Well, that's exactly what happens…when you take a homeopathic remedy.

"Homeopathy represents not just a different type of drug, but a different understanding of and approach to health and medical care—one that not only makes conceptual sense, but is also safer than conventional medicine, and truly works," says Dana Ullman, a homeopath in Berkeley, California, founder of Homeopathic Educational Services (*www.homeopathic.com*), and author of several books on homeopathy, including *Everybody's Guide to Homeopathic Medicines* (Tarcher/Putnam).

How does homeopathy work?

Conventional medicine understands symptoms as problems, and tries to fix them with drugs or surgery, says Ullman. Homeopathy understands a unique set of symptoms as a sign that the body-mind is trying to defend and heal itself. (For example, the pain and redness of inflammation is a sign of the immune system activating itself to heal the area.)

And it uses a particular homeopathic medicine—repeatedly diluted preparations of herbs, minerals and other natural substances—to stimulate the "vital force" of the body-mind, so that the specific set of symptoms can complete itself, leading to full recovery.

As for the minuscule dosages of homeopathy (often no more than a couple of molecules), Ullman compares them to *nanotechnology*—the use of microscopic but powerful components, such as the nanoparticles in sunscreens. Homeopathy, he says, is nanopharmacology.

And a new study shows that nanopharmacology can help relieve low back pain…

50% Less Pain Medication

Doctors at the Charité University Medical Center in Berlin, Germany, evaluated 128 people with chronic back pain (an average of more than nine years) who had been treated with homeopathy.

Their pain levels "showed marked and sustained improvements," wrote the doctors, in the *Clinical Journal of Pain.*

They also had better quality of life, a more positive outlook and their use of drugs for back pain was reduced by 50%.

"Homeopathic treatment represents an effective treatment for low back pain," concluded the doctors.

The Right Remedy for You

For chronic back pain, it's best to see a professional homeopath, says Ullman. (The patients in the study were all treated by professional homeopaths.)

Resource: To find a qualified homeopath near you, visit the Web site of the National Center for Homeopathy (*www.homeopathic. org*) and under "Services" on the home page click "Find A Homeopath."

For acute pain, consider the following remedies, all of which are widely available over-the-counter.

● **Rhus toxicodendron.** This is for a backache or sprain that hits when you first get up in the morning but limbers up after you move around. It's also for back pain from overexertion.

● **Byronia.** This is for a backache that is aggravated by any type of motion. It's also the type of pain that feels relief when deep pressure or hot applications are applied. The person with this type of backache is very irritable and wants to be left alone.

● **Hypericum.** This is for a backache with some type of shooting pain.

● **Arnica.** You can take this remedy for a sore, bruised back, after an injury or trauma. You can also use an arnica cream on the injured area.

Resource: Traumeel, from Heel, is an arnica cream.

Suggested dosage: For all of the above oral remedies, take 30C, three times a day, until you see improvement. (30C is an indication of the degree of "potentization" of the remedy, a homeopathic term indicating the level of dilution.)

Dana Ullman, homeopath in Berkeley, California, founder of Homeopathic Educational Services (*www.homeopathic. com*) and author of *Everybody's Guide to Homeopathic Medicines* (Tarcher/Putnam).

The Right Bed Can Ease Back Pain

People with back pain often think that a very firm mattress is best. Not true. In a study published in *The Lancet*, 313 individuals with low-back pain slept on either a firm or a medium-firm coil mattress. After 90 days, the participants with the medium-firm mattresses had less pain in bed, upon rising and during the day than those with firm mattresses. *Other misconceptions about beds and back pain...*

Misconception: Everyone with back pain feels the pain when he/she first wakes up—so you can't tell if the mattress is a problem or not.

Fact: Most back pain is mildest in the morning, before you get out of bed and begin moving. If you wake up stiff and sore, your mattress may be to blame. Try sleeping on a different mattress—in the guest room, at a friend's, in a hotel—and see if you notice an improvement when you get up.

Misconception: Heavier people with back pain need soft beds.

Fact: Everyone needs enough support during the night to keep the spine in a normal position. If the spine sinks into a sagging bed, the muscles are strained. Heavier people and those who sleep on their backs tend to need firmer mattresses. Side and stomach sleepers need softer beds.

Misconception: A foam pad or an entire mattress made of foam helps relieve back pain.

Fact: There are two kinds of foam generally available—egg-crate and memory foam. Egg-crate foam creates a layer of softness but does not change the support beneath. Memory foam is sensitive to temperature and conforms to the body. However, there is no scientific evidence that either kind of foam reduces back pain.

Misconception: Adjustable beds can ease back pain.

Fact: Some adjustable beds are filled with air or water that can be pumped in or out. Other types have joints that allow parts of the bed to be propped at different angles. There are no authoritative studies showing that adjustable beds help reduce back pain.

Misconception: You can't tell in the store if the mattress is right for you.

Fact: Trying out a mattress in the store can help you determine if it's comfortable. Lie on each mattress for at least five minutes. Start on your back, without a pillow. Your hand should fit snugly in the small of your back. Lying on your side, you shouldn't notice significant pressure on your hips or shoulders. Choose a retailer that will allow you to return a mattress if it isn't comfortable. These include Sleepy's and 1800Mattress.com. (You may have to pay an exchange fee.)

Baljinder Bathla, MD, cofounder of Chicago Sports & Spine, a pain-management practice. He is certified in physical medicine, rehabilitation and pain management. *www. chicagosportsspine.com.*

The Simple 25¢ Remedy —A Quick Fix for Pain

Millions of Americans live with chronic pain in their backs, hips, legs and feet. Many self-medicate with ibuprofen or other analgesics…or they undergo batteries of expensive tests to identify the underlying problem.

Do this first: Take off your socks and look at your toes. If the second toe is even slightly longer than the big toe, you might have Morton's toe, a condition that disrupts normal alignment and can cause pain throughout the body, particularly in the back, legs and feet.

The condition is named after Dudley J. Morton, MD, of Yale Medical School, who first wrote about it causing foot problems. Janet Travell, MD—White House physician to former presidents Kennedy and Johnson— took the concept further by explaining that Morton's toe could cause pain all over the body.

It's estimated that up to 15% of Americans have Morton's toe. Among those with chronic musculoskeletal pain, the prevalence might be as high as 80%. People are born with Morton's toe, but it usually takes decades of accumulated stress and the age-related loss of tissue elasticity to start producing symptoms that can develop into chronic pain.

Why It Hurts

When we walk and our feet push off from the ground, the big toe typically touches before the other toes. For a fraction of a second, it absorbs virtually all of the body's weight. Then as the foot rolls forward, some of the pressure is shifted to the adjoining, weaker toes.

In patients with Morton's toe, the first metatarsal bone (in the big toe) is abnormally short and the longer second metatarsal bone typically touches the ground first and absorbs most of the body's weight. The second metatarsal bone isn't strong enough for this much pressure. To compensate, the foot overpronates—it rolls in the direction of the big toe to support the excess weight.

Overpronation makes the foot unstable. It also prevents the big toe from pushing your weight upward. This means that other muscles and joints have to compensate.

The result: Decades of abnormal stress that can disrupt your posture and potentially damage joints throughout the body, causing pain.

The 25¢ Fix

The simple, inexpensive remedy for Morton's toe is a toe pad. It will act like a shim under the first metatarsal bone and cause the big toe to meet the ground a fraction of a second sooner. This will prevent overpronation and help keep the foot stable. It often relieves symptoms within a few weeks—and sometimes right away.

Exception: Because a toe pad changes the body's alignment, some people experience a temporary increase in pain. This usually diminishes within a few days.

Once the pain goes away, you still will need to wear a toe pad every day, just as someone with sight problems needs to wear glasses or contact lenses every day. *To make a toe pad…*

●**Buy a package of inexpensive foam shoe inserts.** I have found that Dr. Scholl's Molefoam is a good product for making a toe pad (one pack provides six to eight toe pads). Just about any product will work—

even no-name brands available at most pharmacies and discount stores, usually for less than $2.

● **Cut out a rectangle about one-inch wide and two-and-a-half inches long.** That's about the size of a stick of chewing gum or a Band-Aid. Put it over the first metatarsal head, the bulge on the bottom of the foot that is below the point where the big toe joins the foot. Position the pad so that the longer dimension runs lengthwise with the foot. If the insole doesn't have an adhesive backing, tape it to the foot with duct tape, electrical tape or even Scotch tape. It does not have to look pretty.

You can take the toe pad off at night and put it back on the foot in the morning. One toe pad usually lasts two to four days.

Helpful: If you don't have a foam insert, a quarter can work. Anything that adds thickness to the first metatarsal head will help restore proper alignment.

Apply Heat

If a toe pad doesn't eliminate the pain right away, you might want to apply heat. Rest your feet on a heating pad or soak them in warm water for about 15 minutes, once or twice a day.

If after two to three weeks you still have pain, see your physician.

Burton S. Schuler, DPM, podiatrist and director of the Ambulatory Foot Clinic at the Podiatric Pain Management Center in Panama City, Florida. He is author of Why You Really Hurt (La Luz). www.whyyoureallyhurt.com.

How to Prevent Shin Splints

"Shin splints" is a general term for muscle pain along the shins, usually caused by a muscle imbalance—strong calf muscles and weaker shin muscles. *Solution…*

Thread a 24-inch–long shoestring through the center hole in a two- to five-pound weight plate. Tie the ends together so you have one big loop with the weight on it (like a key on a key ring). Sit on a countertop with your knees bent and feet dangling about 12 inches above the floor.

Wrap the loop of string several times around the toe box of one sneaker so the weight dangles below your toes. Let your toes point down…then flex your foot to bring your toes up as high as you can. Point again, then flex while angling your foot slightly to lead with your little toe. On your third repetition, lead with your big toe. Do 15 reps, then switch sides. Work up to three sets every other day.

Wayne L. Westcott, PhD, fitness research director, South Shore YMCA, Quincy, Massachusetts, and author of Building Strength & Stamina (Human Kinetics).

Stop Nighttime Calf Cramps

An imbalance of *electrolytes* (minerals needed for normal body fluid function) may bring on nighttime calf cramps, so eat more foods rich in potassium (sweet potatoes, bananas)…magnesium (nuts, spinach)…and calcium (dairy foods, sardines). Drink enough clear fluids (water, broth, light tea) to keep urine pale yellow.

Also, stretch your calves before bed.

How: Stand with toes pointed straight ahead. With your left foot, step forward about 18 inches. Keeping both heels on the ground and your right leg straight, bend your left knee until you feel a stretch in your right calf. Hold for 30 seconds. Repeat on the other side.

Timothy W. Flynn, PhD, PT, president, American Academy of Orthopaedic Manual Physical Therapists and associate professor of physical therapy, Regis University, Denver.

Insoles Ease Foot Pain

Researchers who reviewed 11 studies involving 1,332 people with foot pain found that custom-made orthotics (prescription shoe inserts that are molded to a cast of the foot) relieved pain within three months for adults with rheumatoid arthritis (chronic inflammation of the lining of the joints) and within three to six months for patients with highly arched feet or overly prominent big toe joints.

If you suffer from chronic foot pain: Ask your podiatrist if custom-made orthotics (costing about $300 to $500) would benefit you. Over-the-counter orthotics were not studied.

Fiona Hawke, researcher, associate lecturer, School of Health Sciences, University of Newcastle, Ourimbah, Australia.

Fast Relief for Burning Feet

Burning feet, the feeling that your feet are uncomfortably hot, can be a minor nuisance or a very painful condition, sometimes causing sleeplessness. There are several possible causes. Some people experience burning and achy feet from standing much of the day or from being overweight. Try using an orthotic support in your shoes, preferably custom made by a podiatrist, so that your feet have better biomechanical support (and, of course, lose weight, if necessary).

Burning feet also can be caused by athlete's foot, a fungal infection of the skin. In this case, apply a tea tree oil salve, such as Desert Essence Tea Tree Oil Skin Ointment (*www. desertessence.com*, $7.49 for one fluid ounce), to the foot twice daily. Burning feet also is a common complaint among those with diabetes who have nerve damage, known as diabetic neuropathy. For this condition, try the antioxidant alpha-lipoic acid (take 600 mg twice daily) and the nutrient acetyl-L-carnitine (1,500 mg twice daily), which can reduce pain and repair damaged nerves. Both are safe for everyone at these doses.

Mark A. Stengler, NMD, naturopathic medical doctor in private practice, La Jolla, California, and author of the *Bottom Line/Natural Healing* newsletter. *www.drstengler.com.*

Pumps Today, Foot Pain Tomorrow

Foot problems are common as we age—four out of five 50-year-olds have at least one foot problem serious enough to see a podiatrist or MD.

You can probably blame bad shoes, says a recent study.

Sandals Lack Support

Researchers at the Institute for Aging Research in Boston interviewed more than 3,300 people with an average age of 66.

Results: Nearly 30% of the women and 20% of the men experienced regular foot pain.

But women who regularly wore good shoes (sneakers, athletic shoes) in the past were 67% less likely to have pain in their hind-foot (heel, ankle and/or lower Achilles tendon) than women who regularly wore bad shoes (heels, pumps, sandals, slippers) when they were younger. (Only 2% of the men regularly wore bad shoes in the past, and there was no correlation with current foot pain.) The findings were in *Arthritis Care & Research*.

"High heels, pumps and sandals lack support and sound structure and may damage the foot," concluded Alyssa B. Dufour, the study leader and a graduate student at the Institute's Musculoskeletal Research Program.

"Pumps and high heels can damage the feet in so many ways," agrees Paul Langer, DPM, a podiatrist, clinical faculty member at the University of Minnesota Medical School, and author of *Great Feet for Life: Footcare and Footwear for Healthy Aging* (Fairview Press). "They elevate the rear foot higher than the forefoot, shortening and stressing the Achilles tendon. They change how the ankle and the heel absorb impact from walking—increasing pressure on the forefoot by 70 to 90%. And most high heels are narrow and squeeze the toes into an unnatural shape."

Comfort Should Come First

"Many young women buy shoes that are uncomfortable or even the wrong size, because they like them," Dufour says. "Young women should make careful choices regarding their shoe types, to avoid foot pain later in life."

If you do wear high heels, consider adding gel inserts or insoles, says Dufour.

And after you take off the high heels, stretch the back of each calf and heel by reaching down and gently pulling the top of the foot toward your knee for a few seconds, she advises.

Other shoe-smart advice from Dr. Langer and from the Institute for Aging Research...

● **Comfort—rather than style or fashion—should rule shoe selection.** "A big part of comfort is finding a shoe that provides both cushioning and stability," says Dr. Langer. "A shoe that's too soft or 'cushy' increases strain on the joints and soft tissue. A shoe that's too hard doesn't absorb enough impact when you're walking."

To test for comfort...when you've found a shoe with a proper width and length, walk around the store, advises Dr. Langer. Does the shoe feel comfortable and supportive?

Smart idea: Studies show that people who compare shoes in the store are better at determining whether or not new shoes are truly comfortable, says Dr. Langer. "Bring a comfortable shoe with you. Wear that shoe and then wear the new shoe, and compare."

● **Don't assume you know your foot size—it increases with age.**

● **Most people have one foot that is larger than the other.** Have both feet measured when you purchase shoes, and fit shoes to your longer foot.

● **Fit shoes at the end of the day,** when your feet have expanded slightly from walking.

● **Shoe sizes vary by brand and style.** Judge shoes not only by the size marked on the box, but on how they fit. "Check the fit of the shoe while standing," says Dr. Langer. "Press your thumb to the right of the little toe to make sure there's a thumbs-width of extra space in the toe box." Also wiggle your toes to ensure that you can move them freely. "The toe box shouldn't be too pointed or narrow," he says.

● **Avoid high-heels and pumps.** "Look for a shoe that elevates the heel less than an inch," says Dr. Langer.

Bottom line: "The shoe should have a shape that's similar to the foot," he says.

Alyssa B. Dufour, researcher, Institute for Aging Research, Boston.

Paul Langer, DPM, podiatrist, clinical faculty member at the University of Minnesota Medical School, and author of *Great Feet for Life: Footcare and Footwear for Healthy Aging* (Fairview Press).

Press Here for Relief— Sciatic Nerve Press Banishes Pain

Many people associate the word *sciatic* with the painful lower leg condition known as sciatica. It's ironic, then, that several recent studies have demonstrated that placing pressure on the sciatic nerve can provide pain relief from a wide variety of problems. In one study, researcher Jiman He, PhD, assistant professor of medicine at Brown University, found that this sciatic nerve press reduced pain in about 80% of dental patients and about 60% of patients with kidney pain.

How to Do It

This intriguing method is loosely based on acupressure. Dr. He says that by applying pressure for just two minutes, you can achieve relief that can last for 30 minutes to two hours. (The amount of relief will vary somewhat from person to person and also from disease to disease, he says, and it does not work for everyone.) Since the pain will eventually return, Dr. He believes this technique is especially useful while waiting for pain medication to take effect.

You need a partner willing to perform the sciatic press on you—the position makes it virtually impossible to do on yourself. The pressure spot is located in the middle rear thigh, three or five inches below the buttocks. This area should be pressed for about two minutes using either the flat of the palms, one on top of the other, or with the flat area of the fingers tucked into fists (so fingertips and knuckles don't protrude). Pain relief should be instantaneous—that's how you'll know the location is right. Dr. He says the pressure should be from 24 to 44 pounds per hand, so that the weight of the person applying the pressure is supported by his two hands. After repeated applications, 10 or so in the same day, the analgesic properties of the sciatic press start to fade, says Dr. He. In that case, stop its use for a time…doing so will revive its effectiveness if you need it a few days later.

Jiman He, PhD, assistant professor of medicine, Brown University, Providence, Rhode Island.

Heal Your Pain Without Drugs or Surgery

Most conventional doctors' approach to orthopedic pain and injuries is "medicate or cut." But there are alternatives.

Before resorting to powerful drugs or surgery, people who suffer from aching knees, backs, shoulders, hips or necks owe it to themselves to first try physical therapy.

Secret to permanent pain relief: A specialized form of physical therapy that focuses on *fascia* (the tough sheet of connective tissue found in all parts of your body) is one of the most effective—yet underused—cures for joint pain.

Why Does It Work?

Over time, the fascia (pronounced fash-ee-uh) throughout your body can become less flexible from lack of exercise. Repetitive movements, such as typing, knitting, golfing or tennis playing…bad posture…or trauma, including bruising or surgery, also affect the fascia. When the fascia tightens, your muscles no longer contract properly. This results in muscle weakness that can lead to aches and pains in other parts of the body.

Important: If the fascia is injured, it won't show up on a *magnetic resonance imaging* (MRI) scan, which doctors routinely use to diagnose orthopedic problems. But unhealthy fascia often is the underlying cause of joint and muscle pain.

The Key to Healthy Fascia

To check the resilience of your fascia, place your palm flat on a table and spread your fingers as wide as possible. Using the thumb and index finger of your other hand, pinch a fold of skin on the back of your flattened hand. Pull it up and hold it for five seconds. Then let go. If the skin snaps back and becomes completely flat instantaneously, your fascia is highly elastic and healthy. If it takes longer than two seconds, your fascia has lost some elasticity.

For the health of your fascia…

• **Stay hydrated.** The fascia in your body is 70% water. For proper hydration, drink at least 64 ounces of filtered water or purified bottled water per day if you're male or 48 ounces daily if you're female.

• **Eat an anti-inflammatory diet by limiting sugar consumption (including fruit juices and sweets),** trans fats ("partially hydrogenated oils" found in many packaged and fast foods) and fried foods.

• **Take supplements to further reduce inflammation.** For example, ask your doctor about taking 1.5 g to 2.5 g of fish oil per day (taken with meals)…and a daily joint-support supplement that combines glucosamine and chondroitin (components of joint tissue and cartilage, respectively)—consult a naturopathic or integrative medicine physician for advice on specific dosages and any precautions that should be taken when using these supplements.

Stretching Tight Fascia

The following three fascial stretches address some especially common problem areas.

Important: Always warm up with two minutes of continuous movement, such as jogging in place or performing arm circles, before stretching.*

• **Hip flexor stretch.** This stretch affects the *psoas*, a muscle that runs down either side of the pelvis, connecting the base of the spine to the hip bones. Tight psoas muscles are a major—and under-recognized—cause of low-back pain as well as hip and knee pain.

What to do: Place a chair on each side of your body. Kneel on your right knee and place your left leg in front of you with your left foot flat on the ground and your left knee bent 90 degrees. Place the palm of each hand on the seat of each chair.

Next, tilt your entire torso to the left. While maintaining this tilt, rotate your torso to the right.

Lift your chest and tuck your chin to your chest. Clench your buttocks to press your right hip forward. To avoid arching your back, contract your abdominal muscles.

Finally, while pressing your right foot downward, imagine that you're dragging your right knee forward and contract the muscles you would use to do this. You should feel a deep stretch in the front of your right hip. Hold for 20 seconds, keeping your buttocks firmly contracted. Relax for 10 seconds, then hold for 30 seconds more. Switch legs and repeat on the other side.

• **Shrug muscle stretch.** This stretch affects the *trapezius* muscle, which runs from the lower back to the outer shoulder and base of the skull. The stretch can help relieve neck stiffness, which is often due to a tight trapezius.

What to do: While seated or standing, hold your right arm five inches out from your hip, elbow straight. Bend your wrist slightly behind your body and drop your chin to your chest. Rotate your chin to the right about 30 degrees, and hold it there while you tilt the upper part of your head to the left. Press your right shoulder down hard, away from your ear and hold for 20 seconds. You should feel a stretch from the back of your head to the outer edge of your right shoulder. Rest for 10 seconds, then hold for 30 seconds more. Repeat on the left side.

• **Biceps stretch.** This stretch helps with a range of problems, including shoulder pain, tennis elbow and golfer's elbow. It also strengthens muscles in the mid-back, which helps improve posture. For this stretch, you'll need a chair and a low table.

What to do: Place the chair back against the table and sit with your feet flat on the floor. Put both arms on the table behind you with the backs of your hands facing down. Pull both shoulders backward and lift your chest. Next, walk both feet slightly leftward so your torso is rotated to the left. Straighten your right elbow and bend your right wrist up, touching the fingers and thumb of your right hand together in a point (your left hand should remain flat on the table).

Next, tilt your head to the left, and rotate it to the left so that the right side of your neck feels a stretch. Then drop your chin to your left collarbone. It should feel like a strap is being pulled from the top front of your shoulder to your elbow. Hold for 20 seconds. Rest for 10 seconds, then hold for 30 seconds more. Switch sides and repeat.

Ming Chew, PT, a physical therapist with a private practice in New York City, *www.mingmethod.net.* He is author of *The Permanent Pain Cure* (McGraw-Hill).

Illustrations by Shawn Banner.

*These stretches should not be performed by pregnant women or people with bone cancer, acute pain or recent muscle tears or strains.

A Warm Cozy Way to Ease Fibromyalgia

One out of every 50 Americans suffers from *fibromyalgia*—chronic muscle pain and "tender points" (spots on

15

the body where even slight pressure causes pain). The condition is often accompanied by a constellation of other complaints, including joint pain, fatigue, headaches, digestive upset, dry eyes and brain fog.

"Fibromyalgia is an energy crisis, in which the body spends more energy than it can make," explains Jacob Teitelbaum, MD, medical director of the Fibromyalgia and Fatigue Centers and author of *From Fatigued to Fantastic!* (Avery).

The crisis targets the muscles, locking them in shortened positions, he says. "Your muscles are tight and hurt, and you have widespread pain."

Fibromyalgia often baffles physicians, some of whom even question its existence. But a nurse in Turkey—herself a fibromyalgia sufferer—is feeling bullish about beating fibromyalgia. Or maybe sheepish. Because the new and simple remedy she's discovered for reducing fibromyalgia pain (particularly during the muscle-tightening months of winter) is—woolen underwear and bedding.

The Wonder of Wool

Emine Kara Kiyak, PhD, at the School of Nursing at Atatürk University in Turkey, studied 50 people with fibromyalgia, dividing them into two groups.

Staring in January, one group wore woolen underwear, or "long johns"—underwear that covered the body from the shoulders to the thighs. (It was a combination of 75% merino wool and 25% acrylic fiber.)

They also used woolen bedding—a woolen bed liner (between the mattress and the cover sheet), a woolen pillow case, and a woolen quilt.

"It's worth noting that, before the study, the patients using wool had worn cotton underwear, and had used synthetic bedding materials," says Dr. Kiyak.

The other group didn't use woolen underwear or bedding.

Results: After six weeks, those wearing and sleeping in wool "reported significant improvements in their condition, including a reduction in pain levels, in tender points and

in the interference of fibromyalgia with their daily life," says Dr. Kiyak. Specifically…pain decreased by 84%...tender points by 51%... muscle stiffness by 86%...morning tiredness by 91%...overall fatigue by 80%...depression and anxiety by 64%...and the impact of fibromyalgia on daily life decreased by 74%. Dr. Kiyak called the level of relief "remarkable."

"The use of wool in patients with fibromyalgia should be recommended as an inexpensive and easy way to mitigate and reduce the symptoms of the disease," she concluded, in *The Journal of Alternative and Complementary Medicine.*

Why it works: "We think the reason for the lower pain level and reduction in the tender point count was the warmth of the wool, which led to increased local blood flow, which in turn reduced the pain," says Dr. Kiyak.

The reason for less morning tiredness and fatigue? "The patients maintained a constant and balanced body temperature during sleep because of wool bedding, and experienced more restorative sleep," she says.

The reason fibromyalgia interfered less in daily life, and there was less depression and anxiety? "The reduction in physical impairment, the increase in the number of days the patients reported feeling good, the reduction in the number of work days missed, the reduction in the number of days the patients reported experiencing work impairment, and a concomitant reduction in anxiety and depression levels, may be attributed to an overall reduction in pain and fatigue and an overall improvement in the quality of sleep," Dr. Kiyak wrote.

Winter Wellness

"Fibromyalgia pain worsens in the winter, and this simple tool—wearing wool for warmth—is very helpful," says Dr. Teitelbaum.

• **Underwear.** He favors long underwear that covers your chest and trunk, at least to your knees.

• **Bedding.** He also suggests a woolen bed liner ("It will make your sleep much more comfortable"), a woolen blanket or quilt and a woolen pillowcase.

"During wintertime, I would add all of these in combo, if you can," he says.

"The woolen bedding can be used year round, including summer," adds Dr. Kiyak. "Woolen underwear is too heavy for hot summer months."

"A company called Cuddle Ewe makes the best sheepskin bed liners and other types of bedding," says Dr. Teitelbaum. Visit *www.cuddleewe.com* or call 800-290-9199.

You can find Australian-made woolen underwear in many varieties at *www.wool-underwear.com*.

Emine Kara Kiyak, PhD, School of Nursing, Atatürk University, Turkey.

Jacob Teitelbaum, MD, medical director of the Fibromyalgia and Fatigue Centers and author of *From Fatigued to Fantastic!* (Avery). *www.endfatigue.com*.

Pain Remedies That Won't Harm You

More than 30 million Americans take conventional painkillers daily for a variety of ailments, including arthritis, headaches, sore muscles and back or neck pain. While these drugs are good at temporarily relieving pain, they all have unhealthful side effects, particularly when used over time for chronic conditions. They can irritate the stomach, cause stomach and intestinal ulcers and increase heart disease risk.

Fortunately, there are natural pain relievers that work as well as, or better than, these drugs, and they are much gentler on your body.

Caution: Women who are pregnant or breast-feeding should not take these remedies, because they have not been studied in these populations.

Strategy: For chronic pain involving any of the conditions in the table on the next page, take the first painkiller listed for that condition for four weeks. If you notice an improvement, stay with it. If not, try the next one (if there is one).

Try the following herbs—which are all available at health-food stores or online—for the conditions listed...

Devil's Claw

Devil's claw (*Harpagophytum procumbens*), a shrub found in southern Africa, works similarly to many pharmaceutical pain relievers—by blocking the action of pain-promoting compounds in the body—but without damaging the digestive tract. In studies involving people with chronic low back pain, devil's claw extract proved as effective as prescription pain relievers.

Dose: Devil's claw extract is available in capsules. Look for 1.5 to 2.0% harpagoside, one of the active ingredients. Take 1,000 milligrams (mg) three times daily of a standardized extract.

Recommended brand: Nature's Way Standardized Devil's Claw Extract (800-962-8873, *http://natureway.com*). The only significant potential side effect is diarrhea.

Curcumin

Curcumin (*diferuloylmethane*), a constituent of turmeric, is the pigment compound that gives the spice its distinctive yellow coloring. In one study of rheumatoid arthritis patients, 1,200 mg daily of curcumin extract improved morning stiffness and sporadic joint swelling.

Dose: Take 500 mg of standardized turmeric extract (containing 90 to 95% curcumin) three times daily.

Recommended brands: New Chapter Turmericforce (800-543-7279, *www.newchapter.com*) and Life Extension Super Curcumin (888-771-3905, *www.lifeextensionvitamins.com*). It has blood-thinning properties, so do not take curcumin if you take blood-thinning medication, such as warfarin, unless monitored by a physician.

Avoid this: If you have gallstones, because curcumin can cause gallstones to block bile ducts.

Natural Pain Relievers

Condition	Pain Relievers To Try*
Headache (tension or migraine)	White willow bark
Inflammatory bowel disease	Boswellia, Curcumin
Low back pain	Devil's claw, White willow bark Curcumin
Muscle aches and pain	White willow bark, Curcumin
Menstrual pain	Boswellia, White willow bark, Devil's claw
Osteoarthritis	Boswellia, Curcumin, Devil's claw
Rheumatoid arthritis	Boswellia, Curcumin, Devil's claw
Tendonitis	Devil's claw, Curcumin, White willow bark

*Take the first painkiller listed for your condition for four weeks. If it doesn't work, try the next one (if there is one).

White Willow Bark

This pain reliever has anti-inflammatory and blood-thinning benefits similar to those of aspirin, but unlike aspirin, it doesn't appear to damage the stomach lining. For centuries, the bark of the white willow (*Salix alba*), a tree found in Europe and Asia, was noted for its pain-relieving qualities. Its active ingredient is *salicin*, which the body converts to *salicylic acid*, a close cousin of aspirin (*acetylsalicylic acid*).

Dose: Take 120 mg daily of white willow bark extract capsules. If this amount does not reduce pain, try 240 mg.

Recommended brand: Solaray White Willow Bark (800-579-4665).

Avoid this: If you have an aspirin allergy and for one week before undergoing surgery. White willow bark is a blood thinner, so take it only while being monitored by a physician if you take blood-thinning medication.

Boswellia

Part of India's Ayurvedic healing tradition, *boswellia* (Boswellia serrata) comes from a tree found in India, Northern Africa and the Middle East. The tree yields a milky resin containing boswellic acids, substances that inhibit the body's synthesis of inflammatory leukotrienes. A study of patients with knee arthritis found that boswellia extract relieved pain and stiffness as well as daily doses of the prescription drug *valdecoxib* (Bextra). And boswellia's benefits persisted for one month longer than those of Bextra.

Dose: Take 750 mg of a standardized extract containing 60 to 65% boswellic acid two to three times daily for as long as symptoms last.

Recommended brand: Solgar Boswellia Resin Extract (877-765-4274, *www.solgar.com*). While generally safe, boswellia has been known to cause occasional mild digestive upset.

Mark A. Stengler, NMD, naturopathic medical doctor in private practice, La Jolla, California, and author of the *Bottom Line/Natural Healing* newsletter. *www.drstengler.com*.

Cherry Juice Relieves Muscle Pain

Runners who drank pure tart cherry juice immediately after a long run had 23% less pain than those who drank a placebo cherry drink. Tart cherry juice has strong anti-inflammatory properties that also could help fight arthritis and heart disease. Tart cherry juice comes from the Montmorency, or sour pie, cherry and may have properties similar to anti-inflammatory medications.

Study by researchers at Oregon Health & Science University, Portland, Oregon, presented at the American College of Sports Medicine Conference.

Try Self-Hypnosis for Drug-Free Pain Relief

Chronic pain is the leading cause of disability in the US, affecting more than 90 million Americans. Painkillers, including morphine and related drugs, invariably cause side effects (ranging from constipation to confusion), can be addictive and are only marginally effective for many patients.

Better: Self-hypnosis. It doesn't eliminate pain, but it improves your ability to cope with it. It also lowers levels of pain-causing stress hormones and increases the body's production of *endogenous opioids,* substances with morphinelike effects. With self-hypnosis, you can alter your relationship with pain. The pain is still there, but the suffering is controlled.

The practice of hypnotism has been distorted in movies and stage shows. You can't be hypnotized against your will, and you can't be made to do things that you don't want to do.

A hypnotic trance is merely an altered state of consciousness. It involves entering a physical and mental state of relaxation from which you redirect your attention to achieve certain goals—including the reduction of pain.

Simple Method

Once you've learned to induce hypnosis, you can do it on your own once or twice a day—preferably for 10 minutes in the morning and 10 minutes at night (if you have trouble judging the time, set a timer with a quiet alarm). You might need more frequent hypnosis sessions if you are in severe pain. Most people notice a significant reduction in pain within two months—some improve after a single session.

One common technique to induce hypnosis is The Zarren Marble Method, developed by the noted hypnotist Jordan Zarren...

• **Sit in a comfortable chair, and hold a marble between your thumb and other fingers.** Roll it around and notice the texture, colors, patterns and tiny imperfections.

• **Notice how relaxed you are.** You're probably blinking more...your eyelids are getting heavy.

• **At this point, close your eyes and close your hand around the marble so that it doesn't drop.** Now you are in a state of deep relaxation. If you find that you're thinking of something else, just bring your mind back to the marble.

Once you've entered this hypnotic trance, you can use a number of mental techniques to reduce pain. *Try the techniques below and see which ones work best for you...*

Deep Relaxation

No one can consciously experience multiple sensations simultaneously. When the sensation of relaxation is dominant, you'll feel less pain.

How to do it: First, before you enter a hypnotic state, choose two or three positive thoughts that you want to implant in your mind. These might include things such as *My body is relaxed* or *With each breath that I take, I relax more and more.*

Then go into a hypnotic state, and mentally focus on the thoughts that you've chosen. If your mind drifts, bring it back to the thoughts.

Dwelling on the positive produces physical changes in the body, including a reduction in muscle tension and lower levels of *cortisol* and other stress hormones. Even when the pain isn't gone, you'll react to it less strongly.

Decatastrophizing

Nearly everyone with chronic pain feels, at one time or another, that there's little hope for the future. Negative thinking increases pain sensations and intensifies suffering.

Decatastrophizing means to stop blowing things out of proportion. This helps separate pain from suffering.

Example: Someone might feel that life is worthless because of the pain. You can decatastrophize by limiting these negative thoughts or feelings. This can stop the transmission of pain signals.

How to do it: While under hypnosis, reframe how you think about pain. Rather than dwelling on hopelessness, for example, consider the possibility that pain has a purpose—that it can alert you that you need to do something to heal. Dwelling on pain's purpose can make you feel stronger and more in control.

You also can practice *disputation*—interrupting negative thoughts about pain by redirecting your attention to a thought that reduces stress. Say to yourself, *My pain is bad today, but I'm still going to get a lot done.*

Direction

During self-hypnosis, dwell on thoughts that emphasize your sense of control. *Examples...*

● **When you notice an increase in pain,** tell yourself, *I know I can handle this. I've dealt with worse before.*

● **If the pain gets stronger,** repeat positive thoughts, such as, *I will not let the pain get the best of me. I know I can do things to make it more tolerable.*

● **Handle the worst moments with thoughts such as,** *This is only temporary. I will get through it.*

When the pain subsides, remind yourself that you coped well—and that you now have a plan to help make it easier the next time.

Important: Minimize physical "pain behaviors," such as grimacing, groaning and complaining. These reinforce the pain and increase disability.

Distraction

Because the mind can process only a limited amount of information at one time, you can introduce sensations that compete with pain sensations.

How to do it: Create physical sensations (such as rubbing the place where it hurts) that are more pleasant than the pain sensations. Or distract yourself with mental exercises, such as listening to the sound of your breathing.

Try this: Go into a hypnotic trance, and pay attention only to your breathing. Listen to the sounds. Note the rhythm and the ways in which your breathing naturally changes.

The mental activity will reach your brain ahead of the pain sensations. This can close the "pain gate" so that you experience less pain.

Dissociation

Again, focus your mind on something other than the pain. The idea is to take advantage of the divide between the conscious and unconscious minds. Your unconscious mind will be aware of the pain, but the pain will be unable to dominate your consciousness.

How to do it: Imagine that your consciousness is floating out of your body—that it is hovering overhead looking down. Think, *When my conscious mind floats away to a pleasant place, I leave the discomfort behind.*

More Help

If you want to consult with a professional hypnotist, you can find one in your area by contacting the American Society of Clinical Hypnosis (ASCH), 630-980-4740, *www.asch. net.* (For more information on hypnosis as a healing therapy, see appendix page 349.)

Bruce N. Eimer, PhD, psychologist and owner/director of Alternative Behavior Associates in Huntingdon Valley, Pennsylvania and author of *Hypnotize Yourself Out of Pain Now!* (Crown House). *www.bestwaytostop.com.*

Swear at Your Pain— You'll Feel Better

He accidentally hit his hand with a hammer while building a garden shed—and swore.

His wife was in the most difficult part of his daughter's birth—and she swore. A lot. (The midwives told him it was a normal part of the process.)

After those two events, Richard Stephens, PhD, a lecturer in the School of Psychology at Keele University in England, started wondering why the readiest words out of our mouths when we're suddenly in pain usually contain four letters. Does swearing soothe the hurt?

To find out, he conducted a first-of-its-kind study, involving buckets of freezing water and a lot of expletives…

The Cursing Cure

Dr. Stephens recruited 64 students for his study, asking them to keep one hand in a bucket of ice-cold water for as long as possible, and swear away, using their favorite expletive.

Then they were asked to repeat the process—this time, saying a word they'd typically use to describe a table. (Flat, brown, hard, etc.)

Cursing was curative…

Results: When the students swore, they could keep their hands in the icy water for an average of two minutes. When they didn't swear, the average was one minute and 15 seconds. Later, the students rated the intensity of their pain during the two immersions—and there was less self-perceived pain when they swore. The findings were published in *NeuroReport*.

Why it works: Dr. Stephens admits that he doesn't know. But he has a theory. Those who swore had a higher heart rate. That means swearing might help trigger the fight-or-flight response, the body's automatic response to immediate threat, which includes increased heart rate, decreased respiration, tighter muscles, slower digestion—and lower sensitivity to pain.

Don't Wear Out Swearing

Dr. Stephens has two recommendations if you want to use swear words to help decrease pain.

●**Relief is a four-letter word.** "If you hurt yourself, swear." That's obvious. *But this isn't…*

● **Don't swear all the time.** "If you want to use the pain-lessening effect of swearing to your advantage, you need to do less casual swearing," he says. "Swearing is an emotion-al language. But if you overuse it, it loses its emotional significance. Without emotion, all that's left is saying the swearword itself—and that's unlikely to reduce anyone's pain."

Richard Stephens, PhD, lecturer in the School of Psychology at Keele University in England.

How Acupuncture Works to Puncture Pain

Studies show that acupuncture, an ancient healing technique from China, can help relieve all kinds of pain—headaches and back pain, joint pain and cancer pain, pain after injury and pain after surgery.

Ask a practitioner of Traditional Chinese Medicine (TCM) how acupuncture relieves pain, and he/she might say that the precisely inserted needles stimulate and balance *qi*, the life-energy that flows through the body along invisible channels called *meridians*.

Ask a scientist who has conducted a study on acupuncture how the needles relieve pain, and he/she might say they stimulate *endorphins*, opiatelike chemicals manufactured by the brain that help turn off pain receptors in nerve cells.

But lately, those scientists have become confused. Four large studies showed that real acupuncture and sham (fake) acupuncture worked equally well to relieve pain. (In sham acupuncture, needles are used to mimic the prickling sensations of acupuncture, but they aren't inserted into the skin. They're also placed in non-acupuncture locations.) How could both real and sham acupuncture do the job? Is acupuncture nothing more than a placebo, a healing technique that works only because a person believes it works?

To find out, scientists at the University of Michigan Medical School conducted a study to locate a brain-based difference between the effects of real and sham acupuncture…

Fake vs. Real Acupuncture

The scientists studied 20 women with *fibromyalgia*, a condition of chronically tender and painful muscles. Over a month, half were given nine treatments of real acupuncture and half were given sham. Before and after the first acupuncture treatment, the researchers took PET scans of the brains of the women, using a special dye to highlight receptors on brain cells that play a role in pain. The women had another set of PET scans after the last acupuncture treatment. And, at the beginning and end of the study, the women filled out questionnaires accessing their pain levels.

After the first treatment, sham acupuncture and real acupuncture both increased endorphins. And they both relieved pain. *But real acupuncture also affected the brain in an entirely different way than sham…*

Why it works: The surface of cells contains receptors that are like loading docks for biochemicals that do their work inside cells. Many brain cells contain *mu-opioid receptors,* which are targeted by opioid painkillers such as morphine and codeine. The mu receptors process and dampen pain signals. And the amount of space on the mu receptors was significantly increased by acupuncture treatments. There was no similar increase from sham acupuncture.

"Interestingly, women in both the acupuncture and sham acupuncture groups had similar reductions in pain," says Richard E. Harris, PhD, an assistant professor, Department of Internal Medicine, at the University of Michigan Medical School and the study's lead researcher. "But the mechanisms leading to pain relief were distinctly different."

"We still haven't found the exact physiological mechanism that explains acupuncture—and we may never find it," comments David W. Sollars, LAc, medical director of FirstHealth of Andover, Massachusetts (*www.firsthealthofandover.com*), and author of *The Complete Idiot's Guide to Acupuncture and Acupressure* (Alpha). "But this is a technology that is thousands of years old, with a proven history of effectiveness, and patients love it. It is a reasonable therapeutic option for a variety of different health conditions, including many pain problems."

A Panacea for Pain

However acupuncture works, the newest research once again shows that it can help relieve many different types of pain problems…

• **Tension headache.** Researchers in Germany analyzed the results of eleven studies on headache and acupuncture, involving more than 2,300 people. "Acupuncture could be a valuable non-pharmacological tool in patients with frequent, episodic or chronic tension-type headaches," they concluded.

• **Migraine.** In a similar analysis, the German researchers looked at 22 studies on using acupuncture to prevent migraines, involving more than 4,400 people. "Acupuncture is at least as effective as, or probably more effective than [preventive] drug treatment, and has fewer adverse effects," they concluded.

• **Chronic low back pain.** Researchers studied more than 600 people with chronic low back pain, with some receiving acupuncture and some receiving standard medical care. After two months, those receiving acupuncture had 40% more improvement in "back-related dysfunction" and 64% greater improvement in "symptom bothersomeness." The findings were in *Archives of Internal Medicine.*

• **Chronic neck pain.** Researchers in Hong Kong studied 49 people with chronic neck pain, treating half with real acupuncture and half with sham. Those receiving the real acupuncture had a 79% greater improvement in their condition, compared with those who had sham acupuncture.

• **Chronic shoulder pain.** Researchers at the Johns Hopkins Bayview Medical Center in Baltimore, Maryland, studied 31 people with chronic shoulder pain, dividing them into three groups. One received a general acupuncture treatment, one received an acupuncture treatment customized for shoulder pain and one received sham treatment. After 12 treatments over six weeks, only the first two groups had pain relief. "Acupuncture may be an effective treatment for chronic shoulder pain," concluded the researchers, in the *Journal of Alternative and Complementary Medicine.*

● **Post-tonsillectomy pain.** After a tonsillectomy, people usually have acute pain on swallowing. German doctors at the Heidelberg University studied 123 people after tonsillectomy, dividing them into two groups. During the first five days after the operation, one group received standard pain medication, and the other received medication and acupuncture. "Acupuncture led to a significant additional pain relief," said the researchers.

● **Rheumatoid arthritis.** Researchers in Japan used acupuncture to treat women with rheumatoid arthritis. "Acupuncture relieves symptoms, remedies physical function, and improves quality of life," they concluded.

● **Carpal tunnel syndrome (CTS).** Researchers in Taiwan studied 77 people with CTS, dividing them into two groups. One group was treated with *prednisolone*, an anti-inflammatory steroid drug; the other group received acupuncture. After two months, both groups were evaluated for several hand symptoms of CTS, including pain, numbness, tingling and weakness. Both groups improved in all those symptoms. "Short-term acupuncture treatment is as effective as short-term low-dose prednisolone for mild to moderate carpal tunnel syndrome," concluded the researchers, in the *Clinical Journal of Pain.*

● **Chronic prostatitis/chronic pelvic pain syndrome (CP/CPPS).** Korean researchers studied 39 men with CP/CPPS, dividing them into three groups. One group received advice about the problem and an exercise program (advice and exercise, or AE); one group received AE and electroacupuncture (mild electricity is run through the inserted needles); one received AE and sham electroacupuncture. After six weeks, all the men in the real electroacupuncture group had a significant improvement in the condition, compared with two men in the sham group and three men in the AE group. Electroacupuncture had therapeutic effects in CP/CPPS, "particularly for pain relief," concluded the researchers, in *Urology.*

● **Joint pain in postmenopausal breast cancer survivors.** Postmenopausal breast cancer survivors who take hormone-blocking drugs called *aromatase inhibitors* often develop severe pain in one or more joints. Researchers at the University of Pennsylvania studied a dozen women with the problem, providing 10 acupuncture treatments around the painful joints, over two months. Pain severity decreased by an average of 65% and stiffness by 66%. There was also an 83% decrease in joint pain interfering with daily life. And a large decrease in fatigue and anxiety.

What to Do

To find an acupuncturist who can effectively treat your pain, follow these recommendations from Sollars…

● **Ask a good friend.** "How do you find a good mechanic or restaurant?" he says. "You ask a friend. It's the same with acupuncture. Find out if a friend you know and respect has been to or heard of a qualified acupuncturist in your area. That's the best and most reliable way to locate a qualified acupuncturist."

Also helpful: "Doctors are often trying to find good solutions for their patients—and your doctor may know a competent acupuncturist."

● **Check for credentials.** "A certified acupuncturist ensures competency," says Sollars.

Resource: Visit the Web site of the American Association of Acupuncture and Oriental Medicine, *www.aaaomonline.com*, where you can use their "Find an Acupuncturist" search function to find a certified acupuncturist near you.

● **Call the acupuncturist.** "Ask him/her if he or she has experience in treating your particular condition," says Sollars, who also advises that you follow your instincts. "Are you reassured by his/her voice and manner? Do you feel confident about the acupuncturist after your phone call? If not, don't see that practitioner."

● **Make an appointment.** "Going to your first appointment will often help you decide if this is a practitioner you want to use regularly," says Sollars.

•Tell your MD what you're doing. "I believe it's essential that you give your doctor a written list of all the healthcare practitioners that you see," says Sollars. "You can even have your acupuncturist make a phone call or send a note to your doctor, letting the physician know that he or she is seeing you as a patient."

•Enjoy the treatments. "Once you've found an acupuncturist you're comfortable with, enjoy the process of healing that a good practitioner can provide." (For more information on acupuncture, see appendix page 354.)

Richard E. Harris, PhD, assistant professor, Department of Internal Medicine, University of Michigan Medical School.

David W. Sollars, LAc, medical director of FirstHealth of Andover, Massachusetts, and author of *The Complete Idiot's Guide to Acupuncture and Acupressure* (Alpha). *www.firsthealthofandover.com.*

Meditate Your Pain Away

Research shows that training in *mindfulness-based stress reduction* (MBSR) can help you manage pain. The training includes learning "mindfulness meditation," in which you sit quietly and focus on your breath, while acknowledging but not judging thoughts and feelings.

Problem: The mindfulness program is eight weeks long, includes daily homework assignments and a full day of silent retreat and requires a trained professional to teach you the technique. In other words, it takes a lot of time, and you can't do it on your own.

Solution: Three, 20-minute sessions of mindfulness meditation may accomplish the same result, says a new study.

More Mindfulness, Less Pain

Led by Fadel Zeidan, PhD, researchers at the University of North Carolina, Charlotte, conducted three experiments on 22 people.

First—since everyone's perception of pain is different—they figured out pain levels for each participant by administering an electric shock to the forearm at several levels of intensity and asking each participant to rate the pain on a scale, with 2 being "low pain" and 4 being "high pain."

Then, they divided the students into two groups.

One group was taught a simple form of mindfulness meditation in three 20-minute training sessions, each of which included a period of meditation.

Next, they again administered the electric shocks to both groups.

The nonmeditators had the same level of pain perception—a 2 was still a 2 and a 4 was still a 4. But the meditators now required a much higher level of electric shock to create the same pain perception of 2 and 4.

"The short course of meditation was very effective on pain perception," says Dr. Zeidan, a post-doctoral researcher at Wake Forest University School of Medicine, in North Carolina. "In fact, it was kind of freaky. I was ramping up the shocks to what was previously perceived as a high level of pain, and their arms would be jolting back and forth because the current was stimulating a motor nerve, yet they would still be asking, 'Is that a 2?' It was very surprising."

The researchers then tested whether or not the distraction of doing a difficult math problem or practicing a relaxation technique could match the decreased pain perception from mindfulness meditation.

Again, the meditators had a lower perception of pain—both at the low and high levels—than those doing the math problem or relaxing. And those who were the most mindful (as measured by a questionnaire called the Freiburg Mindfulness Inventory) perceived the least pain. The meditators also had significantly less anxiety.

"These data suggest that a decrease in anxiety and the ability to sustain focus on the present moment can attenuate the feeling of pain," wrote Dr. Zeidan and his colleagues, in *The Journal of Pain.*

But not only did the meditators have a lower perception of pain while meditating.

The researchers found the meditators continued to have a lowered awareness of pain, outside of meditation. In short, they had lessened pain's ability to distract and disturb.

"This was totally surprising," says Dr. Zeidan. "We did not expect to find a change in general sensitivity to pain."

"This is the first study to demonstrate the efficacy of such a brief intervention on the perception of pain," he continues. "We already knew that meditation has significant effects on pain perception in long-term practitioners whose brains seem to have been completely changed—but we didn't know you could do this in just three days."

Why it works: "It's attention," says Dr. Zeidan. "Mindfulness training lessens the awareness of and sensitivity to pain because it trains a person's brain to pay attention to sensations in the present, rather than anticipating future pain or dwelling on emotions caused by pain. It teaches you that distractions, thoughts and feelings are momentary and don't require a label or judgment, because the moment is already over. With the meditation training, you can acknowledge the pain, realize what it is, but just let it go and bring your attention back to the present, without anxiety."

A Simple Way to Meditate

This study shows that meditation is a much easier way to manage pain than previously thought, says Dr. Zeidan. In fact, even self-taught mindfulness might work to reduce the perception and burden of pain, he says.

Here are instructions to practice a simple mindfulness meditation...

1. Sit comfortably.

2. Close your eyes.

3. Focus on the feeling of the breath as it flows in and out of the nostrils.

4. Non-judgmentally become aware of your thoughts, sensations and feelings, while maintaining focus on the breath in the nostrils.

5. If you are distracted by thoughts, sensations or feelings, simply acknowledge and release the distraction, and bring attention back to the breath.

6. Practice for 15 or 20 minutes, once a day.

Resources: On the second day of the study, the meditators had a guided mindfulness meditation, listening to a 20-minute tape by Jon Kabat-Zinn, PhD, author of *Full Catastrophe Living* (Delta), the classic text on mindfulness-based stress reduction.

You can purchase guided mindfulness meditation CDs and tapes at *www.mindfulnesstapes.com*.

You can also find mindfulness meditation training on the Internet, says Dr. Zeidan. The Web site *www.youtube.com* has several videos that explain mindfulness and/or that guide you through a session of meditation.

Bottom line: "Use mindfulness to change your perception of pain—and that should help alleviate the feeling of that pain," says Dr. Zeidan.

Fadel Zeidan, PhD, post-doctoral researcher at Wake Forest University School of Medicine, North Carolina.

How to Prevent Boomeritis

They're called Baby Boomers—but many of them aren't babying their bodies.

In a recent year, more than 166,000 people between the ages of 45 and 64—in other words, Boomers—were treated in emergency rooms, clinics and doctors' offices for exercise-related injuries, says a new report from the US Consumer Products Safety Commission.

What happens: "When you're 50 or so, your joints, muscles, and tissues may not be as flexible as they used to be, and you can injure your body more easily than when you were 20," says Ray Monto, MD, a spokesperson for the American Academy of Orthopedic Surgeons (AAOS) (*www.aaos.org*).

This situation causes many different types of exercise-related injuries, which some experts are collectively calling "Boomeritis."

"Among boomers—particularly men in their fifties who aren't as fit or flexible as they once were—I'm seeing more tendonitis, tennis elbow, knee pain, back pain, shoulder injuries and neck injuries," says Vinod So-mareddy, PT, DPT, a physical therapist and owner of Reddy-Care Physical Therapy in Great Neck, New York.

"As boomers age, they should take extra steps to protect themselves from injuries when exercising," advises Dr. Monto.

Easy Ways to Avoid Injury

Here are some recommendations for staying active without injuring yourself, from Kathi Casey, a yoga teacher, Pilates instructor and owner of the Healthy Boomer Body Center in Otis, Massachusetts.

• **Stretch before and after exercising.** "I highly recommend stretching for at least two to three minutes before and after exercising," says Casey.

Example: "This simple exercise stretches the muscles from the hips all the way down the legs," says Casey. "The grief it can save—in injury and pain—is priceless."

1. Kneel on the floor in the "table position"—on both knees, and on the palms of your hands.

2. Bring your right knee forward and place it between your hands.

3. Stretch your left leg out straight behind you.

4. Relax and breathe deeply, for 1 minute.

5. Return to the table position.

6. Repeat with the other leg.

• **Stretch your shoulders regularly.** "A shoulder roll once a day takes a couple of minutes, and can help prevent shoulder, neck and back injuries," says Casey. *The exercise...*

1. Lie on the floor on your side with your knees bent and your arms perpendicular to your body, with your hands stacked on top of each other.

2. Stretch your top arm out and gently slide it along the floor in a half circle above your head and around toward your back, as far as it will go without pain.

3. Slide it back, until your hands are stacked again.

4. Breathe deeply.

5. Repeat four times, breathing deeply.

6. Switch to the opposite side, and repeat the entire exercise with the other arm.

More recommendations from the AAOS. Other ways to prevent boomeritis include...

• **Check with your doctor before beginning an exercise program.**

• **Avoid being a "weekend warrior"—** moderate exercise every day or every other day is healthier.

• **Don't be afraid to take lessons.** An instructor can help ensure you're using the proper form, which can prevent overuse injuries such as tendonitis and stress fractures.

• **Develop a balanced fitness program** that includes aerobic exercise, strength training and stretching.

• **When introducing new exercises, start gradually,** so you don't try to do too much at once.

• **Take calcium and vitamin D supplements daily,** to maximize the health of your bones.

• **Schedule regular days off from exercise.**

Ray Monto, MD, spokesperson for the American Academy of Orthopedic Surgeons (AAOS). *www.aaos.org.*

Vinod Somareddy, PT, DPT, physical therapist and owner of Reddy-Care Physical Therapy in Great Neck, New York. *www.reddycare.net.*

Kathi Casey, yoga teacher, Pilates instructor and owner of the Healthy Boomer Body Center in Otis, Massachusetts. *www.healthyboomerbody.com.*

Post-Workout, Pain-Free

After your workout, take a hot shower for five minutes, then turn the water as cold as you can stand for one minute. Repeat this for at least three cycles, and end with cold water. Alternating between hot and cold water dilates your blood vessels and helps facilitate circulation, reducing inflammation and pain, which helps you recover faster.

Men's Journal, 1290 Avenue of the Americas, New York City 10104, *www.mensjournal.com.*

Chapter 2

AGING & LONGEVITY

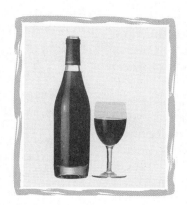

Have a Goal and Live Longer

I f you want to increase your chances of living longer, you probably know what to do—eat healthy foods, exercise regularly, handle stress, get enough sleep, don't smoke.

Well, you can add another item to that list—have a purpose in life.

Researchers at the Rush University Medical Center in Chicago studied more than 1,200 people with an average age of 78. Over a five-year period, they found that those with a greater purpose in life (the sense that life has meaning and direction, and that one's goals and potential are being achieved or are achievable) had a 57% lower risk of dying.

Study Details

It didn't matter whether the study participants were male or female, rich or poor, healthy or sick, happy or depressed, fully functioning or disabled—purpose in life stood out as a major determining factor in whether they lived or died.

Specifically, the researchers found that those who did agree with the following statements were 57% more likely to die than those who didn't agree...

- I sometimes feel as if I've done all there is to do in life.

- I used to set goals for myself, but that now seems like a waste of time.

- My daily activities often seem trivial and commonplace.

"Statistically, this was a very robust finding," says Patricia Boyle, PhD, the study leader.

She also notes that purpose in life has been linked to several biomarkers of healthy aging, such as lower levels of the stress hormone cortisol, lower levels of disease-causing inflammatory factors, higher HDL "good" cholesterol and better waist-hip ratios (a widening waistline is a risk factor for heart disease and diabetes).

Maximize Meaning

"Purpose and meaning in life is a very personal construct," says Dr. Boyle. "What brings you a sense of purpose might be very different from how I derive purpose." *Her recommendations for customizing a more purposeful life...*

● **Think about what makes your life more meaningful.** Is it spending time with family and friends? Educating yourself? Improving the lives of others? "Take the time to sit down and think, 'What is important to me?'" says Dr. Boyle. Make a list of those activities.

Helpful: Many people find purpose and meaning by making a contribution beyond their own lives that also establishes connections with other people. "You may decide that you want to spend time with younger grandchildren, teaching them to read...or work with the homeless...or teach English as a second language—something that allows you to know you've touched someone else and changed his or her life," says Dr. Boyle.

● **Ask yourself, "Am I doing what's meaningful to me?"** Review your list of meaningful activities to see if you're actually doing them. "If family is important to you, for example, ask yourself if you're communicating with them as much as you'd like to," says Dr. Boyle. "If education is your priority, ask yourself if you're truly learning and improving your mind."

● **Set goals.** Once you've determined how much you're participating in meaningful activities, set goals that will involve you in more of those activities.

"Set small, realistic goals," advises Dr. Boyle. "Write them down. Be very intentional and exacting about how you're going to achieve them, and then monitor your progress."

For example, you may decide to spend one hour every week as a volunteer at a local hospital. Or to sign up for a class at your community college next semester. Or to call each of your children at least once a month.

● **Review the day.** At the end of every day, ask yourself, "Have I spent significant time today doing things that were important to me and gave me personal meaning and satisfaction?" If you haven't, write down something you'll do tomorrow to increase your sense of meaning and satisfaction.

● **Don't believe the myth that aging is a time when purpose and meaning is diminished or lost.** "Aging is not a time of inevitable decline—that's the common view, and it's incorrect," says Dr. Boyle. "The more we study older people, the more we find that they are engaged and connected.

"Older people can thrive and they can contribute to society—including the contribution of qualities that younger and middle-aged people often don't possess, such as wisdom and experience, and the balance and emotional stability that comes with them."

Patricia Boyle, PhD, assistant professor, Department of Psychology, Rush University Medical Center in Chicago.

Lessons for Living Longer From the People Who Live the Longest

The average life expectancy in the US is 78.1 years, an age that is far less than our potential maximum life spans.

On the Japanese island of Okinawa, there are approximately 50 centenarians (those who reach 100 years or more) per 100,000 people. In the US, at most 20 per 100,000 people reach this impressive milestone.

A long life is not an accident. Writer and longevity expert Dan Buettner, in conjunction with the National Institute on Aging and the nation's top gerontologists, has studied what he calls the world's Blue Zones, areas where people live unexpectedly long and healthy lives. In addition to Okinawa, the Blue Zones include Sardinia, Italy...Loma Linda, California (home to many Seventh-day Adventists)...and the Nicoya Peninsula in Costa Rica.

Important finding: Only about 25% of longevity is determined by genetics. The other 75% is largely determined by the choices that we make every day. *The average American could live up to 14 more good years by putting the following habits to work...*

Choose Activity, Not "Exercise"

In Sardinia, where the rate of centenarians is 208 per 100,000, many men work as shepherds. They hike for miles every day. Similarly, people in Okinawa get hours of daily exercise in their gardens. California's Seventh-day Adventists, one of the longest-living groups in the US, take frequent nature walks.

What these groups have in common is regular, low-intensity physical exercise. They don't necessarily lift weights or run marathons. They merely stay active—and they do it every day throughout their lives.

Daily physical activity improves balance and reduces the risk for falls, a common cause of death among seniors. It lowers blood pressure and improves cardiovascular health. It increases the odds that people will be functionally independent in their later years.

Recommended: 30 to 60 minutes of moderate physical activity daily. This could include riding a bicycle or walking instead of driving.

Eat Less

Okinawan elders intone this adage before eating—*hara hachi bu*—a reminder to stop eating when their stomachs are 80% full.

People who quit eating when they're no longer hungry (rather than eating until they feel full) find it easy to maintain a healthy weight, which reduces the risk for heart disease. This approach is more natural than conventional diets. *Helpful...*

• **Serve yourself at the kitchen counter, then put the food away.** People who do this tend to eat about 14% less than those who don't.

• **Use smaller plates and bowls.** Doing so makes servings look larger, which helps you eat less. In one study, people who ate from a 34-ounce bowl took in 31% more than those who used a 17-ounce bowl. Similarly, people drink at least 25% more when they use short, wide glasses instead of tall, narrow ones.

• **Buy small.** Most people consume about 150 more calories when they take food from large packages than when they take it from smaller ones.

Limit Meat

In every Blue Zone, meat is consumed, at most, a few times a month. People in these communities live mainly on beans, whole grains, vegetables and other plant foods. These foods are high in fiber, antioxidants and anticancer compounds. Traditional Sardinians, Nicoyans and Okinawans eat what is produced in their gardens supplemented by staples—durum wheat (Sardinia), sweet potato (Okinawa) and maize (Nicoya). Strict Adventists avoid meat entirely.

Studies of Seventh-day Adventists show that a relatively high proportion eat nuts (any kind). Those who eat about two ounces of nuts five or more times a week have heart disease rates that are only half those who rarely eat nuts.

Consider Wine

Studies of long-lived people suggest that drinking alcohol in moderation is a powerful factor in living longer. It is consumed in three of the Blue Zones (Okinawa, Sardinia and Costa Rica). In Sardinia, the shepherds drink about one-quarter bottle of red wine a day. Their wine has two to three times more flavonoids than other wines (because of the hot climate and the way the wine is made). Flavonoids reduce arterial inflammation. Inflammation has been linked to atherosclerosis, diabetes and Alzheimer's disease.

Cultivate a Sense of Purpose

A study funded by the National Institutes of Health (NIH) found that people who are excited by life and feel that they're making a difference tend to live longer (and healthier) lives than those who just "get by."

Okinawans call it *ikigai* and Nicoyans call it *plan de vida*, but in both cultures, the phrase essentially translates to why I wake up in the morning. Anything that gives you a sense of purpose—even something as simple as taking pleasure in watching your children or grandchildren grow up well—can add years to your life.

De-Stress

Many people don't realize that the 24/7 American lifestyle is literally toxic. It produces a chronic increase in stress hormones that triggers inflammation throughout the body.

Most of the world's longest-lived people incorporate some form of meaningful downtime into their daily lives. Nicoyans take a break every afternoon to socialize with friends. For Adventists, the Saturday Sabbath is a time to rest.

Embrace Your Spiritual Side

Faith is a key element that most centenarians have in common. The Sardinians and Nicoyans are mostly Catholic. Okinawans have a blended religion that stresses ancestor worship. The Adventists form a strong religious community. People who attend religious services are about one-third less likely to die in a given period than those who don't. Even among people who don't go to church, those with spiritual beliefs have less depression, better immunity and lower rates of heart disease.

Put Family First

In the Blue Zones, a great emphasis is placed on family—and people who live with or maintain close ties with their families get sick less often than those without these ties. They also are more likely to maintain better mental and social skills throughout their lives.

Dan Buettner is founder of Blue Zones, an organization that studies the regions of the world where people commonly live active lives past the age of 100, and author of The Blue Zones (National Geographic). www.bluezones.com.

The Six Lifesaving Super Foods in the Mediterranean Diet

Nearly 1,800 scientific studies have been conducted on the Mediterranean diet, showing that it can prevent (and sometimes stop or reverse) a wide variety of health problems, including heart disease, diabetes, overweight, high blood pressure, depression and several cancers.

Latest development: Researchers at the University of Athens and Harvard School of Public Health evaluated the Mediterranean diet and think they have discovered exactly which foods in the diet contribute to longevity, publishing their results in BMJ (formerly the *British Medical Journal*).

Red Wine Good, Red Meat Bad

The researchers studied 23,000 people for nine years, evaluating their diets with a "Mediterranean diet score" of 0 to 9, with 9 being frequent consumption of each of the nine food factors in the Mediterranean diet and 0 being infrequent consumption.

They found that increasing adherence to a Mediterranean diet by a factor of 2—for example, from 5 to 7—was linked to a 14% lower risk of dying. But when they analyzed the data more closely, they found that only six of the nine food factors in the Mediterranean diet were linked to a lower risk of dying, while three others weren't. They also found that some food factors were more protective than others. *Specifically, they found...*

●**24% lower risk**—Moderate alcohol intake (mostly in the form of red wine during meals)

●**17% lower risk**—Low intake of meat and meat products

●**16% lower risk**—High intake of vegetables

●**11% lower risk**—High intake of fruits and nuts

● **11% lower risk**—High intake of monounsaturated fats compared with saturated fats, mostly from olive oil

● **10% lower risk**—High intake of legumes (beans and peas)

Three other elements of the Mediterranean diet—whole grains, fish and seafood, and low intake of dairy—had little or no effect on the risk of dying.

Super Foods at the Supermarket

Stella Metsovas, CN, a nutritionist in Laguna Beach, California, with both parents from Greece, has these recommendations for incorporating more Mediterranean super foods into your diet...

1. More wine. "If you want to follow the Mediterranean diet in terms of alcohol consumption, drink red wine on social occasions, with your family and friends, at meals."

2. More vegetables. Try *horta*, or "greens". "In Crete, literally half the dietary intake is from wild greens," says Metsovas. Comparable greens in the US would be dandelion greens, mustard greens, collards or beet greens.

Try this: Boil for three to six minutes in water with a pinch of salt, drain, eat at room temperature, use the following dressing...

3. More olive oil. "In Greece, a simple dressing of about two tablespoons of olive oil, one tablespoon of lemon juice, sea salt and pepper is added to horta, and to just about every vegetable that's served," says Metsovas.

Also try: Italians prefer horta with pine nuts and Romano cheese.

4. More fruit. For a wonderful Mediterranean-style salad dressing, throw berries in a blender and add a teaspoon of olive oil, and a pinch of sea salt and pepper, says Metsovas.

5. More nuts. Put raw nuts, such as pecans or walnuts, on top of salads or fish.

6. More beans. "A bean salad is one of the main menu items in the tavernas—the small, family-owned restaurants in Greece that specialize in the Mediterranean diet," says Metsovas. In the summertime, you'll find black-eyed beans or fava beans served cold and drizzled with olive oil. In the wintertime, you'll find the beans warmed.

Try this: Metsovas advises her clients to make a big bowl of beans in the beginning of the week, and then add them to salads or to sauces for chicken or fish.

Stella Metsovas, CN, nutritionist in private practice in Laguna Beach, California. *www.w8lessnutrition.com.*

Extra Pounds = Extra Years?

We're in the midst of what experts are calling an "obesity epidemic"—34% of Americans are overweight (and 33% are obese).

Experts link this epidemic to a rising incidence of many conditions and diseases, including high cholesterol and heart disease, high blood pressure and stroke, type 2 diabetes, several cancers, arthritis, heartburn, sleep apnea, gallbladder and liver disease and infertility.

So how can new research show that being overweight might increase your lifespan?

Don't Lose Weight?

In a recent study in the journal *Obesity*, Canadian researchers analyzed 12 years of health data from more than 11,000 people.

To understand their surprising results, you need to understand the "Body Mass Index," or BMI, a formula that calculates body fat based on a person's weight and height.

According to the BMI, a 5-foot, 5-inch adult would be considered...

● Underweight at 110 pounds or less (BMI less than 18.5)

● Normal weight at 111 to 149 pounds (BMI from 18.5 to 24.9)

● Overweight at 150 to 179 pounds (BMI from 25 to 29.9)

31

●Obese at 180 to 210 pounds (BMI from 30 to 34.9)

●Extremely obese at 211 pounds (BMI of 35 or greater).

In the study, the researchers found that people who were overweight had a 17% lower risk of dying from any cause, compared with those of normal weight.

People who were obese had a 5% lower risk of dying.

People who were underweight had a 73% higher risk of dying.

And people who were extremely obese had a 36% higher risk of dying.

"Our results are similar to those from other recent studies," write the researchers, "showing that...overweight appears to be protective against mortality."

And in another recent study, researchers in England found that weight loss in overweight people caused a 9% increase in death rate.

"The available evidence does not support advising overweight or obese individuals who are otherwise healthy to lose weight as a means of prolonging life," say the researchers, in *Nutrition Research and Reviews*.

What's that again? If you're overweight, you shouldn't lose weight if you want to live longer? How could that be?

The Myth of Healthy Thinness

Linda Bacon, PhD, a nutrition professor at the City College of San Francisco, thinks she knows the answer. The author of *Health at Every Size: The Surprising Truth About Your Weight* (BenBella), Dr. Bacon has rigorously analyzed the scientific data on overweight, health and longevity—and found that what the experts are telling us about weight and health are mostly myths, supported by our cultural obsession with thinness and bias against fatness, and by the economic pressures of the multi-billion dollar weight-loss industry.

"The scientific evidence is clear—body fat is not the killer it's portrayed as," she says. "No one has ever proven that losing weight prolongs life. And the idea that weight plays a large causative role in disease is also unproven."

What the scientific evidence really shows, she says, is that several other lifestyle factors—for example, physical activity, stress and social support from family and friends—are far more important in determining longevity.

"Focusing on weight as a factor in longevity or even disease prevention is not useful," says Dr. Bacon.

Partner with Your Setpoint

Dr. Bacon says that each of us is genetically "wired" to maintain a healthy weight—that each of has a "setpoint" that automatically keeps our weight at a healthy level if we don't interfere with it, by trying to override or control our natural weight through the deprivations of dieting (which can peel off pounds in the short-term but never works in the long-term).

Here's how to partner with your setpoint to maintain the weight that's right for you...

●**Trust your setpoint.** Like every other genetically determined human trait—for example, shortness or tallness—there is a wide range of natural weights, from thin to fat, with the majority of us in the middle range. If your setpoint is genetically programmed to fatness, there is nothing you can do about it—you can guiltlessly carry a few more pounds than "normal" and still be healthy!

"Everybody is genetically predisposed to look a certain way, and the majority of us are not going to look like the models in magazines and on TV," says Dr. Bacon. "As a culture, we need to accept the diversity of body sizes, including one's own body size."

●**Lighten up—about the fact that your weight may not be perfect.** Like everyone in our society, if you're so-called overweight you've been encouraged to seek the Holy Grail of weight loss. "That search causes endless emotional pain, as you fail to maintain weight loss and blame yourself," says Dr. Bacon.

"Instead, trust that you will maintain the weight that's right for you if your diet emphasizes wholesome foods and you exercise regularly."

●**Don't diet.** Dieting has been shown to be the quickest way to gain weight, as you deprive yourself and then compensate by eating large amounts of food. Research shows that if you don't diet, weight tends to stay stable, says Dr. Bacon.

●**Accept your body.** "If you hate your body, and you're always looking at it as if something's wrong with it, you have no incentive to take good care of it," says Dr. Bacon. "Instead, appreciate your body. If you honor it, it's easier to make better nutritional and other lifestyle choices."

Self-acceptance has to come before weight loss, she emphasizes. "People think, 'When I lose weight, I'll accept myself.' But research shows the opposite is true—change happens when you feel good about yourself, and empower yourself to make better choices."

●**Watch out for foods that fool your body.** The prevalence of processed, high-calorie foods has contributed to "fooling" the body, causing us to overeat, says Dr. Bacon.

"Foods come from nature packaged with 'information' such as fiber that tells us our body is getting calories," says Dr. Bacon. "When you process that food, throwing away the information, the body doesn't register that it's getting everything it needs and continues to eat."

Example: High-fructose corn syrup, found in many processed foods. "If you get those calories in the form of corn, you can eat an ear or two and you're full," says Dr. Bacon. "If you get them in the form of corn syrup, you get an infusion of sweetness that activates your appetite's pleasure signals that say 'Keep eating!' but not its fullness signals that say 'Stop eating!'"—making it all-too-easy to eat much more than your body needs.

Best: Emphasize whole, natural foods such as fruits, vegetables, whole grains, beans, lean meat and fish, nuts and seeds and dairy products.

Bottom line: "Eat attentively, listen to your body, and you can arrive at a healthy weight for you, whatever that is," says Dr. Bacon. "What's important is a healthy lifestyle—weight loss may be a result of that, and it may not."

Linda Bacon, PhD, nutrition professor, Department of Biology, City College of San Francisco and author of *Health at Every Size: The Surprising Truth About Your Weight* (BenBella).

Anti-Aging Secrets From China

We all know that a nutritious diet is one of the keys to living a long, healthy life.

Problem: Even health-conscious individuals get stuck in a rut of consuming the same foods and drinks all the time.

Solution: Traditional Chinese Medicine (TCM) offers a wide variety of healthful, delicious foods and drinks that have been consumed for their disease-fighting properties for thousands of years.

Ancient anti-aging favorites…

●**Orange peel for cholesterol.** As we age, LDL "bad" cholesterol often accumulates in the arteries, leading to heart disease and stroke. Orange peel actually may lower cholesterol better than some medications, such as statin drugs, without the side effects.

Studies show that compounds called *polymethoxylated flavones* (PMFs), found in pigments of oranges and tangerines, can reduce bad cholesterol—without decreasing the level of HDL "good" cholesterol.

Advice: Grate or chop the peel of an orange or tangerine (preferably organic to avoid potentially toxic pesticides). If cooking a 12-ounce serving of meat or chicken, use the whole rind. As an alternative, use low-sugar marmalade, which contains orange rind, in your sauce.

●**Papaya for allergies.** Papaya is rich in the enzyme bromelain and has long been used by the Chinese to help reduce the inflammatory process that promotes allergic reactions. Other bromelain-rich foods include pineapple and kiwifruit.

Advice: Try eating two to three cups of the bromelain-rich fruits mentioned above daily—and add cherries and grapes (all types), which are rich in phytochemicals that also fight the inflammation that results from the body's immune response to allergens. Bromelain is also available in supplement form. If you suffer from hay fever or other allergies, take 200 mg daily.

• **Chicory for heart health.** Chicory, a vegetable that is popular in China and parts of Europe, contains a compound called inulin that helps strengthen the heart muscle—and may even be useful in treating congestive heart failure (a condition that causes inadequate pumping action of the heart).

One study found that chicory helps regulate an irregular heartbeat—a potentially dangerous condition that can lead to heart failure. Other research shows that chicory helps lower cholesterol levels and may slow the progression of hardening of the arteries.

Advice: In the US, chicory root is most often roasted for use as a brewed coffee substitute that can be found in most organic food markets. For heart health, drink one to two cups daily of chicory coffee substitute.

Recommendation: Teeccino Java Mediterranean Herbal Coffee. Radicchio, a type of leafy chicory, is also widely available. Eat it two to three times weekly (in salads, for example).

• **Chinese asparagus root for increased energy and brain function.** This close cousin to the asparagus found on Western dinner tables contains many phytonutrients, including quercetin, an antioxidant and anti-inflammatory compound. It has been used in China to promote longevity for more than 2,000 years. Chinese asparagus root can be found online, in health food stores and at the offices of TCM practitioners.

Advice: Consume as a brewed tea (one to two cups daily) or in capsule form (300 mg to 500 mg daily).

• **White willow bark tea for pain relief and blood-thinning properties.** This tree bark contains *salicin*, a compound found in aspirin. Aspirin was originally discovered in—and extracted from—this bark. White willow bark, unlike its pharmaceutical cousin aspirin, does not cause gastric upset and erode the stomach lining.

Besides its pain-relieving properties, white willow bark acts as an anticoagulant, which helps prevent the formation of blood clots and thickening of blood that can lead to heart attacks and strokes.

Advice: If you have pain caused by arthritis, muscle strain or *tendinitis* (tendon inflammation) or are at increased risk for heart disease or ischemic stroke (from a blockage)—due to family history, high blood pressure or smoking—drink one to two cups of white willow bark tea daily. If you take daily aspirin therapy for heart attack and/or stroke prevention, ask your doctor about taking supplemental white willow bark (100 mg daily) instead.

Caution: If you have a bleeding disorder or take a blood thinner, such as *warfarin* (Coumadin), do not use white willow bark.

Mao Shing Ni, LaC, DOM, PhD, a Santa Monica, California–based licensed acupuncturist and doctor of oriental medicine. *www.taoofwellness.com.* He is author of *Secrets of Longevity* (Chronicle).

Eat Fiber, Live Longer

P revious studies have linked dietary fiber intake with a reduced risk of dying from coronary heart disease, but little was known about fiber and mortality. Now a study from the Netherlands has found that every additional 10 grams (g) daily of dietary fiber reduced the risk for death from all causes by 9% and heart disease mortality by 17%.

Americans have long been told to increase their intake of fiber—and this study shows why. A 9% reduction in deaths from all causes by ingesting an extra 10 g of fiber daily is significant. Fiber reduces the risk for several diseases, including heart disease, hypertension and diabetes. Whole grains, fruits and vegetables are the primary sources of dietary fiber. Add salads and fruit to your diet—and reduce your risk for an early death.

Mark A. Stengler, NMD, naturopathic medical doctor in private practice, La Jolla, California, and author of the *Bottom Line/Natural Healing* newsletter. *www.drstengler.com.*

Wine Extends Life Span for Men

In a study of 1,373 men, those who drank wine—on average, less than one-half glass daily—lived an average of five years longer than alcohol abstainers and two-and-a-half years longer than beer and spirits drinkers.

Theory: Wine's cardiovascular benefits may account for the added longevity. More research is needed to assess whether these findings would also apply to women.

Marinette Streppel, PhD, researcher, Division of Human Nutrition, Wageningen University, Wageningen, the Netherlands.

Coffee May Boost Life Span

When dietary data for 127,950 healthy middle-aged men and women were tracked for 18 to 24 years, researchers found that those who drank two to three cups of caffeinated coffee daily had an 18% lower rate of death from all causes—especially deaths related to cardiovascular disorders—compared with people who did not drink coffee. Those who consumed two to three cups of decaffeinated coffee daily had an 11% lower risk of dying from heart disease.

Theory: Antioxidant compounds in coffee curb inflammation that may lead to cardiovascular disease.

Esther López-García, PhD, assistant professor of epidemiology, Universidad Autónoma de Madrid School of Medicine, Spain.

The Fat That Guarantees Longevity

The government's Centers for Disease Control and Prevention (CDC) recently funded an analysis by researchers at the Harvard School of Public Health that ranked from number 1 to number 12 the health activities that could have done the most good in preventing the early deaths of Americans—the 12 most effective actions Americans could have taken to save their lives. But didn't.

Top Eight Ways to Stay Alive

The seven biggest life-saving actions weren't a big surprise.

The analysis—"The Preventable Causes of Death in the United States: Comparative Risk Assessment of Dietary, Lifestyle and Metabolic Risk Factors," published in *PLoS Medicine*—outlined the top ways to prevent death were…

1. Stop smoking. Yearly preventable deaths: 467,000.

2. Control high blood pressure. 395,000.

3. Maintain healthy weight. 216,000.

4. Exercise regularly. 191,000.

5. Control high blood sugar levels. 190,000.

6. Lower LDL "bad" cholesterol. 113,000.

7. Reduce salt intake. 102,000.

But number 8 on the list was a big surprise.

The researchers determined that diets deficient in omega-3 fatty acids cause 84,000 preventable deaths every year in the US.

In fact, a low intake of omega-3s—the EPA (*eicosapentaenoic acid*) and DHA (*docosahexaenoic acid*) found mainly in oily fish such as sardines, anchovies, salmon and mackerel, and in fish oil supplements—may cause more preventable deaths than a high intake of the artery-clogging trans fats found in many baked goods, snacks and crackers. Low omega-3 intake also appears to cause more preventable deaths than a low intake of fruits and vegetables.

"This analysis reinforces the idea that diet has a tremendously powerful impact on health and longevity—and that the consumption of omega-3s by Americans is far from adequate," says Andrew Shao, PhD, senior vice president of scientific and regulatory affairs at the Council for Responsible Nutrition, an industry trade group for supplement manufacturers.

More Omega-3

"Chronic inflammation causes or complicates many diseases, and omega-3 fatty acids have an important effect on reducing chronic inflammation," says Floyd H. Chilton, PhD, a professor in the Department of Physiology and Pharmacology at Wake Forest University in North Carolina, and author of *The Gene Smart Diet* (Rodale). "Omega-3s have been found to prevent and reverse heart disease and stroke, and also produce positive effects in diabetes, arthritis, cancer, age-related cognitive decline, depression, chronic obstructive pulmonary disease, asthma, psoriasis, and inflammatory bowel disease."

● **Take a fish oil supplement daily.** "Unless you eat fish at every meal, it's difficult to get enough omega-3 fatty acids from your diet," says Dr. Chilton. He suggests taking a fish oil supplement.

Red flag: According to Dr. Chilton, many fish oil supplements don't contain as much EPA and DHA as advertised. For example, a study that analyzed 20 fish oil supplements found that EPA concentration was typically 50 to 75% lower than stated on the label.

Recommended: "Buy fish oil supplements that contain at least 500 milligram (mg) each of EPA and DHA per capsule—typically in a 1,000 to 1,200 mg capsule of total oil, which allows you to achieve your targeted omega-3 intake with just one or two capsules a day," says Dr. Chilton.

If you'd rather get your omega-3 fatty acids through the food you eat, your best source is fish. *To get to the recommended daily level of 1,000 mg, Dr. Chilton suggests...*

● **As often as possible, eat fish high in omega-3.**

Analyses in his laboratory show the following fish contain over 500 mg of omega-3s per 3.5 ounce serving: mackerel, coho salmon, sockeye salmon, Copper River salmon, canned wild Alaskan salmon, canned gourmet salmon (prime fillet), canned skinless pink salmon, trout and canned albacore tuna.

● **Occasionally, eat fish with moderate levels of omega-3.**

These fish contain between 150 and 500 mg of omega-3 per 3.5 ounce serving: haddock, cod, hake, halibut, shrimp, sole, flounder, perch, black bass, swordfish, oysters, Alaska king crab and farmed Atlantic salmon.

Resource: Dr. Chilton has studied omega-3 fatty acids for 30 years and has formulated a supplement—Gene Smart Omega-3—that he says is ideal for delivering an adequate daily level of EPA and DHA. You can order the supplement at *www.genesmart.com*, or by calling 888-571-0112.

The Web site also offers a blood test—the Gene Smart Omega 3 Index Home Blood Test Kit—that allows you to find out if you have adequate blood levels of omega-3s to promote optimal health and protect against heart disease and other chronic inflammatory conditions.

Andrew Shao, PhD, senior vice president of scientific and regualtory affairs Council for Responsible Nutrition.

Floyd H. Chilton, PhD, professor in the Department of Physiology and Pharmacology at Wake Forest University in North Carolina and author of *The Gene Smart Diet* (Rodale).

Vitamin D Delays Death

If you skimp on vitamin D, you could double your risk of premature death. *That's the implication of several studies on vitamin D and mortality rates recently published in leading medical journals...*

Recent Research

•*Clinical Endocrinology.* Researchers in Austria looked at the vitamin D levels in more than 600 older people. They found that those with the lowest blood levels of the vitamin had more than double (2.24 times) the risk of dying from any cause, compared with those with the highest levels.

•*European Journal of Clinical Nutrition.* Researchers from Johns Hopkins University School of Medicine analyzed six years of health data from more than 700 women aged 70 to 79. Once again, those with the lowest blood levels of vitamin D had more than double (2.11 times) the risk of dying.

•*Journal of the American Geriatrics Society.* Researchers at the University of Colorado analyzed seven years of nutrition and health data from more than 3,400 people with an average age of 73. Those with the lowest blood levels of vitamin D had an 83% higher risk of dying. "Current vitamin D recommendations for people 65 years and older appear inadequate," the researchers concluded.

50% Are Deficient in D

Those results don't surprise Jack Cannell, MD, the executive director of the Vitamin D Council.

What you may not know: Vitamin D is not technically a vitamin—a nutrient found in food, explains Dr. Cannell. High levels of *cholecalciferol* (vitamin D-3) are produced in the skin when it's exposed to sunlight. D-3 then turns into *calcitriol*, a hormone.

Scientists used to think calcitriol had one function—regulating blood levels of calcium. Now they know that the hormone targets more than 2,000 genes, or 10% of the human genome. "Vitamin D is what your genes require to send the messages that maintain and repair the cells in your body. Without sufficient vitamin D in your system, it is likely your cells will become unhealthy—and you will suffer a premature death."

Warning: Thirty-six percent of so-called healthy adults in the US are vitamin D deficient, as are 57% of people admitted to hospitals. Overall, say experts, the risk for vitamin D deficiency is about 50%—one out of every two people is likely to have blood levels below 20 nanograms per milliliter (ng/mL). "For optimal health and longevity, you want blood levels between 50 to 80 ng/mL," says Dr. Cannell.

•**Get the most healthful dose of vitamin D.** To achieve those levels, Dr. Cannell recommends a vitamin D supplement, at a dosage of 5,000 IU of vitamin D a day. "People need five thousand IU a day to stay healthy," he says. (To get that amount from milk, you'd need to drink 50 glasses a day, he points out.)

But isn't there a risk of vitamin D toxicity, as the nutrient builds up in the system? Not really, says Dr. Cannell. "There is not a single case in the medical literature of vitamin D toxicity while taking regular doses of twenty-five thousand IU or less."

•**Take a blood test.** If you decide to take 5,000 IU a day of vitamin D, Dr. Cannell suggests you take a 25-hydroxyvitamin D test for blood levels of the nutrient, to ensure that your levels are adequately maintained and don't exceed the upper limits of the so-called "reference range" of safety, about 100 ng/mL.

Resource: You can find a link to an in-home vitamin D blood test from ZRT Laboratory at the Web site of the Vitamin D Council, *www.vitamindcouncil.com.*

The ZRT Lab contact information is *www.zrtlab.com*, ZRT Laboratory, 8605 SW Creekside Pl., Beaverton, OR 97008, call 503-466-2445.

Test yourself every six months, says Dr. Cannell.

•**Use the best form of vitamin D.** "I believe *cholecalciferol* (vitamin D-3) is the preferred oral form of vitamin D, as it is the compound your skin makes naturally when you go in the sun," says Dr. Cannell. "It is more potent and perhaps even safer than the synthetic analog, *ergocalciferol* (vitamin D-2), found in many supplements."

Resource: You can order supplements of vitamin D-3 at the Web site of Biotech Pharmacal, *www.bio-tech-pharm.com*, or call 479-443-9148 or 800-345-1199.

Dr. Cannell has also formulated a vitamin D-3 supplement that includes nutritional cofactors such as magnesium and vitamin K-2 that boost absorption. The product is Dr. Cannell's Advanced D, and it is available at *www.purityproducts.com*, or call 800-256-6102.

You can also pump up blood levels of vitamin D with sunlight and artificial light, says Dr. Cannell.

●**Soak up the sun.** Step outside at midday with as much skin uncovered as possible. Try to get 20 minutes of daily exposure, 5 to 10 minutes on each side of the body.

The best times of year to use the ultraviolet light from the sun to produce vitamin D in your body are late spring, summer and early fall, says Dr. Cannell. It doesn't work as well in the winter, when the sun's rays aren't as direct.

Warning: "Don't get sunburned," he adds. "Vitamin D production is already maximized before your skin turns pink and further exposure doesn't increase levels of vitamin D—but may increase your risk of skin cancer."

Fact: "The shorter your shadow when standing upright, the more vitamin D you are making per minute," says Dr. Cannell. "If your shadow is longer than you are, you're not making much vitamin D."

●**Use artificial light.** "Several artificial light sources are commercially available that provide the proper wavelength for vitamin D production," says Dr. Cannell.

Resource: You can find the D-Lite, Renew and SunSplash UV/Tanning System at *www.mercola.com*. "The D-Lite System is the first of its kind," says Dr. Cannell. "It is a 12-lamp system that produces only UVB rays, and is designed for those who want the vitamin D benefits of the sun without tanning."

Follow the exposure recommendations that accompany the artificial light products.

Jack Cannell, MD, executive director of the Vitamin D Council. *www.vitamindcouncil.com.*

Age-Defying Moves

Physical therapy (PT) exercises you can do at home help your body retain youthful vigor. How? By improving posture, balance, flexibility and strength. The anti-aging moves below are quick and simple and require no equipment. For seated exercises, sit in a straight-backed chair, feet flat on floor and hip-width apart.

All exercises: To do a "set," repeat each move three times, breathing slowly and deeply...relax momentarily between each repetition. Aim for two or three sets daily.*

●**Improved Posture.** Poor posture makes your spine curve and jaw jut forward (as shown at right), causing back and neck pain and compressing the lungs. These moves correct head alignment and strengthen mid-back muscles.

●**Chin Tuck.** Sit...without tilting head to the back or side, tuck chin slightly...draw head rearward until neck is elongated and in line with spine...hold 15 seconds.

●**Isometric Elbow Press.** Sit...bend elbows to a 90-degree angle so hands are in front of you, held in relaxed fists. Keeping your back against the chair back, press elbows backward against the chair back, using the pressure to help straighten spine...hold 15 seconds.

●**Better Balance.** Avoiding falls requires keeping your balance while moving.

*Check with a health-care professional before beginning any new exercise routine.

• **Tandem Walk.** Stand straight, abdominal muscles ("abs") tight, head aligned with spine. Stepping forward, place right foot directly in front of left foot, so right heel touches left toes (as if on a tightrope). Walk this way for 15 feet. Start slowly…increase your pace gradually as balance improves.

• **Greater Flexibility.** Being flexible helps prevent muscle and joint injuries. For these moves, sit with hips six to 10 inches from the chair back.

• **Behind-the-Back Shoulder Stretch.** Reach left hand over left shoulder, palm facing your back…bring right hand up behind your back, palm facing away from you. Gently move left hand down and right hand up for 30 seconds, trying to get tips of third fingers of each hand to touch. Switch hand positions and repeat.

• **Sit-and-Reach.** Straighten right knee and place right heel on floor, toes pointed toward ceiling. With one hand on top of the other, lean forward, trying to touch toes of right foot… hold 30 seconds. Switch to left leg. (If you have low bone density or a history of spine fractures, skip this exercise.)

• **Increased Strength.** The stronger you are, the easier it is to do just about anything.

• **Plank Position.** Get down on all fours, hands flat on floor and directly below shoulders. Tightening abs and keeping head aligned with spine, extend one leg and then the other until toes are curled under and on the floor in "push-up" position. Hold position, with body perfectly straight, for 15 to 30 seconds (do not lower yourself into a push-up)… return to hands and knees.

Marilyn Moffat, PT, DPT, PhD, professor of physical therapy at New York University in New York City and coauthor of *Age-Defying Fitness* (Peachtree).

Illustrations by Shawn Banner.

Exercise Keeps Your Brain Young

Aging isn't kind to your brain. Gray matter—the part of the brain that processes information—shrinks. White matter—the part of the brain that controls communication between brain cells—develops lesions.

Theory: Underlying both of these developments are abnormal blood vessels in the brain. With age, you have fewer of those small blood vessels…they shrink…and they develop twists and kinks, a process called tortuosity.

But exercise may protect those blood vessels, say researchers at the University of North Carolina at Chapel Hill, in a study in the *American Journal of Neuroradiology*.

Better Blood Vessels

The researchers took magnetic resonance angiography (MRA) images of the blood vessels in the brains of 14 healthy older people with an average age of 64.

Half of them were regular exercisers—they had participated in a minimum of 180 minutes of aerobic activity a week for the past 10 years. The other half weren't regular exercisers.

When they analyzed the MRA images, the researchers found that those who exercised regularly had…

• *More* blood vessels and

• Fewer twisted blood vessels.

"The blood vessels in the brains of the aerobically active people appeared younger than those of the relatively inactive people," says Elizabeth Bullitt, MD, the study leader.

Work Out Like You're Young

"Wellness is the best antiaging 'drug' and exercise is a key factor in wellness," says John J. Ratey, MD, an associate clinical professor of psychiatry at Harvard Medical School and author of *Spark: The Revolutionary New Science of Exercise and the Brain* (Little,

Brown). "It builds resilience within every cell of the body, including brain cells, allowing us to deal with the inevitable stresses and strains of aging."

Specifically, says Dr. Ratey, exercise works to counter aging by strengthening the cardiovascular system...regulating blood sugar...reducing obesity...elevating stress thresholds...lifting mood...boosting the immune system...fortifying bones...boosting motivation...and fostering a stronger brain.

Dr. Ratey's exercise recommendations for staying young...

• **Aerobic exercise.** Four days a week, from 30 minutes to an hour, at or slightly above 60% of your estimated maximum heart rate, which is 220, minus your age, multiplied by 60%.

Example: If you're 50, that would be 220-50=170 x .60, or 102 beats per minute. "At this level of aerobic exercise, you'll be making anti-aging structural changes in the brain."

Good idea: Try for a more intense pace—70 to 75% of your maximum—for two days a week, for 20 to 30 minutes, perhaps by walking up a hill at a rapid pace.

"The problem with our ideas about exercise for the elderly is that we don't encourage those 65 and over to push themselves very hard," says Dr. Ratey. "Antiaging exercise means going beyond your comfort level. By working out like you're young, you turn on the mechanisms to stay young."

• **Strength training.** "Use weights or resistance machines twice a week," says Dr. Ratey. "Do three sets of your exercises with weights that allow you to do ten to fifteen repetitions in each set. If you don't have experience with resistance training, it's a great idea to get a trainer for the first month—good form is important in avoiding injuries."

• **Balance and flexibility.** "Without balance and flexibility, your ability to stick with an aerobic and strength-training regimen will diminish," says Dr. Ratey. "Focus on these abilities twice a week for thirty minutes or

so." He recommends yoga, Pilates, tai chi, martial arts and dance.

(For more information on yoga and tai chi, see appendix pages 345 and 348.)

Elizabeth Bullitt, MD, Van Weatherspoon Jr. Distinguished Professor of Surgery, University of North Carolina, Chapel Hill.

John J. Ratey, MD, associate clinical professor of psychiatry at Harvard Medical School and author of *Spark: The Revolutionary New Science of Exercise and the Brain* (Little, Brown). *www.johnratey.com.*

Falls—Beware of the Hidden Causes

Anyone can trip and be thrown momentarily off balance. But can you regain your balance—or do you go down? Anything that makes an initial misstep more likely or interferes with a person's ability to self-correct increases the risk for falls. And many such factors become more common with age. *For example...*

• **Muscle weakness.** If you stumble, it requires coordinated actions of your feet, ankles, knees and hips to prevent a fall. Muscle weakness in any of those areas impairs this ability. That's why physical inactivity is a common—though often unrecognized—cause of falls.

Exercise helps slow the loss of muscle mass that occurs with aging. Stair-climbing is an excellent way to strengthen critical thigh muscles.

Also helpful: Leg extensions—while sitting in a chair, raise your lower leg until it is in line with the thigh. Repeat 10 times and switch legs. Perform this exercise three times a day.

• **Impaired nerve function.** The nervous system plays a part in sensing loss of balance early and guiding the self-correction process. Blunted nerve function in the feet often is due to peripheral neuropathy, which can be caused by diabetes, vitamin B-12 deficiency or low thyroid levels (hypothyroidism).

• **Thinning bones.** Bone mass declines with age. If the thinning process goes far enough, osteoporosis can develop—in both women and men—and those dangerously fragile bones are liable to fracture. Osteoporosis can worsen the consequences of a fall, but in some cases, weakened bones are the cause, rather than the effect.

Here's what happens: As bones lose density, the body's center of gravity shifts forward, causing an older person to lean progressively forward. Balance becomes more precarious, so a slip is more likely to become a fall. Small fractures of the vertebrae caused by osteoporosis accentuate the forward shift.

• **Low vitamin D levels.** An analysis of five studies published in *The Journal of the American Medical Association* found a more than 20% reduction in falls in healthy older people who took vitamin D supplements, compared with those who didn't.

Researchers theorize that vitamin D may have an effect on muscle that helps reduce falls. Although the Daily Value (the FDA's reference guideline for daily nutrient intake) for vitamin D is 400 international units (IU), most studies have found that daily doses of 700 IU to 800 IU are needed to prevent falls and fractures.

Vitamin D deficiency is more common than previously believed—it's often due to a lack of regular sun exposure and/or a low intake of foods containing or fortified with vitamin D. If either of these factors applies to you, ask your doctor to check your blood level of vitamin D.

Vision and Hearing Loss

"Silent" vision problems, such as cataracts and glaucoma that have not yet caused difficulties in reading or other activities, can increase a person's risk for falls. Subtle vision changes, such as a decline in the ability to see contrasts in color or light and dark, can be missed as well. This makes tripping over curbs and on stairs or escalators more of a danger.

Correcting nearsightedness or farsightedness with glasses will help but initially can be risky. It takes time to adjust to new glasses—particularly when they have multifocal (bifocal, trifocal or variable) lenses. An Australian study found that in the period just after patients got new glasses, they were more likely to fall.

Even hearing loss may be linked to increased falls—possibly because some hearing problems reflect damage to the eighth cranial nerve, which also controls the inner-ear system that maintains balance.

Dangerous Medications

Any drug that causes sedation can impair alertness, slow reaction time and disable the coordinated interplay of nerves and muscles that protects against falls. Some medications lower blood pressure when you stand up—these can cause weakness and light-headedness that can lead to a fall.

Among the most common culprits: Some antidepressants and anti-anxiety drugs… medications taken for enlarged prostate… painkillers, such as codeine and oxycodone (OxyContin)…and pills for high blood pressure.

Important: The more medications you take, the higher your risk of falling.

Hidden menace: Over-the-counter (OTC) drugs. For example, older OTC antihistamines that can have sedating effects, such as *diphenhydramine* (Benadryl), should not be used by older adults, who may experience confusion when taking such drugs. First try a nonsedating antihistamine, such as *loratadine* (Claritin).

Sleep Problems

Lack of sleep can increase fall risk by impairing alertness and slowing reaction time. However, sleeping pills aren't the solution—their effects often linger, dulling the senses and slowing reaction time. Even newer sleep medications, such as *zolpidem* (Ambien), which are designed to be shorter acting, keep working longer in older people, possibly contributing to falls.

Anything that gets you out of bed in the middle of the night—such as an urgent need to urinate—also increases your fall risk. Keep a clear path to the bathroom, use night-lights and keep a cane or walker easily accessible, if necessary.

Undiagnosed Illness

Falls also can be a harbinger of a new health problem, such as pneumonia, a urinary tract infection, heart attack or heart failure. In some cases, weakness that can lead to a fall is more evident than the usual symptoms for these illnesses.

Small Changes That Help

The exact cause of a fall is often impossible to pin down and may actually be due to several subtle factors working together—such as a slight loss of sensation in the feet, mild sedation due to medication and minor difficulty with balance.

Fortunately, safety is cumulative, too. Slight adjustments can be lifesaving. For example, avoid shoes that don't fit snugly or have slippery soles…instead, wear sneakers or walking shoes. In addition, get rid of any throw rugs…make sure that lighting is adequate and handrails are available where needed…and don't be vain about using a cane or walker if it helps you move about safely.

Rosanne M. Leipzig, MD, PhD, vice chair for education and Gerald and May Ellen Ritter Professor of Geriatrics in the Brookdale Department of Geriatrics and Adult Development at Mount Sinai School of Medicine in New York City.

Age-Proof Your Muscles

As we age, we steadily lose muscle mass. It's a fact that, many falls and bone fractures result not from weak bones, but from insufficient muscle to support ourselves as we go about our lives.

It's easy to preserve muscle or reverse age-related muscle loss, which doctors call *sarcopenia.* You can do this through diet, exercise and supplements or any combination of these. The more you do, the more

you will ensure that you lead an active, independent and productive life long into your 60s…70s…80s…and beyond.

The Power of Protein

For too many years now, doctors and dietitians have warned patients about the dangers of eating too much protein. It turns out that many people, particularly seniors, do not consume enough high-quality protein. High-quality protein foods contain all the essential *amino acids,* the compounds that are the building blocks of protein. Poultry is one example. Fish is another, and it has an added benefit since many cold-water types, such as salmon and sardines, are high in the healthful type of omega-3 fatty acids. Eggs, in moderation, are another option, especially those enriched with omega-3s.

Several recent articles in *The American Journal of Clinical Nutrition* have focused on ideal amounts of dietary protein. One study, conducted at Purdue University in Indiana, found that seniors actually had the same protein requirements as men and women half their age. The researchers calculated that an "adequate" daily intake is 0.39 grams (g) of protein per pound of body weight, or 64 g for a 165-pound man or woman. This is more than the current US Recommended Dietary Allowance (RDA) of 60 g daily for an adult man or woman weighing 165 pounds. Many seniors can benefit from as much as 25% more protein than the RDA. (To determine the amount in grams for you, take 125% of your weight and multiply by 0.39.)

Best: Eat a variety of proteins, including fish, poultry and legumes, such as kidney beans and lentils. A legume might be low in one particular amino acid, but chances are you'll eat another food rich in that amino acid that will make up for it.

Important: Protein is both essential and safe. However, people with kidney disease should consume relatively small amounts of protein daily because high amounts can stress the kidneys. If you have reduced kidney function or any type of kidney disease, speak to your physician first before changing the amount of protein you consume.

The Role of Vegetables

Most plant foods have less protein than fish, poultry, beef and other meats, but they are good protein sources because they are low in fat and high in fiber.

What you might not know: Vegetables and fruits help build muscle, but not because

Eat More Protein Every Day

There are lots of ways to get more protein into your diet. Here are the protein amounts for some common foods. Do the math—you'll see that it's not hard to boost intake.

- **Chicken (white meat)**, 3.5 oz = 31 g protein
- **Turkey,** 3 oz = 28 g protein
- **Beef round roast (preferably grass fed),** 3 oz = 25 g protein
- **Tuna,** 3 oz = 24 g protein
- **Salmon,** Chinook, 3 oz = 21 g protein
- **Pumpkin seeds,** ¼ cup = 19 g protein
- **Pork roast,** 3 oz = 21 g protein
- **Black beans (boiled),** 1 cup = 15 g protein
- **Chickpeas (boiled),** 1 cup = 15 g protein
- **Shrimp,** 6 large = 8.5 g protein
- **Skim milk,** 1 cup = 8 g protein
- **Walnuts,** ¼ cup = 4 g protein
- **Brown rice (cooked),** 1 cup = 4 g protein
- **Peanut butter,** 1 tbsp = 4 g protein
- **Broccoli,** 1 cup = 3 g protein

of their protein content. Plant foods are rich in potassium and bicarbonate, which result in a more alkaline pH (pH is the body's alkaline-to-acid ratio). Most other foods make your body more acidic, and acidosis triggers muscle wasting. A recent Tufts University study found that higher intake of foods rich in potassium, such as fruits and vegetables, can help preserve muscle mass in older men and women.

The Benefits of Exercise

The benefits of regular exercise, particularly resistance activities, such as weight lifting, for preserving and increasing muscle cannot be overstated. Exercise stimulates the conversion of dietary protein to muscle. The more exercise you do, the better. Going for a daily brisk walk is a good way to start. Consider advancing to hand weights, larger weights, cycling or swimming. Alternate activities to avoid boredom. Resistance exercise, such as weight lifting, will reverse sarcopenia even if you consume relatively little protein, according to an article in *Journal of Physiology*, because physical activity stimulates the conversion of protein to muscle.

Take Vitamin D Daily

Vitamin D is needed to make muscle. It ensures that calcium, which is essential for transporting proteins to muscle tissue, is absorbed. If you don't already do so, take 1,000 international units (IU) of vitamin D daily.

Getting Protein from Supplements

Since protein consists of amino acids, think of taking amino acid supplements as a way of getting more protein.

Beware: Not all amino acid supplements are alike. Many of the protein powder supplements that come in huge containers in health food stores or pharmacies have poor-quality proteins (such as soy) and lots of sugar. These are not worth using.

Recommended protein supplements...

●**Multi amino acids.** These supplements, available at most health food stores, provide between eight and 11 different amino acids. Recent studies have shown impressive benefits in seniors after they took these supplements. One of the studies, reported in *The American Journal of Cardiology*, found that people who took daily amino acid supplements had significant increases in muscle after six months—and experienced even more of an increase after 16 months, reaching the normal levels found in peers without sarcopenia. Multi amino acids come closest to being a complete protein (one that contains all of the amino acids). One good example is Country Life's Max Amino Caps (800-645-5768, *www.country-life.com*). Follow instructions on the label.

Alternatives: Use supplements that contain individual amino acids, such as *beta-alanine, l-ornithine* (which seems to help women especially) and *l-leucine*, known to help convert protein to muscle. For each, follow instructions on the label.

Mark A. Stengler, NMD, naturopathic medical doctor in private practice, La Jolla, California, and author of the *Bottom Line/Natural Healing* newsletter. *www.drstengler.com*.

Muscle Keeps You Out of the Hospital

Seniors who had better muscle strength and function were 50% less likely to be hospitalized for any reason than those of the same age with poor physical function, according to researchers from California Pacific Medical Center Research Institute in San Francisco. To keep yourself out of the hospital, follow a regular exercise program or, at the least, walk for 30 minutes daily.

P.M. Cawthon, et al., "Do Muscle Mass, Muscle Density, Strength and Physical Function Similarly Influence Risk of Hospitalization in Older Adults?" *Journal of the American Geriatrics Society* (2009).

Supercharge Your Anti-Aging Defenses

Most people associate aging with an inevitable decline in overall vitality and well-being. Over time, our bodies' major organs just don't seem to work as well, and our bones and muscles weaken.

But what if it were possible to slow down this process before such age-related damage occurred?

Breakthrough thinking: The best way to fight aging may be to attack it on a cellular level. By focusing on the health of our mitochondria (tiny energy-producing structures in each cell of our body), we can minimize age-related decay to our organs and other major bodily systems.

What Are Mitochondria?

There are hundreds of mitochondria within each cell of your body. Each mitochondrion is a miniature energy factory that turns fuel (dietary fat and sugar) into *adenosine triphosphate* (ATP), the primary energy source in every cell.

Though your doctor is unlikely to talk to you about the health of your mitochrondria, you should be aware of various factors that can weaken these important cellular structures…

●**Certain medications.** Cholesterol-lowering statins, for example, block the body's natural production of coenzyme Q10, which plays a crucial role in normal mitochondrial functioning.

●**Inadequate intake of key nutrients.** Low levels of nutrients, such as iron, magnesium or biotin (vitamin B-7), cause damage to mitochondrial DNA.

●**Age-related wear and tear.** To produce the cells' energy source, ATP, mitochondria burn up (oxidize) fuel—a process that generates free radicals, unstable molecules that can damage mitochondrial structures.

If mitochondria are weakened, a domino effect is created, thereby weakening cells, tissues and, eventually, organs.

This harmful process may affect your brain (with poor memory and concentration)... heart (with irregular heartbeats that increase your risk for a heart attack)...muscles (with pain and fatigue) and overall vitality (with energy levels that are only one-fourth to one-half of what you enjoyed in your youth).

Mitochondrial decay also may play a role in the development of cancer, Alzheimer's disease and Parkinson's disease.

How to supercharge your mitochondria...

Must-Have Nutrients

Your mitochondria require most of the roughly 40 essential nutrients to function at optimal levels. *These include...*

●**The Heme Seven.** Seven nutrients are required for the synthesis of heme (an iron-containing molecule that is made in—and used by—mitochondria).

The heme-synthesizing nutrients are riboflavin (vitamin B-2)...pantothenate (vitamin B-5)...pyridoxine (vitamin B-6)...biotin...and the minerals zinc, copper and iron.

Inadequate levels of heme can damage mitochondrial DNA...promote mitochondrial decay...and accelerate cellular aging overall.

Advice: Take a daily multi-vitamin-mineral supplement that supplies most essential nutrients (megadoses aren't necessary).

Caution: Most multis don't contain enough calcium, magnesium, potassium, vitamin K, vitamin D and omega-3 fatty acids—or lack some of those nutrients entirely.

Therefore, it's important to also eat a balanced diet that contains more fish and poultry than red meat, as well as fruits and vegetables, whole grains, legumes and some low-fat dairy products.

●**Magnesium.** About 55% of American adults get inadequate amounts of magnesium in their diets (leafy green vegetables are a good source of this mineral). Low levels of this nutrient can damage mitochondrial DNA.

Magnesium also is a key element in calcium absorption, so the ratio between the two nutrients is important. The body needs more than twice as much calcium as magnesium.

Advice: A good rule of thumb is to take supplements that supply a total daily intake of 500 mg of calcium and 250 mg of magnesium. (These doses can be adjusted depending upon your dietary intake of these minerals.)

Important: Some experts recommend higher daily doses of calcium supplements, but research shows that it's preferable to get these minerals from dietary sources, whenever possible, since foods also contain other important nutrients.

Good calcium sources: Low-fat yogurt (300 mg per eight-ounce serving)...spinach (115 mg per one-half cup, cooked)...and pinto beans (45 mg per one-half cup, cooked).

Bottom line: Get 1,200 mg of calcium daily—from all sources—if you are age 51 and older. Do not exceed 350 mg of magnesium daily (some people may experience diarrhea).

●**Acetyl-L-carnitine (ALCAR).** This nutrient helps move fatty acids into the mitochondria, to produce the cells' energy sources, and helps transport waste products out of the mitochondria.

Important human evidence: In an analysis of 21 studies focusing on the use of ALCAR to help prevent Alzheimer's and mild cognitive impairment (the stage of memory loss before Alzheimer's), researchers found that people who took the supplement had less mental decline, compared with those taking a placebo.

●**Lipoic acid (LA).** This compound performs several functions, including acting as an antioxidant, which protects the mitochondria from free radicals.

Compelling animal research: In studies conducted at the University of California at Berkeley in which older rats were given a combination of LA and ALCAR, the two nutrients reduced the amount of mitochondria-damaging free radicals produced by oxidation...increased mitochondrial oxygen consumption (a sign of increased energy production)…and reversed age-associated decay of mitochondrial structures.

In a study on aged beagles, the dogs improved their ability to learn and remember when taking the nutrients in supplement form.

Advice: Ask your doctor about taking a dietary supplement that combines ALCAR and LA. One such product is Juvenon Cellular Health Supplement,* which contains 1,000 mg of ALCAR and 400 mg of LA. The supplement is available from Juvenon (800-567-2502, *www.juvenon.com*). A 30-day supply costs $39.95.

As an alternative to Juvenon: Consider taking one of two other supplements that contain ALCAR and LA and are specifically formulated for mitochondrial health—Anti-Age/Energy Formula from Body Language Vitamins, available at *www.bodylanguagevitamin. com* ($47 for a 30-day supply)…or MitoForte: Energy, Memory and Anti-Aging Support from Nutritional Biochemistry, Inc., available at 406-582-0034, *www.montanaim.com* and click on "Shop" ($69.95 for a 30-day supply).

For Optimal Results

Exercise is an important adjunct to the use of the supplements listed above. That's because frequent physical activity improves the number and functioning of mitochondria in muscles.

Standout scientific evidence: When researchers studied the effect of regular exercise on mitochondrial health in adults (average age 67), there was a 53% increase in mitochondrial DNA…and a 62% increase in energy-making mitochondrial enzyme activity.

Advice: Follow the standard recommendation for regular exercise—a minimum of 30 minutes of moderate exercise, such as brisk walking, most days of the week.

*Dr. Ames is the volunteer chairman of the scientific advisory board for Juvenon. He accepts no pay from the company.

Bruce Ames, PhD, professor of biochemistry and molecular biology at the University of California, Berkeley, and a senior scientist at the Children's Hospital Oakland Research Institute. *www.bruceames.org*.

Cultivate Optimism For a Long, Happy Life

"There is no sadder sight than a young pessimist," wrote Mark Twain. As for sighting an old pessimist—good luck finding one!

A team of scientists from the University of Pittsburg, Harvard Medical School and other institutions recently studied optimists and pessimists, publishing their results in *Circulation*. *They showed that compared with pessimists, optimists were less likely to die…*

The Tonic of Trust

Led by Hilary A. Tindle, MD, MPH, assistant professor of medicine at the University of Pittsburgh School of Medicine, the researchers looked closely at the attitudes, health and longevity of more than 97,000 postmenopausal women who participated in the Women's Health Initiative.

They found those who were optimistic—defined as the "general expectation that good things, rather than bad things, will happen in the future"—were 14% less likely to die of any cause, and 30% less likely to die of heart disease.

They also found that those with hostile thoughts toward others and a mistrust of people in general were 16% more likely to die, compared with those with more positive thoughts and a trusting attitude.

And those results held up even when the researchers took other risk factors into account, such as age, disease, obesity and smoking.

Dr. Tindle points out that the study *linked* optimism and mortality, but didn't prove a cause-and-effect relationship. Nor did it uncover a mechanism for the link between optimism and death rates.

"If we take pessimists and turn them into optimists through psychological therapy, does their risk of disease go down?" asks Dr. Tindle. "My hypothesis is that it does, but this remains to be tested.

"As a physician, however, I'd like to see people try to reduce their negativity. The totality of evidence from all the medical and psychological literature suggests that sustained, high degrees of negativity are hazardous to physical health. So I tell my patients, 'Try to be positive and forward-looking, and take steps to live joyfully.'"

Practice Positivity

You can cultivate optimism, says Sonja Lyubomirsky, PhD, a professor of psychology at the University of California, Riverside, and author of *The How of Happiness: A New Approach to Getting the Life You Want* (Penguin). (The book's Web site is *www.thehowofhappiness.com.*)

Here are some of her recommendations for developing optimism…

• **Best possible selves diary.** "Sit in a quiet place, and take 20 to 30 minutes to think about what you expect your life to be one, five or 10 years from now," says Dr. Lyubomirsky. "Visualize a future for yourself in which everything has turned out the way you've wanted. You have tried your best, worked hard, and achieved all your goals. Now write down what you imagine.

"This writing exercise puts your optimistic 'muscles' into practice."

• **Identify barrier thoughts.** "Another strategy to increase optimistic thinking involves identifying the pessimistic thoughts, which are also called 'barrier thoughts' because they are barriers to optimism," says Dr. Lyubomirsky.

Examples: "I feel so stupid for giving the wrong advice to my officemate—he'll never ask me again to collaborate." "Ever since my relationship ended, I feel unloving and unappealing."

Write down your barrier thoughts, and then consider ways to reinterpret the situation, she says.

Ask yourself: What else could this situation or experience mean? Can anything good come from it? Does it present any opportunities for me? What lessons can I learn and apply to the future? Did I develop any strengths as a result?

"Practice this exercise when you're in a neutral or positive mood, and consider writing down your answers," says Dr. Lyubomirsky.

• **Practice and persist.** "All optimism strategies involve the exercise of construing the world with a more positive and charitable perspective," she says. "It takes hard work and a great deal of practice. But if you can persist at these strategies until they become habitual, the benefits could be immense. Some optimists may be born that way, but scores of optimists are made with practice."

Hilary A. Tindle, MD, MPH, assistant professor of medicine at the University of Pittsburgh School of Medicine.

Sonja Lyubomirsky, PhD, professor of psychology at the University of California, Riverside, and author of *The How of Happiness: A New Approach to Getting the Life You Want* (Penguin). *www.thehowofhappiness.com.*

Want to Stay Spry? Socialize!

Scientists have located the Fountain of Youth—in the living room of your best friend!

Researchers at Rush University Medical Center in Chicago studied the physical functioning (or "motor function") of nearly 1,000 seniors with an average age of 82, publishing the results in the *Archives of Internal Medicine.* They found that those with lower levels of socializing—less visits to friends or relatives, less attendance at sporting events or religious services, less volunteer work—also had less muscle strength in their arms and legs, slower walking speed, poorer balance and poorer coordination.

Loneliness Ages You

The researchers rated participation in several common social activities using a 1-to-5 scale, with a score of 1 indicating once-a-year participation and a score of 5 indicating daily or near-daily participation.

At the start of the study, a 1-point lower score in the social activity scale correlated with being five years older, in terms of motor function—for example, a 75-year-old with low levels of social activity had the motor function of a typical 80-year-old.

As the five-year study progressed, researchers found that for each 1-point yearly decline in social activity, there was a 33% faster loss of motor function.

"Statistically, that translates into a more than 65% increased risk of disability and 40% increased risk of death" for those with decreasing social activity scores, says Aron Buchman, PhD, the study leader and associate professor of neurological sciences at Rush. "It's not just physical activity that's good for preserving physical health. Our findings suggest that engaging in social activities may also be protective against loss of motor abilities."

Theory: Dr. Buchman is quick to point out that his study only links social activity and motor function, and doesn't prove that low levels of social activity cause loss of function.

But, he adds, if future research does prove the cause-and-effect connection, it also might find that social activity works to improve motor function by energizing brain cells that coordinate and control muscles. In the meantime, you've got little to lose and a lot to gain—including fun—by staying active.

Supercharge Your Social Life

Social activity may also improve motor function because you're more active when you socialize, says Szifra Birke, MS, a social behavior specialist in Massachusetts and author of *Together We Heal* (Infinity Publishing). "You get up and answer the door rather than sit on the couch, you prepare dinner for friends or go out to eat, you dance or bowl—you move."

Want to supercharge your social life and energize your body? *Here are Birke's recommendations…*

● **Override your anxiety.** New social activities can make you anxious because you might be doing new things and meeting new people, says Birke. "If you can push yourself to participate in the new activity in spite of your anxiety, you'll quickly discover that you're fine."

● **Look for extroverts.** Find a friend who enjoys socializing and has his or her own, established network of friends.

● **Volunteer.** "This is one of the best ways for people to create new social networks," says Birke.

Smart idea: Volunteer at a Senior Center, where you'll have the added bonus of participating with peers in the activities there, such as eating lunch or playing bingo.

Also helpful: "I love the idea of inter-generational volunteering, such as Big Brother or Big Sister," says Birke. "Oftentimes, seniors are shocked by how little time kids are spending with adults, and how much the kids need them." Schools always need volunteers, she adds.

● **Share a ride.** If you're concerned about driving at night, ask a neighbor to attend a nighttime activity with you. He or she can drive and you can share the cost of gas.

Also try: Share a taxi with a friend.

Check the activities calendar in your local newspaper. Look for activities that you might enjoy and then invite a neighbor, says Birke.

● **Do activities in a social environment.** Whether it's exercising at a gym, attending adult education classes, or joining a bird-watching group—look for enjoyable activities you can do with others, says Birke.

Aron Buchman, PhD, associate professor of neurological sciences, Rush University Medical Center, Chicago.

Szifra Birke, MS, social behavior specialist in Massachusetts and author of *Together We Heal* (Infinity Publishing). *www.szifrabirke.com.*

Your Mind—The Most Powerful Tool for a Longer and Healthier Life

Remember the cliché "You're only as old as you feel"? A significant body of scientific evidence shows that it may be more accurate to say, "You're only as old as you think."

The Power of the Mind

Much of what we call aging is shaped by mental and cultural cues. Our bodies obviously undergo changes, but many of the "typical" characteristics of age, such as achy joints or memory lapses, are often triggered more by self-perception than by physical changes.

Key lessons in using your thoughts to optimize your health...

Lesson #1. **Change your vocabulary.** Our medical system promotes the use of labels. If you have diabetes, for example, you are a "diabetic." If you are ill, you are a "patient." Such labels encourage us to see ourselves as always being sick.

People who are diagnosed with "chronic" pain are also affected by labeling. Some expect to always be in pain, so they don't notice the times when the pain is absent or less severe. If they did, they might try to figure out why and find a way to control their pain. The chronic pain label can become a detrimental self-fulfilling prophecy, leading those in pain to act as if their lives are only about pain.

Advice: Focus on the healthy parts of your life. Someone with asthma, for example, can enjoy walks when his/her lungs are feeling strong. Someone with arthritis can play nine holes of golf instead of 18, or one hole instead of nine. If you have chronic pain—or any other condition with symptoms that come and go—use the times of day when you are basically pain-free to feel good and do the things that you want.

Lesson #2. **Remember what's important.** Our world is filled with negative stereotypes about aging. Most of us assume, for example, that older adults are forgetful. (Young people forget things all the time, but this doesn't get noticed.) However, the reason we may not remember certain things is that we didn't care to learn the information in the first place.

Scientific evidence: In a three-week study, one group of nursing-home residents were given incentives to remember information—chips that could be exchanged for prizes whenever they recalled certain information, such as nurses' names and when certain activities were scheduled. Comparison groups were not awarded prizes for this task.

In tests of cognitive ability at the end of the study, the "prize group" outperformed the other groups. And in a follow-up study, the death rate was more than four times higher in the comparison groups than in the prize group.

Advice: Get involved so that you care about things. When something has meaning to you, you are more likely to remember it than to recall information that is not relevant to your daily life.

Lesson #3. **Live mindfully.** Being mindful simply means noticing new things. It doesn't matter what they are, as long as they are novel. This entails being engaged in life...cultivating a sense of personal responsibility and control...and staying alert to new experiences and information.

Advice: Stay engaged. People who pursue new interests, make their own decisions and live life on their terms are the ones who live best—and, in many cases, longest.

Lesson #4. **Expect good health.** Nearly everyone can live longer and feel better by being active. Yet about 250,000 deaths annually in the US can be attributed to a sedentary lifestyle. How you think about exercise makes a difference.

Important research: In a study of hotel maids, it was explained to one group that the work they did met the standard recommendations for an "active" lifestyle, while the second group was not given this information.

Result: After four weeks, maids who recognized that their work was good exercise lost an average of two pounds, had a significant reduction in body fat and an average drop in blood pressure of 10 points systolic (top number) and five points diastolic (bottom number). Women in the other group did not get these benefits.

Advice: When striving for a physiological result, engage your mind. People who expect to feel good are more likely to feel good.

Whatever the goal, take the smallest step necessary to get you started. If you've failed to lose 20 pounds, try to lose two pounds…or one pound…or an ounce. You'll feel a greater sense of control once you realize that small changes make a big difference over time.

Ellen J. Langer, PhD, *www.ellenlanger.com*, professor of psychology at Harvard University and author of numerous books, including the recently published *Counterclockwise: Mindful Health and the Power of Possibility* (Ballantine).

To Live Longer, Volunteer

Seniors were asked if they had spent any time in the past 12 months doing volunteer work for religious, educational or other charitable organizations. Even after researchers adjusted for factors such as chronic health conditions, physical limitations and socioeconomic status—as earlier studies had not—volunteers were less than half as likely to die during the four-year study as nonvolunteers.

Theory: Volunteering encourages social networking, physical and mental activity and self-esteem—all of which contribute to good health.

Sei J. Lee, MD, assistant professor of geriatrics, University of California, San Francisco, and leader of a study of 6,360 people over age 65.

Chapter 3

ARTHRITIS

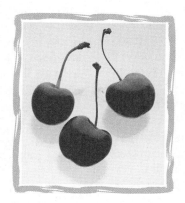

Nine Ways to Keep Joints Young

Exciting developments are occurring in the field of arthritis research. In many cases, even among people who are genetically predisposed to arthritis, unless there also is an environmental or lifestyle trigger (being a smoker, for instance) to spur the onset of the disease, chances are good that arthritis will never develop.

What this means: Far from being an inevitable result of aging or an inescapable fate for those with a family history of the disease, arthritis is quite possibly preventable...and many of the same strategies that guard against the development of arthritis also help slow its progress, making the condition more manageable if you do get it.

What it is: Arthritis is an umbrella term for more than 100 conditions that affect the joints. *Osteoarthritis*, which is by far the most common type, involves the deterioration of the cartilage that covers the ends of

bones, leading to pain and loss of movement as bone rubs against bone. Among young adults, osteoarthritis most often is seen in men—but after age 45, women sufferers outnumber men. Second-most common is *rheumatoid arthritis*, an autoimmune disease in which the immune system attacks and inflames the *synovium* (membrane lining the joints). One of the most severe types of arthritis, it affects women twice as often as it does men.

What to do: Follow the steps below to help prevent various types of arthritis...

1. Reduce the weight load on your knees. The more you weigh, the more likely you are to get arthritis in the knees.

Helpful: Even if genes place you at increased risk, dropping your excess weight—or perhaps even as little as 10 to 12 pounds—makes your arthritis risk drop, too.

2. Guard against joint injury. People who have had any type of knee or shoulder injury are more likely to eventually develop arthritis in that joint than people with no such history of injury.

Prudent: To help prevent neuromuscular injuries that can place added stress on joints, warm up for five minutes before you exercise or perform any strenuous activity (shoveling snow, moving furniture)...and stretch afterward. Watch out for hazards that could lead to falls and bone fractures, such as icy sidewalks and cluttered floors.

3. Avoid repetitive motions. Some evidence suggests a link between osteoarthritis and activities that require repetitive use of specific joints, such as continuous typing or cashiering.

Self-defense: Vary your motions as much as possible...and take frequent breaks.

4. Minimize exposure to infection. Arthritis can develop after a person contracts certain infections, such as salmonella, erythema infectiosum ("fifth disease") or hepatitis B.

Theory: These infections trigger cellular damage, especially in people genetically predisposed to arthritis.

Precautions: Wash hands often...avoid contact with people who have infections.

5. Stay away from cigarettes. Toxic chemicals in smoke appear to damage joint fibers—so refrain from smoking and minimize your exposure to secondhand smoke.

To quit smoking: Visit *www.smokefree. gov* for referrals to quit lines and advice on smoking cessation.

6. Exercise for 75 minutes or more each week. In a recent study, women in their 70s who exercised for at least an hour and 15 minutes weekly for three years reported significantly fewer joint problems than women who exercised less. Doubling that workout time was even more beneficial.

Good options: Walking, tai chi, yoga, swimming, weight lifting.

7. Eat the "Big Three" anti-arthritis antioxidants. Antioxidants neutralize tissue-damaging molecules called free radicals. Some observational studies suggest that three in particular may guard against arthritis.

Findings: In a study of more than 25,000 people, researchers found that those who developed arthritis ate, on average, 20% less *zeaxanthin* and 40% less *beta-cryptoxanthine* than those who did not get arthritis. Both of these antioxidants are found in yellow-orange fruits and vegetables (apricots, pineapple, peppers, winter squash)...zeaxanthin also is found in leafy green vegetables (arugula, chicory, kale, spinach). Another study of 400 people showed that those with the highest blood levels of *lutein*—also found in leafy greens—were 70% less likely to have knee arthritis than those with the lowest levels.

Sensible: Boost your intake of foods rich in these three important antioxidants.

8. Get the "Top Two" vitamins. In one study of 556 people, those with the lowest blood levels of vitamin D were three times more likely to have knee osteoarthritis than participants with the highest levels. A larger clinical study is in progress, so it is too early to make specific recommendations—but it probably is wise to include plenty of vitamin D–rich foods (such as fish and low- or nonfat dairy) in your diet.

Observational studies also suggest that vitamin C helps keep arthritis from progressing—perhaps by stimulating the production of collagen, cartilage and other connective tissues in the joints.

Healthful: Foods high in vitamin C include citrus fruits, guava, peppers and sweet potatoes.

9. Do not neglect omega-3 fatty acids. These natural anti-inflammatories appear to reduce the risk of developing arthritis (especially rheumatoid) and to ease symptom severity in people who already have the disease.

Best: Ask your doctor about taking fish oil supplements that provide the omega-3s *eicosapentaenoic acid* (EPA) and *docosahexaenoic acid* (DHA).

Interesting: You have an advantage if you were born, raised and currently live in the western part of the US.

Recent finding: Compared with women in the West, those in other areas of the country have a 37 to 45% higher risk for rheumatoid arthritis.

Possible influences: Regional differences in lifestyle, diet, environmental exposures and/or genetic factors.

What to do: You can't necessarily change where you live, of course—but if your location suggests an increased risk for arthritis, you can be extra conscientious about following the self-defense strategies above.

Joanne M. Jordan, MD, MPH, professor and chief of the division of rheumatology, allergy and immunology, University of North Carolina, and director of the Thurston Arthritis Research Center, both in Chapel Hill.

Eggshells Can Give You a Break from Arthritis Pain

Why did the chicken cross the road? To provide relief to the arthritis sufferers on the other side.

Well, that could be a new punch line for the old joke—because a recent study shows that a nutritional supplement made from an extract of chicken eggshells can soothe the stiff, painful joints of people with osteoarthritis.

Study Details

Sixty people with osteoarthritis of the knee were divided into two groups. One received a daily supplement of 500 milligrams (mg) of *Natural Eggshell Membrane* (NEM), a hydrolyzed extract of the inner linings of chicken eggshells. (Hydrolysis uses a protein to predigest the membrane, making it easily absorbable by the body.) The other group received a placebo. Researchers evaluated both groups after 10, 30 and 60 days, for pain and stiffness.

After 10 days, the NEM group had 16% less pain and 13% less stiffness than the placebo group. After 60 days, the NEM group had 16% less pain and 27% less stiffness than the placebo group.

"NEM is a safe and effective option for the treatment of pain and stiffness associated with knee osteoarthritis," wrote the researchers, in *Clinical Rheumatology.*

Why it works: In a joint afflicted with arthritis, the cartilage that covers and cushions the ends of bones degenerates, allowing bones to rub together. The result—pain and stiffness.

NEM contains several compounds—including glucosamine, chondroitin sulfate, hyaluronic acid and collagen—that help maintain and restore healthy cartilage. Animal studies also show NEM alleviates inflammation by reducing the number of pro-inflammatory immune factors called *cytokines.*

A Less Toxic Therapy

Nonsteroidal anti-inflammatory drugs (NSAIDs) for arthritis, such as *ibuprofen* (Motrin, Advil) and *naproxen* (Aleve, Naprosyn) relieve symptoms only about 30 to 40% of the time, says Anne Winkler, MD, PhD, a rheumatologist in Missouri, and a study researcher. NSAIDs also cause gastrointestinal bleeding, hospitalizing 200,000 people a year and killing 15,000 to 20,000.

"If a person wants to try a less toxic therapy, NEM is a good choice," says Dr. Winkler. "It works for a majority of people and—if it works for you—it provides significant relief from pain and stiffness in just 10 days. I recommend it to my patients."

Suggested intake: With the approval and supervision of your primary care physician or rheumatologist, take 500 mg of NEM daily, says Dr. Winkler.

Warning: Don't take NEM if you are allergic to eggs.

Resource: You can order JOINThealth, an NEM-containing product, at *www.membrell. com,* or call 800-749-1291. The Web site also includes a "Store Locator"—enter your zip code to find the store nearest you that sells JOINThealth.

Anne Winkler, MD, PhD, rheumatologist practicing in Missouri, and a study researcher.

Get Fit in the Water!

Many people avoid exercise because they assume that they are too out of shape to get started or fear that they will get injured or their muscles will ache after workouts. Sound familiar?

If so, water exercise could be your solution. It involves much more than swimming. A good water workout may include jogging, pushing and pulling—all in the water.*

Key advantage: The buoyancy of water reduces your "weight" by 90 to 100% (depending on the depth of the water), so there's far less stress on your joints and muscles.

This makes water exercise an excellent option for people with osteoarthritis, rheumatoid arthritis or back problems. It's also ideal for those with peripheral arterial disease (reduced blood flow to the extremities) or other circulatory problems—the force of water against your body stimulates blood circulation.

Don't assume that you can't get a good workout from water exercises. When done properly, this form of exercise can boost your cardiovascular fitness.

Water exercise also improves muscular strength, endurance and flexibility—all of which help with daily activities ranging from grocery shopping to gardening.

A Tough Workout That Doesn't Hurt

Water exercise is safe and comfortable. Water's natural buoyancy—it resists downward movement and assists upward movement—allows you to virtually eliminate any jarring physical impact on your lower body, especially your hips, knees and ankles.

The gravity-defying effects of water also eliminate any risk of falling during your workout. In addition, water's natural resistance—currents push and pull against the body—strengthen your "core" muscles (the abdominals and back) to improve your pos-

*Check with your doctor before starting any new exercise program. Water exercise may not be recommended if you have a skin condition, such as psoriasis, or have recently undergone surgery.

ture, promote better balance and reduce low back pain.

Best Water Workouts

The following workout, which is a good introduction to water exercises, is best performed in a water depth slightly above the navel. Perform the workout at least twice weekly—ideally, in addition to exercises on land, such as walking.

● **Jog and Scull boosts heart health.**

What to do: Begin by moving your hands across the water's surface as if smoothing sand. This movement, called sculling, helps promote balance. While keeping your ears, shoulders and hips in a straight line, jog up and down with your knees raised high, as if marching, and continue to scull with your hands just beneath the water's surface.

Jog up and down the lanes of a lap pool. (If the pool ranges from shallow to deep, run side to side across the shallow end.) Continue for three to five minutes, increasing to 10 minutes or more as you build stamina. In addition, aim to gradually increase your speed and the height of your knees as you jog.

● **Tandem Stand promotes balance and reduces your risk of falling on land.**

What to do: Stand with one foot in front of the other as if walking on a line. Move your arms so that you alternate with one arm in front and the other one behind the hips. As you move your arms, the water currents will challenge your balance and strengthen your core. Continue for 30 seconds to one minute, then switch feet front to back. Repeat three to four times.

● **Rock Forward, Rock Back improves posture and back strength.**

What to do: While standing on one leg, tilt your upper body forward with your other leg

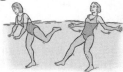

bent at the knee and your hands held flat in front of you for balance.

Then rock back and pull your arms slightly back, while squeezing your shoulder blades together and keeping your hands turned so that your thumbs are pointed upward. Switch legs and repeat. Perform one to three sets (eight to 15 repetitions each).

Mary E. Sanders, PhD, associate professor of health education at the University of Nevada School of Medicine in Reno. She has developed water exercise programs based on research that she has conducted for more than 15 years.

Illustrations by Shawn Banner.

Soak Arthritis Away—in Warm Mineral Water

A warm bath is almost guaranteed to provide temporary relief from aching, arthritis joints. Now, researchers have discovered that a couple of warm baths a week—in water loaded with minerals—might soothe those aching joints for months.

Study Details

Researchers in Israel studied 44 people with osteoarthritis of the knee, dividing them into two groups. One group soaked for 20 minutes, twice weekly, in a pool filled with heated (95° to 98°F) water from the Dead Sea, which is rich in many minerals, including sodium (with levels ten times higher than any other sea or ocean in the world). The other group soaked in a Jacuzzi filled with heated tap water. The treatment lasted six weeks.

Results: The Dead Sea group had a significant decrease in pain and stiffness for six months after the therapy. The Jacuzzi group enjoyed those same benefits for only one month after the six weeks of soaks.

"The results of the study are very encouraging," wrote the authors, in the *Israeli Medical Association Journal*.

Theory: No one knows exactly why heated mineral water is so effective at relieving joint pain and stiffness, says Shaul Sukenik, MD, a professor of medicine at Ben-Gurion

Don't Have a Pool?

You don't need your own backyard swimming pool to perform water exercise. Nonprofit organizations, such as the YMCA/YWCA and Jewish Community Centers, operate approximately 4,000 swimming pools across the US. Memberships, which range from $30 to $90 monthly depending on location, are often less expensive than those at for-profit health clubs. Municipal pools also are common in the US. Many do not charge admission, and some offer water exercise classes.

University in Be'er Sheva, Israel, and the study leader. But there are several theories, he says.

Bathing in warm mineral water triggers the excretion of several hormones, including anti-inflammatory cortisol and pleasure-inducing endorphins. It also increases cardiac output (the amount of heart the blood pumps into circulation), which may decrease swelling of the joints.

More standout scientific evidence: Researchers analyzed nine studies that used mineral water soaks to treat knee osteoarthritis in more than 500 people. Most of the studies found improvement in pain and everyday functioning, often lasting as long as six months. Thermal mineral waters are safe and effective for treating patients with OA, concluded the researchers, in *Clinical Rheumatology*.

Spa Therapy

●**Spa therapy in the US.** "We hear from many people with arthritis that a soak in our warm mineral waters relieves pain for days afterward—probably by reducing inflammation, relaxing muscles around the joint, and decreasing stiffness in the joint itself," says John C. Gray, founder of Glen Ivy Hot Springs, in Corona, California (*www.glenivy.com*). "A warm bath is always relaxing—but when the heat comes from the earth itself, it's a gift from nature, and there's something special about it."

Resource: To obtain a list of spas in the US with warm mineral springs, visit the International Spa Association Web site *www.experienceispa.com* (click "Spa-Goers" and "Search for a Spa") or e-mail *ispa@ispastaff.com.*

Address: 2365 Harrodsburg Road, Suite A325 Lexington, KY 40504, or call 888-651-4772.

•**Spa therapy overseas.** "Travel to the Dead Sea and stay at least 10 days—and two weeks is much better," says Dr. Sukenik.

The high level of sodium and other minerals in the Dead Sea...the consistently warm climate...the highest barometric pressure in the world (low barometric pressure increases joint pain)...make the treatment ideal for anyone with osteoarthritis, he says.

Recommended: The DMZ Medical Spa. "This is the best medical spa in the Dead Sea area," says Dr. Sukenik. Web site: *www.dmz-medical-spa.com.*

•**Home therapy.** "We have conducted a study which shows that using salt from the Dead Sea in a bathtub is an effective way to relieve the symptoms of arthritis," says Dr. Sukenik.

Study: Twenty-six people with osteoarthritis of the knees were divided into two groups—for two weeks, one group bathed daily for 20 minutes in warm water with Dead Sea salt; the other group bathed in warm water with regular salt. After two weeks, both groups had a significant decrease in the severity of the disease. But one month later, only the group that had bathed in the Dead Sea salt continued to experience relief.

Resource: You can find true Dead Sea salts from Israel at *www.deadseapremium.com.*

Follow the directions on the product label, bathing in Dead Sea salt for 20 minutes at least twice a week, says Dr. Sukenik.

Shaul Sukenik, MD, professor of medicine at Ben-Gurion University in Be'er Sheva, Israel.

John C. Gray, founder, Glen Ivy Hot Springs, Corona, California. *www.glenivy.com.*

Breakthrough Research On Beating Arthritis Pain Naturally

Osteoarthritis has long been considered a "wear-and-tear" disease associated with age-related changes that occur within cartilage and bone.

Now: A growing body of evidence shows that osteoarthritis may have a metabolic basis. Poor diet results in inflammatory changes and damage in cartilage cells, which in turn lead to cartilage breakdown and the development of osteoarthritis.

A recent increase in osteoarthritis cases corresponds to similar increases in diabetes and obesity, other conditions that can be fueled by poor nutrition. Dietary approaches can help prevent—or manage—all three of these conditions.

Key scientific evidence: A number of large studies, including many conducted in Europe as well as the US, suggest that a diet emphasizing plant foods and fish can support cartilage growth and impede its breakdown. People who combine an improved diet with certain supplements can reduce osteoarthritis symptoms—and possibly stop progression of the disease.

A Smarter Diet

By choosing your foods carefully, you can significantly improve the pain and stiffness caused by osteoarthritis. *How to get started...*

•**Avoid acidic foods.** The typical American diet, with its processed foods, red meat and harmful trans-fatty acids, increases acidity in the body. A high-acid environment within the joints increases free radicals, corrosive molecules that both accelerate cartilage damage and inhibit the activity of cartilage-producing cells known as chondrocytes.

A Mediterranean diet, which includes generous amounts of fruits, vegetables, whole grains, olive oil and fish, is more alkaline. (The body requires a balance of acidity and alkalinity, as measured on the pH scale.) A predominantly alkaline body chemistry inhibits free radicals and reduces inflammation.

What to do: Eat a Mediterranean-style diet, including six servings daily of vegetables... three servings of fruit...and two tablespoons of olive oil. (The acids in fruits and vegetables included in this diet are easily neutralized in the body.) Other sources of healthful fats include olives, nuts (such as walnuts), canola oil and flaxseed oil or ground flaxseed.

Important: It can take 12 weeks or more to flush out acidic toxins and reduce arthritis symptoms after switching to an alkaline diet.

• **Limit your intake of sugary and processed foods.** Most Americans consume a lot of refined carbohydrates as well as sugar-sweetened foods and soft drinks—all of which damage joints in several ways. For example, sugar causes an increase in *advanced glycation end products* (AGEs), protein molecules that bind to collagen (the connective tissue of cartilage and other tissues) and make it stiff and brittle. AGEs also appear to stimulate the production of cartilage-degrading enzymes.

What to do: Avoid processed foods, such as white flour (including cakes, cookies and crackers), white pasta and white rice, as well as soft drinks and fast food. Studies have shown that people who mainly eat foods in their whole, natural forms tend to have lower levels of AGEs and healthier cartilage.

Important: Small amounts of sugar—used to sweeten coffee or cereal, for example—will not significantly increase AGE levels.

• **Get more vitamin C.** More than 10 years ago, the Framingham study found that people who took large doses of vitamin C had a threefold reduction in the risk for osteoarthritis progression.

Vitamin C is an alkalinizing agent due to its anti-inflammatory and antioxidant properties. It blocks the inflammatory effects of free radicals. Vitamin C also decreases the formation of AGEs and reduces the chemical changes that cause cartilage breakdown.

What to do: Take a vitamin C supplement (1,000 mg daily for the prevention of osteo-arthritis...2,000 mg daily if you have osteoarthritis).* Also increase your intake of vitamin C–rich foods, such as sweet red peppers, strawberries and broccoli.

• **Drink green tea.** Green tea alone won't relieve osteoarthritis pain, but people who drink green tea and switch to a healthier diet may notice an additional improvement in symptoms. That's because green tea is among the most potent sources of antioxidants, including *catechins*, substances that inhibit the activity of cartilage-degrading enzymes.

For osteoarthritis, drink one to two cups of green tea daily. (Check with your doctor first if you take any prescription drugs.)

• **Eat fish.** Eat five to six three-ounce servings of omega-3–rich fish (such as salmon, sardines and mackerel) weekly. Omega-3s in such fish help maintain the health of joint cartilage and help curb inflammation. If you would prefer to take a fish oil supplement rather than eat fish, see the recommendation below.

Supplements That Help

Dietary changes are a first step to reducing osteoarthritis symptoms. However, the use of certain supplements also can be helpful.

• **Fish oil.** The two omega-3s in fish—*docosahexaenoic acid* (DHA) and *eicosapentaenoic acid* (EPA)—block chemical reactions in our cells that convert dietary fats into chemical messengers (such as *prostaglandins*), which affect the inflammatory status of our bodies. This is the same process that's inhibited by nonsteroidal anti-inflammatory drugs (NSAIDs), such as *ibuprofen* (Motrin).

What to do: If you find it difficult to eat the amount of omega-3–rich fish mentioned above, ask your doctor about taking fish oil supplements that supply a total of 1,600 mg of EPA and 800 mg of DHA daily. Look for a "pharmaceutical grade" fish oil product, such as Sealogix, available at FishOilRx.com, 888-966-3423, *www.fishoilrx.com*...or RxOmega-3 Factors at iherb.com, *www.iherb.com.*

*Check with your doctor before taking any dietary supplements.

If, after 12 weeks, you need more pain relief—or have a strong family history of osteoarthritis—add…

● **Glucosamine, chondroitin and MSM.** The most widely used supplements for osteoarthritis are glucosamine and chondroitin, taken singly or in combination. Most studies show that they work.

Better: A triple combination that contains *methylsulfonylmethane* (MSM) as well as glucosamine and chondroitin. MSM is a sulfur-containing compound that provides the raw material for cartilage regrowth. Glucosamine and chondroitin reduce osteoarthritis pain and have anti-inflammatory properties.

What to do: Take daily supplements of glucosamine (1,500 mg)…chondroitin (1,200 mg)…and MSM (1,500 mg).

Instead of—or in addition to—the fish oil and the triple combination, you may want to take…

● **SAMe.** Like MSM, *S-adenosylmethionine* (SAMe) is a sulfur-containing compound. It reduces the body's production of TNF-alpha, a substance that's involved in cartilage destruction. It also seems to increase cartilage production.

In one study, researchers compared SAMe to the prescription anti-inflammatory drug *celecoxib* (Celebrex). The study was double-blind (neither the patients nor the doctors knew who was getting which drug or supplement), and it continued for four months. Initially, patients taking the celecoxib reported fewer symptoms—but by the second month, there was no difference between the two groups.

Other studies have found similar results. SAMe seems to work as well as over-the-counter and/or prescription drugs for osteoarthritis, but it works more slowly. It usually takes at least three months for patients to see effects.

What to do: Start with 200 mg of SAMe daily and increase to 400 mg daily if necessary after a few weeks.

Peter Bales, MD, a board-certified orthopedic surgeon and author of *Osteoarthritis: Preventing and Healing Without Drugs* (Prometheus).

Natural Medicine Speeds Joint Recovery

Sometimes, even the best medicines (natural or pharmaceutical) are no match for a badly degenerated hip or knee joint. Joint-replacement surgery is often the best way to go.

Of course there are risks associated with these procedures, including failure of the joint replacement and, as with any surgery, a risk for blood clots. But, in most cases, these remarkable surgeries can literally change your life if you have an aching joint that has become increasingly painful with age but has not improved with the use of natural therapies, physical therapy and/or pharmaceutical medications.

Here's some advice for patients going through the joint-replacement process…

● **Eat healthfully for at least one month prior to your surgery.** We should be eating nutritious foods all of the time, but it's especially important before an operation. Eat several daily servings of vegetables and fruits, whole grains and lean meats or fish and/or poultry, and drink lots of water (one-half ounce per pound of body weight). This eating plan is good for your liver and digestive tract, which break down and eliminate anesthetics and medications used during surgery.

● **Tell your surgeon about any natural medicines you take.** Many doctors want patients to discontinue all natural medicines a week or so before surgery. That's because some natural remedies, such as ginseng and ginkgo biloba, may increase bleeding risk or have other adverse effects. However, ask your surgeon how quickly you can start taking three key supplements—vitamin E (400 international units daily)…vitamin C (1,000 mg daily)…and fish oil (2,000 mg daily). These supplements are anti-inflammatory and promote healing. Take them for at least one month after your surgery. If your surgeon approves, also take the supplements for one month prior to surgery.

• **Take a single oral dose of arnica 200C as soon as possible immediately after surgery.** (Check first with your surgeon.) This homeopathic remedy, which is often used after any kind of physical trauma, speeds recovery time and will not interfere with conventional medications. Use the single dose, under the tongue, 20 minutes before or after eating food.

•**Apply arnica ointment to the area where your surgery was performed,** three times a day for one week, to reduce pain and speed local healing.

Caution: Do not apply any kind of ointment directly to your incision.

• **Follow your doctor's orders for physical therapy and post-surgery posture** (the way you sit, stand and move). Failure to do so can result in dislocation of the newly fitted joint, an excruciatingly painful experience that requires immediate medical treatment and possibly repeat surgery.

Jamison Starbuck, ND, naturopathic physician in family practice in Missoula, Montana.

Cherry Pills Ease Arthritis Pain

In a new study of 20 patients with osteoarthritis of the knee, more than half the patients experienced significant improvement in knee pain after taking tart-cherry supplements daily for eight weeks.

Theory: Cherry extracts contain flavonoids and anthocyanins, which have been shown to have anti-inflammatory effects.

If you have osteoarthritis: Ask your doctor about trying tart-cherry supplements.

John J. Cush, MD, rheumatologist, Baylor Research Institute, Dallas.

Moderate Drinking May Reduce Arthritis Risk

Risk for rheumatoid arthritis was about 40 to 50% lower among people who consumed more than three alcoholic beverages per week than among those who consumed less or no alcohol, according to a recent study.

Henrik Kallberg, PhD, researcher, Karolinska Institute, Stockholm, and leader of an analysis of Swedish and Danish studies of 2,750 people, published in *Annals of the Rheumatic Diseases*.

Reduce RA Pain—Brush Your Teeth

Rheumatoid arthritis (RA) is an autoimmune disease—for unknown reasons, your immune system mistakes the lining of your joints for a foreign invader and attacks them.

The inflammatory condition, which afflicts 2.5 million Americans, causes severe pain and disability—tender, stiff and swollen joints that eventually become deformed.

But scientists have discovered two new tools you can use to reduce the discomfort of RA.

A toothbrush and a string of floss.

Flossing for Pain Relief

Researchers in the Department of Periodontics at Case Western Reserve University in Cleveland, Ohio, studied 40 people with RA and gum disease (*periodontitis*), a chronic bacterial infection of the gums that eats away both gum tissue and underlying bone. Twenty patients received dental care consisting of instructions on better home oral hygiene and a form of deep cleaning of the gums and teeth called scaling and root planing. The other twenty didn't.

Six weeks later, those with better oral care had a significant decrease in the symptoms of RA—less pain, fewer swollen joints and less morning stiffness. They also had a decrease in *tumor necrosis factor-alpha* (TNF-alpha), an inflammation-causing component of the immune system.

Those whose oral care didn't change had no improvement in RA symptoms or levels of TNF-alpha.

"Nonsurgical periodontal therapy had a beneficial effect on the symptoms and signs of RA," wrote the researchers, in *Periodontology*.

"It was exciting to find that if we eliminated the infection and inflammation in the gums, then patients with rheumatoid arthritis reported improvements in the symptoms and signs of the disease," says Nabil Bissada, DDS, professor and chair of the department of periodontics at the Case Western Reserve University School of Dental Medicine.

What happens: Local inflammation in the gums sparks more inflammation in the joints—just as a local burn raises levels of inflammatory factors throughout the body. In addition, bacteria and other inflammatory factors from a periodontal infection travel to the joints, worsening inflammation there.

The Best At-Home Oral Hygiene

"New questions for patients with RA should include, 'Have you seen your dentist lately?' 'Do you have periodontal disease?'" says Dr. Bissada.

"If so, your dentist should treat the infection with deep cleaning—scaling, which removes plaque and bacteria from tooth surfaces and beneath your gums; and root planing, which smoothes the surfaces at the root of the tooth, making them less susceptible to plaque buildup. You should also have a regular program of oral hygiene at home."

Here are at-home hygiene instructions from Thomas E. Van Dyke, DDS, director of the Clinical Research Center and professor in the Department of Periodontology and Oral Biology at Boston University's Goldman School of Dental Medicine.

● **Brush at least twice a day.** Gum disease is fueled by biofilm, or plaque—a multilayered, mineral-encrusted bacterial ecosystem.

It re-forms every 12 hours. "Brushing twice a day helps keep it in check," says Dr. Van Dyke.

● **Use the best toothbrush.** Studies show that a power toothbrush is more effective than a manual brush at reducing plaque, he says.

However: Any toothbrush works if you use it twice a day, and use it correctly—with the bristles at a 45-degree angle to the gums, wiggling rather than scrubbing.

● **Floss twice a day.** Flossing helps you clean between-teeth areas that a toothbrush can't reach. Use the same twice-a-day timing. After flossing in the evening, rinse with an antiseptic mouthwash, such as Listerine.

Helpful: For an excellent step-by-step refresher course on brushing and flossing, visit Dental Health Topics (specifically "Dental Floss" and "Oral Care and Hygiene") at *www.oralb.com*.

● **See your dentist regularly.** Twice a year is optimal for reducing plaque, says Dr. Van Dyke.

Nabil Bissada, DDS, professor and chair, Department of Periodontics, Case Western Reserve University School of Dental Medicine, Cleveland, Ohio.

Thomas E. Van Dyke, DDS, director of the Clinical Research Center and professor in the Department of Periodontology and Oral Biology at Boston University's Goldman School of Dental Medicine.

Strong Thighs Prevent Painful Knees

Every year, hundreds of thousands of older people are diagnosed with knee *osteoarthritis* (OA), the most common form of the disease, joining the 10 million people already afflicted.

Knee OA is not only incredibly common. It's also the most common cause of disability in the US, with knee pain, stiffness and limited mobility that hinders everyday activities.

But knee OA isn't inevitable. Doctors have discovered a new and unique way to help prevent it. *Strengthen your thighs...*

Study Details

Researchers in the Department of Orthopaedics and Rehabilitation at the University of Iowa evaluated more than 3,700 people (average age 62) who were participating in a study tracking the development of knee osteoarthritis.

Results: They found women with the greatest thigh (quadriceps) strength had the lowest risk of developing knee OA—30% lower than those with the weakest thighs.

However: The study didn't prove thigh strength caused lower rates of knee OA. It only links the two, says Neil Segal, MD, director of the Clinical Osteoarthritis Research Program at the University of Iowa, and the study's lead researcher.

But it seems to be a very strong link.

What happens: "The strength of the muscles of the thigh is a really important factor on how much stress is placed on the knee joint," says Dr. Segal. "The stronger the muscles, the lower the level of stress, and the more the knee joint is protected from injury and damage."

And the exercises called squats are one of the best ways to strengthen your thigh muscles, he says.

Squats for Stronger Thighs

Here are three thigh-strengthening squats recommended by exercise therapist Suzanne Andrews, host of the *Functional Fitness* show on PBS and creator of the DVD *Functional Fitness Arthritis*. Do this exercise routine two to three times a week, she says.

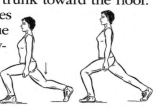

- **Resist knee squat.** Stand on both legs. Hold a two-pound weight in each hand. Bend knees to 90 degrees, keeping torso erect as possible and head in line with spine. Straighten knees. Wait four seconds. Repeat. Perform three sets, of 12 repetitions each. Rest one minute between sets.

- **Knee wall slide.** Lean on the wall, with your feet approximately one foot from the wall and shoulder distance apart. Place a

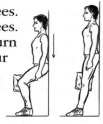

pillow between your knees. Bend knees to 45 degrees. Hold for five seconds. Return to starting position. Wait four seconds. Repeat. Perform three sets of 12 repetitions each. Rest one minute between sets.

- **Lunge squat.** Step forward and bend knees until in a lunge position. Slowly bend both knees to lower trunk toward the floor. Slightly straighten knees to raise up. Continue to lower and raise every four seconds while in lunge position. Perform three sets of 20 repetitions, every other day. Rest one minute between sets.

Also helpful: Regular aerobic exercise, such as biking, swimming or walking, can also help strengthen the thigh muscles, says Dr. Segal. "Pick an exercise that you enjoy and that you'll participate in regularly," he advises.

Neil Segal, MD, director of the Clinical Osteoarthritis Research Program at the University of Iowa.

Suzanne Andrews, host of *Functional Fitness* on PBS and creator of the DVD *Functional Fitness Arthritis*. *www.healthwiseexercise.com.*

Illustrations by Shawn Banner.

For Healthier Knees, Try a Little Electromagnetism

The earth's electromagnetic field extends tens of thousands of miles from the north and south poles, like two massive wings from the body of a bird. The forces in the field—electrical charges and the magnetism they generate—shield the earth's surface (and the earthlings on it) from the cosmic strafing of gamma rays and other forms of lethal radiation.

Well, new research shows that electromagnetism can also shield *you*—from the everyday limitations in activity caused by osteoarthritis of the knee. *The restricted walking…the difficulty climbing stairs…the hobbled housework…*

Better Than Painkillers

Researchers at Harvard Medical School analyzed data from nine studies that used *pulsed electromagnetic field therapy* (PEMF) for osteoarthritis of the knee—a series of 20- to 30-minute treatments with a machine that safely generates a pulsed electromagnetic current.

They found that six weeks of treatment significantly improved the so-called activities of daily living, or ADL.

And when they ranked a wide range of nonsurgical therapies for knee arthritis, they found that PEMF was more effective than *acetaminophen* (Tylenol) or physical therapy for pain relief, and just as effective as corticosteroid shots for improving ADL, pain and stiffness.

They also note that—unlike medications—there have been no reports of long-term side effects with PEMF, giving it a "clearly superior safety profile."

"PEMF might be a useful and effective addition to…management of osteoarthritis of the knee," wrote the researchers, in the *Journal of Rehabilitative Medicine*.

Theory: PEMF may improve arthritis by activating *chondrocytes*, the cells that produce and maintain the cushions of cartilage that protect joints, says Patrick Vavken, MD, the study leader. It may also aid in the production of glucosamine and hyaluronic acid, two key components of the cartilage. And it increases blood flow, which brings more nutrients to the knees and carries away waste products.

An Effective Option

Talk to your doctor about PEMF, says Dr. Vavken.

"There are other ways to improve arthritis than taking painkillers, and PEMF is one of those ways" he says. "Arthritis patients and their doctors should consider it a viable and effective option, perhaps using it as one therapy among others in the day-to-day management of the disease."

Resources: If you want to find a health practitioner near you who uses PEMF, you can contact a company that manufactures PEMF devices for medical and personal use. (The personal devices typically sell for several thousand dollars.)

Those companies include:

● **Bemer 3000,** distributed in the US by Bemer USA. 407-628-0511…*www.bemeramerica.com*

● **MRS2000+,** from EnergyWays Corporation. 800-900-5556…*www.mrs2000.com*

● **ONDAMED,** from Ondamed Inc. 845-534-0456…*www.ondamed.net*

● **PER 2000,** from Pulsed Energy Technologies. 877-785-7330…*www.pulsedenergytech.com*

● **Quantron Resonance System,** distributed in the US by Body Fields USA. 877-354-7152…*www.quantronmedicine.com*.

Patrick Vavken, MD, clinical researcher, Harvard Medical School and research fellow, Department of Orthopedic Surgery, Children's Hospital, both in Boston.

Thunder God Vine—the Herb That Beat the Drug

If you have *rheumatoid arthritis* (RA)—a chronic inflammatory condition with painful, swollen joints—your doctor might prescribe the anti-inflammatory drug *sulfasalazine* (Azulfidine). But if you're like nine out of 10 people who use the medication, you'll stop taking it soon after you start.

For one thing, it often doesn't work. For another, it can have a lot of side effects during the first week or so, such as stomach upset, nausea, vomiting, diarrhea, drowsiness, dizziness and insomnia.

Good news: New research shows that there's a natural alternative to sulfasalazine and other anti-inflammatory drugs used for RA—an extract of the root of the Thunder God Vine (*Tripterygium wilfordii Hook F*, or *TwHF*), a Chinese herb that has been used for thousands of years to treat inflammatory conditions such as RA.

Relief in Two Weeks

Researchers at the National Institutes of Health and the University of Texas, working with nine rheumatology clinics around the US, studied 121 people with RA, all of whom had six or more swollen joints. They divided them into two groups—one group took two daily doses of 1 gram of sulfasalazine; the other group took three daily doses of 60 milligrams (mg) of TwHF.

Results: The researchers measured results using a scale devised by the American College of Rheumatology (ACR). The scale scores for tender joints, swollen joints, pain, everyday functioning and general health. A 20% recovery is called an ACR20 response; a 50% recovery, an ACR50 response; and a 70% recovery, an ACR70 response.

Six months later, 65% of those taking TwHF had an ACR20 response, compared with only 33% of those taking sulfasalazine.

The researchers also noted that improvements in functioning and general health with TwHF were very rapid—typically occurring two weeks after patients started taking the herbal extract.

TwHF also outdid sulfasalazine in slowing the disease. X-rays showed that, on average, the patients on TwHF had "no progression of...joint space narrowing and erosion"—two markers of advancing disease. Those taking sulfasalazine had progression.

And those taking TwHF had a six-fold greater decrease in *interleukin*, an inflammatory biomarker.

"Patients with active rheumatoid arthritis can be effectively treated with a standardized extract of the roots of TwHF," concluded Raphaela Goldbach-Mansky, MD, the study leader, in the *Archives of Internal Medicine*. TwHF, she continued, is an attractive and affordable alternative to currently available drugs.

Why it works: The active ingredients in the extract are three powerful anti-inflammatory compounds called *diterpenoids*, says Dr. Goldbach-Mansky. And TwHF has other effects that directly relieve pain.

However: Like sulfasalazine, TwHF also has gastrointestinal side effects in the first days of use. While 59% of people in the study stopped taking sulfasalazine because of side effects, so did 38% of those taking TwHF.

Find a TCM Practitioner

"Historically, practitioners of TCM (Traditional Chinese Medicine) have used Thunder God Vine to deal with what's called 'painful obstruction syndrome,' which includes many arthritic conditions," says Michael Yang, LAc, DOM, a doctor of oriental medicine and director of the Pacific Medical Group in Los Angeles, California. "Thunder God Vine has what TCM calls cooling, bitter qualities, both of which help treat rheumatoid arthritis—the coolness counteracts the heat of the pain, and the bitterness tends to drain the swelling."

But even though Thunder God Vine is available without a prescription, Dr. Yang says not to use it without proper medical supervision.

Best: Work with a reliable practitioner of TCM, who will probably combine Thunder God Vine with other herbs in a formula customized for the individual.

"For example, a practitioner of TCM might combine the herb with detoxifiers such as licorice or ginger, to decrease its toxic effects," says Dr. Yang. "An herb like licorice is also anti-inflammatory, allowing the practitioner to use smaller doses of both herbs, minimizing the risk of side effects."

Dr. Yang treated one of his RA patients with a combination of Thunder God Vine and other herbs, as well as dietary changes.

"She had decreased pain and swelling, increased mobility, and has continued to do quite well," he says.

Bottom line: "An herb that is strong enough to help you is also strong enough to hurt you," warns Dr. Yang. "Use Thunder God

Vine only with the guidance and supervision of a qualified health practitioner."

Resource: To find a qualified practitioner of oriental medicine near you, visit the Web site of the National Certification Commission for Acupuncture and Oriental Medicine (NC-CAOM) at *www.nccaom.org*, and click "Find a Practitioner" on the home page.

Raphaela Goldbach-Mansky, MD, rheumatologist at the National Institute of Arthritis and Musculoskeletal and Skin Diseases, Bethesda, Maryland.

Michael Yang, LAc, DOM, a doctor of oriental medicine and director of the Pacific Medical Group in Los Angeles, California. *www.pacificmedicalgrouponline.com.*

The Chinese Secret of Effortless Healing

Qi (pronounced chee) is the Chinese word for energy or life force—in traditional Chinese medicine, when your qi is flowing freely, you're healthy; when it's stagnant or blocked, you're ill.

Gong is the Chinese word for cultivation, practice or work.

Qigong—an ancient Chinese method for health and healing—is a way to "cultivate your life force," an approach that combines movement, breathing exercises and visualization to invigorate and balance qi.

A master of qigong can control the flow of qi in his own body and can also send intensified life force into another person's body to remove blockages and speed up healing.

And that's exactly what happened recently—not in China, but in Piscataway, New Jersey, at the UMDNJ-Robert Wood Johnson Medical School, where 112 people with osteoarthritis of the knee were treated by a Qigong master.

49% More Pain Relief

The people with arthritis were divided into two groups—60 received real qigong, while the other 52 received a look-alike but fake (sham) therapy.

After several treatments over three weeks, the group receiving real qigong experienced 49% more pain relief and had a 53% greater improvement in knee functioning, compared with those receiving sham qigong. Three months later, those treated with real qigong continued to experience less pain and an increase in joint strength and mobility.

"Qigong therapy may be a safe and effective modality for knee osteoarthritis," wrote study leader Kevin Chen, PhD, in *Clinical Rheumatology.*

But, added Dr. Chen, the study didn't take full advantage of qigong therapy. "Qigong is considered mostly a self-care tool in health, and active self-practice is one of the key concepts of qigong therapy."

Cultivate Your Qi

Shoshanna Katzman, MS, LAc, couldn't agree more. Katzman, the first woman president of the National Qigong Association, is the Director of the Red Bank Acupuncture and Wellness Center in New Jersey, and author of the book and DVD, *Qigong for Staying Young: A Simple 20-Minute Workout to Cultivate Your Vital Energy* (Avery).

"I prefer to see someone cultivate his or her own qi, rather than receive someone else's qi in a healing treatment," she says. Why? "If you cultivate your own qi, you're not dependent on someone else for health and healing."

However, if you decide to use a qigong healer, Katzman has the following suggestions...

● **Find out about the healer's training.** You don't want someone who has taken a weekend course in qigong. You want someone who has been practicing qigong for years, if not decades.

● **Find out about the healer's reputation.** Do they have published testimonials from people they have treated? Do they have satisfied students? Have they written a book?

Example: Effie Poy Yew Chow, PhD, RN, coauthor of *Miracle Healing from China—Qigong* (MediPress), a National Diplomate in Acupuncture from the National Commission for Certification in Acupuncture and Oriental Medicine (NCCAOM), and founder and president of East West Academy of Healing Arts, the American Qigong Association and World Qigong Federation. Her Web site is *www.eastwestqi.com.*

• **Make sure you feel comfortable with the healer.** Before your treatment, the healer should talk to you and tell you what he/she plans to do, says Katzman. If something about the healer and his/her approach doesn't feel right to you, don't proceed with the treatment.

• **Try qigong for yourself.** "Basically, arthritis is the blockage of qi and blood in the affected joint," says Katzman. "The best way to get that qi and blood moving is with movement—not high-impact exercises that can further stress the joint, but gentle and powerful exercises. And that's where qigong comes in. It really moves qi in the body and releases blockages in the joint."

"Qigong is easy to learn from a book or DVD," she says. *To sample the technique, here is a qigong exercise Katzman says can release "stagnant energy" in all the joints and stiff areas of your body...*

• **Shaking Like a Tree.** Stand comfortably, and simply shake your body out in any way you see fit. Be spontaneous and creative as you shake out your legs, your arms, your hands, your wrists—one at a time, together or separately. Next move your torso and head. Move in any way that you like, creating natural gyrations throughout your body, releasing your own unique blockages. And remember to maintain an "inner smile"—a sense of enjoyment and fun—throughout this spontaneous Qigong exercise.

Resource: You can find a certified local teacher of qigong at the Web site of the National Qigong Association, at *www.nqa.org.* (Click on "Find Members" on the home page.)

(For more information on energy healing and qigong, see appendix pages 343 and 357.)

Kevin Chen, PhD, associate professor, Center for Integrative Medicine, University of Maryland School of Medicine.

Shoshanna Katzman, MS, LAc, director of the Red Bank Acupuncture and Wellness Center in New Jersey and author of the book and DVD, *Qigong for Staying Young: A Simple 20-Minute Workout to Cultivate Your Vital Energy* (Avery). *www.healing4u.com.*

Douse Inflammation With an Herbal Fix

For those who know about and use herbs for health and healing, milk thistle is the classic treatment for chronic liver diseases, such as hepatitis C and cirrhosis.

But now doctors have discovered a new use for the herb—easing the inflammation of osteoarthritis.

Milk Thistle for Arthritis

Doctors in the Middle East recently conducted two experiments with *silymarin*, the herbal extract found in most milk thistle supplements.

In the first, they gave silymarin to laboratory animals, to see if it reduced experimentally induced inflammation—the same type of redness, swelling and pain that is a hallmark of osteoarthritis.

The herb worked. In fact, it reduced inflammation to the same degree as an anti-inflammatory drug, the corticosteroid *dexamethasone*. "Silymarin exerts anti-inflammatory activity," concluded the researchers.

In the second, the researchers studied 220 people with knee osteoarthritis, dividing them into several groups. One group received 300 milligrams (mg) a day of silymarin. Another received an anti-inflammatory drug—either *piroxicam* (Feldene) or *meloxicam* (Mobic). Another received silymarin and an anti-inflammatory drug.

Results: The researchers found that silymarin significantly reduced a number of inflammatory *biomarkers* (compounds that indicate whether inflammation is high or low), such as interleukins. So did the combination of silymarin and piroxicam. The groups receiving a single drug had no significant reduction of inflammatory biomarkers.

The herb is a possible treatment for OA, concluded the researchers.

Other Herbal (and Nonherbal) Options

A daily supplement of 300 mg of silymarin is one herbal option for easing the inflammation of osteoarthritis.

But there are many others, says Michael Tierra, LAc, OMD, an herbalist, acupuncturist, and doctor of oriental medicine in Santa Barbara, California, and founder of the American Herbalists Guild (AHG) (*www.americanherbalistsguild.com*), the leading US organization for the training and certification of herbalists.

"Osteoarthritis is one of the easier conditions to treat with herbal medicine," he says. *His recommendations…*

• **Guggul.** This herbal preparation from India is the most all-around effective single herb for osteoarthritis, says Dr. Tierra. It works by relieving liver congestion, the root cause of inflammation. "When the liver is functioning normally, it filters out toxins, so they don't settle in the joints and contribute to inflammatory diseases such as arthritis," he explains. It also promotes blood circulation—and poor circulation is another underlying cause of the inflammatory process.

Suggested intake: Guggul is widely sold over the counter—follow the dosage recommendation on the label.

Try this: Guggul Cholesterol, a formula designed by Dr. Tierra for treating arthritis or for lowering cholesterol. Take 2 or 3 tablets a day, he says.

"I recommend that everyone from the age of 50 on use guggul as part of their daily health program. It is the best treatment to rid toxic buildup from the body and improve circulation."

You can purchase it at *www.planetherbs.com.*

• **Red clover tea.** "In most people who I've treated with inflammation from osteoarthritis, drinking red clover relieves pain within a week," says Dr. Tierra.

Like other anti-arthritis herbs, it works by reducing inflammation, increasing circulation, and detoxifying the liver.

Suggested intake: Use an ounce of the herb to one pint (two cups) of boiling water, instructs Dr. Tierra. Pour water over the herb. Steep for a few minutes, and strain. Drink two or three cups a day.

Try this: Red Clover Cleanser Complex, a formula designed by Dr. Tierra, which also includes sarsaparilla, yellow dock, echinacea, lonicera, goldenseal, forsythia, cinnamon twigs, ginger and American ginseng. "It's better to use a formula than a single, symptom-specific herb, because reversing any disease process involves addresses many underlying problems," he explains. "The symptom is just the end result of those problems."

Start at the dose recommended on the label, and then double or triple the dose within three to four days, under the supervision of a qualified herbalist or other qualified health professional, says Dr. Tierra.

Another formula Dr. Tierra devised to address arthritis is the Flex-Ability Formula, which includes several Chinese herbs. For best results, use it in the same way as the Red Clover Formula, starting at the dose on the label and tripling the dose after several days, under the supervision of a qualified health professional.

You can also purchase these herbal formulas at *www.planetherbs.com.*

• **Alfalfa tea.** "It used to be that a lot of people knew that drinking alfalfa tea daily would limber up their joints and relieve arthritis," he says. "It's in the same family as red clover—it thins the blood."

Suggested intake: As with red clover, use one ounce of herb to one pint of water, drinking two cups a day.

• **Magnets—a nonherbal treatment.** Dr. Tierra has found that the use of a small magnet worn on the area of arthritis pain is "phenomenally effective" in providing relief. "I've had hundreds of patients at my clinic whom I've treated this way," he says.

He recommends the product Accu-Band, which uses full strength (9000 Gauss) but pea-sized magnets that are attached with an adhesive.

How to use: "Find the ouch point—the trigger point for your pain—and apply the magnet on it," he recommends. "The more precise you are, the more effective the treatment." After applying, tap on the magnet 10 to 20 times, which helps activate it. Keep the magnet on until you achieve pain relief.

"I have a bit of arthritis at the tip of my thumb from years of playing the piano," says Dr. Tierra, who is in his seventies. "If I put the magnet on there and tap it, the pain is gone in a minute or two. I take it off after four or five days. The pain stays away for weeks or even months."

You can find Accu-Band magnets at *www. amazon.com.* (Don't confuse them with a similarly named product, the Acuband bracelets worn around the wrist to relieve nausea.)

Resource: Dr. Tierra's book *Biomagnetic and Herbal Healing* (Lotus Press).

Michael Tierra, LAc, OMD, an herbalist, acupuncturist and doctor of oriental medicine in Santa Barbara, California, and founder of the American Herbalists Guild (AHG). *www.americanherbalistsguild.com.*

Combine Fish with Dairy for Better RA Heart Health

It's bad enough that you have *rheumatoid arthritis* (RA)—the flare-ups with fever and fatigue…the painful, swollen joints…the hours of morning stiffness…the warped, eroding bones.

But the systemwide inflammation of RA can also cause high cholesterol, high blood pressure and other circulation-damaging metabolic changes.

Problem: People with RA have a 59% increased risk for death from a heart attack and a 52% increased risk of death from stroke.

Solution: New research shows that a glass of milk can help lower your risk. *But only if there's some fish in it…*

Increasing "Good" Cholesterol

It's well-known that the anti-inflammatory omega-3 fatty acids found in fish oil can help manage the symptoms of RA and lower the risk of heart disease. So an international team of researchers from Germany and Sweden decided to find out if omega-3s could also lower the risk of cardiovascular disease (CVD) in people with RA. And they decided to combine those omega-3s with calcium, to not only reduce inflammation, but also protect cartilage and bone.

Their approach—enrich dairy products with omega-3s. (They also felt people were more likely to regularly consume dairy products than fish.)

So for 3 months, 39 people with RA consumed omega-3–enriched dairy products— six ounces of yogurt, an ounce of cheese and 1½ tablespoons of butter.

Results: The consumption of the omega-enriched dairy products…

• Increased "good" HDL (high-density lipoprotein) cholesterol;

• Lowered lipoprotein-A, a dense form of cholesterol linked to higher risk of heart attack and stroke;

• Lowered diastolic blood pressure and

• Decreased inflammation.

The omega-enriched dairy products had "cardioprotective effects," concluded the researchers, in the *British Journal of Nutrition.*

Why it works: "The improvement of cardiovascular risk factors is caused by the beneficial nutrients in dairy products—such as conjugated linoleic acids, or CLA, oleic acid, and bioactive proteins—and by the omega-3 fatty acids," says Christine Dawczynski, the study leader, from the Department of Nutritional Physiology at Friedrich Schiller University of Jena, in Germany.

Milk That Heals

"My colleagues and I recommend the daily consumption of omega-3 enriched dairy products to reduce cardiovascular risk factors in RA," says Dawczynski.

There are several omega-3 supplemented brands of milk that are distributed nationally. *They include...*

●Kemps Plus Healthy Lifestyle 1% Milk with Omega-3 (*www.kemps.com*)

●Farmland Dairies Special Request 1% Plus with Omega-3 (*www.farmlanddairies.com*)

●Horizon Organic Whole Milk Plus DHA Omega-3 and Horizon Organic Reduced Fat Milk Plus DHA Omega-3 (*www.horizondairy.com*).

Christine Dawczynski, study leader, the Department of Nutritional Physiology at Friedrich Schiller University of Jena, Germany.

Yoga Chases Away the Arthritis Blues

Rheumatoid arthritis (RA) doesn't only destroy joints—it can also drown your mind in depression.

Fact: Approximately 20% of people with RA are depressed—and they experience more pain from their disease than their non-depressed counterparts.

Good news: A new study shows there's a drug-free way to chase away the RA blues—yoga, the gentle stretching, breathing and mental exercises that can relax the body and calm the mind.

25% Less Depression

Researchers at A.T. Still University in Arizona and Arizona State University studied post-menopausal women with RA. (The disease typically strikes around age 50, and is three times more common in women than in men.) They divided them into two groups—one group took three, 75-minute yoga classes a week for 10 weeks; the other didn't.

Before and after the 10 weeks, the researchers evaluated both groups for depression, as well as pain levels, balance (a

problem for some people with RA of the feet, knees or hips), and general disability from the disease. *The results were published in Alternative Therapies in Health and Medicine...*

●**Depression.** The yoga group had a 25% decrease in the symptoms of depression, such as sadness, loss of interest in everyday activities, guilt, fatigue and insomnia. The non-yoga group had almost no change.

●**Pain.** The yoga group had a significant decrease in pain; the non-yoga group stayed the same.

●**Disability.** The yoga group had a 35% decrease in disability; the non-yoga group had a 16% increase.

This improvement suggests that yoga "offers promise for slowing the progressive disability" of rheumatoid arthritis, says Pamela R. Bosch, PhD, PT, the study's lead researcher.

And she notes that this improvement in disability might lower levels of depression. "In a previous study, high levels of disability affecting physical function were the major factors in explaining depression in people with RA. This suggests that depression is caused by the physical devastation of the disease, including the inability to perform valued activities."

●**Balance.** The yoga group had improved balance; the non-yoga group didn't.

"The improved balance among yoga participants provides further evidence of enhanced physical function as a result of yoga," says Dr. Bosch. "Two participants who initially required assistance getting down to the floor and back up during yoga classes could do so independently after 10 weeks of yoga classes."

Bottom line: "This study provides evidence that participating in a structured yoga program may improve physical function and decrease disease activity in women with rheumatoid arthritis," says Dr. Bosch. "It should be considered as a treatment option for people with RA."

Increase Strength and Balance

"The yoga group loved participating in the classes," says Dr. Bosch. "Many reported no longer being afraid to leave their homes, more self-confidence and that yoga was even more effective in relieving the symptoms of RA than other programs they had participated in, such as strength training.

"I would definitely recommend yoga for anyone with RA. It's a way to gain control over the disease by increasing strength and balance. And because it's relaxing, it also helps people control stress from the disease."

Want to take a yoga class? Here are recommendations from Dr. Bosch, and from Andrea Marcum, a yoga instructor and owner of U Studio Yoga in Los Angeles (*www.ustudio yoga.com*). (Marcum's mother has RA, and follows a program designed by her.)

● **Find the right teacher.** Individuals with RA should seek out a yoga teacher who understands their limitations and special needs, says Dr. Bosch. "The instructor should offer alternative ways to perform a pose, or props and equipment that make the pose easier. And they shouldn't encourage people to 'work through' the pain of a pose."

"Back off any sharp pain immediately," adds Marcum. "Today's yoga should feel good tomorrow."

● **Find the right class.** "Some yoga classes are like competitive events, with each person trying to do the pose more perfectly, and that's not helpful for people with RA," says Dr. Bosch. "They need a teacher—and a class—that provides a safe, protective, supportive environment."

"You need to find a yoga class that respects you have pain and limited mobility—otherwise, you can do more harm than good," adds Marcum. "Look for a class that advertises itself as 'Gentle Yoga" or 'Yoga Therapy.'"

You may also want to attend a class in the mid-morning, afternoon or evening, since many people with RA are very stiff early in the day, says Dr. Bosch.

Recommended: For the study, classes were developed and taught by Ginnie Livingston, RN, a registered nurse and certified yoga therapist at Arthritis Health in Scottsdale, Arizona (*www.arthritishealth.net*).

Here is the general structure of her class, which you may want to share with your yoga therapist...

1. **Tadasana** (Mountain pose)
2. **Centering**
3. **Deep breathing**
4. **Shoulder range of motion and release**
5. **Half moon with modification** (one arm overhead)
6. **Half sun salutations** (4 rounds)
7. **Balance poses**
   ● One leg balance with toe lift on opposite leg
   ● Crane pose
   ● Toe rolls
   ● Eagle preparation
   ● Eagle modified
   ● Triangle (begin using the wall for support and gradually progress to free standing)
   ● Shallow Triangle
   ● Warrior
   ● Tree pose
8. **Poses while lying on the floor**
   ● Sphinx (or cobra, if capable)
   ● Half locust, each leg
   ● Locust pose
   ● Half boat, each side
   ● Side leg lifts
   ● Yoga sit-ups (3 sets of 15)
   ● Piriformis stretch (each side)
   ● Hip flexor lifts (each side)
   ● Bridge pose (2 sets)
   ● Reclining spinal twist to each side
   ● Knee down twist
   ● Relaxation pose

9. Guided imagery, relaxing each body part

10. Positive affirmations

11. Silence, while following the breath with the mind

The sequence above may need to be modified to make it appropriate for you. Those whose joints are acutely inflamed need to avoid strenuous practices that could make the inflammation worse.

● **Practice regularly.** "As long as you've chosen poses that won't hurt you, doing any yoga is better than none," says Marcum. But for maximum benefit, she encourages those with RA to practice a routine of gentle poses a few times a week.

Resources: Yoga teachers who specialize in teaching yoga as a way to treat disease are called yoga therapists, and they have their own organization—the International Association of Yoga Therapists. To find a yoga therapist near you, visit its Web site at *www. iayt.org*, and click "Find a Member" on the home page.

You can also find a yoga therapist at the Web site of *Yoga Journal* magazine, *www. yogajournal.com*. Click "Yoga Directory" on the tab at the top of the Home page. You can browse by state or by style category (search "yoga therapy"). (For more information on yoga, see appendix page 345.)

Andrea Marcum, yoga instructor and owner of U Studio Yoga in Los Angeles. *www.ustudioyoga.com.*

Ginnie Livingston, RN, registered nurse and certified yoga therapist at Arthritis Health in Scottsdale, Arizona. *www.arthritishealth.net.*

Pamela R. Bosch, PhD, PT, associate professor, A.T. Still University, Mesa, Arizona.

Drink Water to Curb Gout

When researchers reviewed data (including water consumption) for 535 adults with gout (a form of arthritis), the higher the water intake in the prior 24-hour period, the lower the risk for a gout attack. Even two to four glasses of water had an effect…five to eight had a significant effect.

Theory: Dehydration may be an under-recognized risk factor for acute gout attacks.

Tuhina Neogi, MD, PhD, assistant professor of medicine, Boston University School of Medicine, Boston.

Gout—No Longer a Rich Man's Disease

Brought on by overindulging in food and drink, gout was once considered a disease of the monied classes. Nowadays those of a lower socioeconomic status may be more likely to have the disease, due to overindulgence in fast food and sugary drinks. Research suggests that the number of cases here in the US doubled from 1977 to 1997, with an estimated six million Americans suffering this painful, debilitating form of arthritis.

Gout is characterized by sudden, severe attacks of pain, redness and tenderness typically affecting the big toe, but potentially other joints, such as the ankles, knees, fingers, wrists and elbows as well. Gout incidence is more common in men, although women are increasingly susceptible after menopause.

Hyon Choi, MD, DrPh, professor of medicine at Boston University and an expert on the condition, says that the reason behind the resurgence of gout is obesity and certain western lifestyle factors. Eating the kinds of foods that lead to being overweight, including red meat, particularly in combination with sugary soda, is the key factor behind this trend, according to Dr. Choi. He notes that gout is also a red flag for metabolic syndrome. Sixty percent of those with gout also have metabolic syndrome, he adds. "It's not just about having gout, it is also about associated serious medical conditions in the future."

All About Gout

Gout develops from a buildup of uric acid, a chemical in the blood formed by the breakdown of *purines*, which are found in meat, seafood and in some beers. Consuming lots of these means that your body has more purines to break down—and more purines lead to higher levels of uric acid. This can cause the formation of uric acid crystals (a solid form of uric acid), which accumulate in the joints, causing inflammation, swelling and pain.

The good news is that changing your ways usually reduces symptoms and also can prevent recurrence of gout altogether. Step one, of course, is to lose weight. "Being overweight is the most important of all the risk factors," emphasizes Dr. Choi. "Increased fat cell mass increases uric acid production, decreases uric acid excretion and increases risk for metabolic syndrome." In addition to maintaining a healthy weight, gout sufferers should limit alcohol and sugary drinks and reduce consumption of purine-rich foods, such as animal proteins.

In addition to altering your diet, natural remedies include...

● **If you're a coffee drinker, keep at it.** Both regular and decaffeinated coffees have been found helpful in lowering uric acid levels and reducing risk for gout. Experts believe an antioxidant in coffee decreases insulin sensitivity, and insulin resistance is strongly linked to elevated uric acid levels. Drinking coffee black is best.

● **Take vitamin C.** Supplements of 500 to 1,500 milligrams increase the excretion of

Vitamin C Cuts Gout Risk for Men

Gout risk was 17% lower for men who took in 500 mg to 999 mg of vitamin C daily...34% lower for those who took in 1,000 mg to 1,499 mg...and 45% lower for those who took in 1,500 mg or more. Vitamin C appears to lower blood levels of uric acid. Buildup of uric acid leads to the pain and inflammation associated with gout.

Gary C. Curhan, MD, ScD, associate professor, Department of Medicine and Epidemiology, Harvard Medical School, Boston.

uric acid. Research reported in *Archives of Internal Medicine* found that people who took vitamin C supplements reduced their risk of developing gout by up to 45%.

● **Choose low-fat dairy products.** Research has suggested that choosing low-fat dairy products, such as skim milk and low-fat yogurt, over the higher-fat products increases uric acid secretion.

● **Eat cherries or drink cherry juice concentrate,** both of which seem to help reduce symptoms for some people.

● **Soothe sore joints with a comfrey poultice application,** which has been used since 400 BC. (Grind comfrey leaves and mix with distilled water to apply as a paste, then wrap the afflicted area in gauze or an ace bandage.)

Hyon Choi, MD, DrPh, professor of medicine, Boston University.

Chapter 4

CANCER

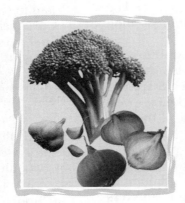

The Anticancer Diet From a Doctor Who Survived Cancer

At any given time, the average person might have thousands of cancer cells in his/her body. Individually, these abnormal cells are harmless, but any one of them could potentially proliferate and form a mass of cells (a tumor) that damages normal tissues and can spread to other parts of the body. About one-third of us eventually will get full-fledged cancer.

Often people who get cancer have created impairments in their natural defenses, allowing cancer cells to survive and proliferate. About 85% of all cancers are caused by environmental and lifestyle factors. We can't always control our environments, but we can control what we eat. Diet is one key factor that determines who gets cancer and who doesn't.

Example: Asian men have just as many precancerous microtumors in the prostate gland as American men, yet they are as much as 60 times less likely to develop prostate cancer. It's not a coincidence that their diets are far healthier, on average, than those consumed by men in the US. Asian men eat far more fruits and vegetables than Americans and relatively little red meat. They also tend to eat more fish and soy foods, and they drink more tea, especially green tea. These and other dietary factors allow their immune systems and other natural defenses to prevent cancer cells from proliferating.

David Servan-Schreiber, MD, PhD, was a physician in Pittsburgh when he was first diagnosed with a brain tumor in 1992. With the benefit of hindsight—and years of research into the origins and development of cancer—he came to understand that his previous lifestyle, particularly his poor diet, fostered a procancer environment. For example, a typical lunch for him was chili con carne, a plain bagel and a can of Coke.

Causes of Cancer

It can take years for cancer cells to turn into tumors—assuming that they ever do. This lag time means that we have many opportunities to create an anticancer environment in our bodies.

There are three main factors that promote the development of cancer...

●**Weakened immunity.** The immune system normally patrols the body for bacteria and viruses, as well as for cancer cells. When it spots something foreign, it dispatches a variety of cells, including natural killer cells, to destroy the foreign substance. In people who eat an unhealthy diet—not enough produce, too much alcohol, very little fish and so on—the immune system works less efficiently. This means that cancer cells can potentially slip under the radar and eventually proliferate.

●**Inflammation.** Millions of Americans have subclinical chronic inflammation. It doesn't cause symptoms, but it can lead to heart disease and cancer. Chronic inflammation can be caused by infection, a diet low in antioxidant nutrients and even emotional stress. It's accompanied by the release of cytokines and other inflammatory chemicals. Inflammation also prevents the immune system from working efficiently.

●**Angiogenesis.** Cancer cells, like other cells in the body, need blood and nourishment to survive. They send out chemical signals that stimulate the growth of blood vessels that carry blood to and from the cancer.

This process is called *angiogenesis*—and it can be strongly influenced by what we eat.

Example: People who eat no more than 12 ounces of red meat weekly can reduce their overall risk for cancer by 30%. Red meat stimulates the release of inflammatory chemicals that inhibit *apoptosis*, the genetically programmed cell death that prevents uncontrolled growth.

Cancer Fighters

Here's Dr. Servan-Schreiber's list of best cancer-fighting foods...

●**Fatty fish.** The omega-3 fatty acids in fish reduce inflammation. Oncologists in Scotland have measured inflammatory markers in the blood of cancer patients since the 1990s. They have found that patients with the lowest levels of inflammation are twice as likely to live through the next several years as patients who have more inflammation.

Laboratory studies indicate that a high-fish diet can reduce the growth of lung, breast, colon, prostate and kidney cancers. And naturally, people who eat more fish tend to eat less red meat.

Important: The larger fatty fish, such as tuna, are more likely to be contaminated with mercury and other toxins. The best sources of omega-3s are smaller fatty fish, such as sardines, anchovies and small mackerel.

●**Low-glycemic carbohydrates.** The glycemic index measures the effects of the carbohydrates in foods on blood glucose levels. Foods with a high glycemic index, such as white bread and table sugar, cause a rapid rise in insulin as well as a rise in *insulin-like growth factor* (IGF). IGF stimulates cell growth, including the growth of cancer cells. Both insulin and IGF also promote inflammation.

Data from the Harvard Nurses' Health Study indicate that people who eat the most high-glycemic foods (these same people tend to be sedentary and overweight) are 260% more likely to get pancreatic cancer and 80% more likely to get colorectal cancer.

Recommended: Unprocessed carbohydrates that are low on the glycemic scale, such as whole-grain breakfast cereals and breads (with whole wheat, barley, oats, flaxseeds, etc.)...cooked whole grains, such as millet, quinoa and barley...and vegetables, such as broccoli and cauliflower.

Also important: Reduce or eliminate refined sugar as well as honey.

Better: Agave nectar, available at most health-food stores. Extracted from cactus sap, it's sweeter than sugar or honey, yet it has a glycemic index four to five times lower. You can use agave nectar just as you would sugar or honey—by adding it to cereals, tea and so on. Because of the liquid content of the syrup, you'll generally want to reduce the amount of other liquids in baked goods. Substitute three-quarter cup of agave nectar per one cup of any other sweetener.

•**Green tea.** Between three and five cups daily can significantly reduce your cancer risk. A chemical in green tea, *epigallocatechin gallate* (EGCG), inhibits angiogenesis. Green tea also contains polyphenols and other chemical compounds that reduce inflammation and activate liver enzymes that break down and eliminate potential carcinogens.

In men who already have prostate cancer, consuming five cups or more of green tea daily has been associated with reduced risk of progressing to advanced cancer by 50%. In women with certain types of breast cancer, three cups daily reduced relapses by 30%. Because black tea is fermented, it has a lower concentration of polyphenols and is less protective than green tea.

•**Soy foods.** The isoflavones in tofu, soy milk, edamame (green soybeans) and other soy foods help prevent breast cancer, particularly in women who started eating soy early in life. These compounds, known as phytoestrogens, have estrogen-like effects. They occupy the same cellular receptors as the body's estrogen yet are only about one-hundredth as active. This means that they may slow the development of estrogen-dependent tumors.

Recommended: Three servings of soy per week—but only for women who are cancer-free. Avoid soy if you have or had cancer—there's some concern that the estrogen-like compounds in soy might promote tumor growth in women who have a type of breast cancer that is sensitive to estrogen's effects.

•**Turmeric.** No other food ingredient has more powerful anti-inflammatory effects. In laboratory studies, the active ingredient curcumin in the spice turmeric inhibits the growth of many different cancers. It helps prevent angiogenesis and promotes the death of cancer cells.

In India, people consume an average of one-quarter to one-half teaspoon of turmeric daily. They experience one-eighth as many lung cancers as Westerners of the same age… one-ninth as many colon cancers…and one-fifth as many breast cancers.

•**Asian mushrooms, such as shiitake, maitake and enokitake.** They're available in most supermarkets and gourmet stores and are one of the most potent immune system stimulants. Among people who eat a lot of these mushrooms, the rate of stomach cancer is 50% lower than it is among those who don't eat them. One to two half-cup servings weekly probably is enough to have measurable effects.

•**Berries.** Berries contain ellagic acid, which strongly inhibits angiogenesis. Aim for one-half cup per day.

•**Dark chocolate.** One ounce contains twice as many polyphenols as a glass of red wine and almost as much as a cup of green tea. Laboratory studies indicate that these compounds slow the growth of cancer cells.

Look for a chocolate with more than 70% cocoa. The lighter milk chocolates don't contain adequate amounts of polyphenols—and the dairy component of milk chocolate blocks the absorption of polyphenols.

David Servan-Schreiber, MD, PhD, neuroscientist and clinical professor of psychiatry at University of Pittsburgh School of Medicine and author of *Anticancer: A New Way of Life* (Viking). *www.anticancerbook.com.*

How Gender Affects Your Cancer Risk

Beyond the gender-specific cancers, such as prostate and ovarian, most people assume that other malignancies affect men and women equally—but that's not true.

Recent development: Researchers are increasingly identifying gender-related differences in genes, environmental exposures and behavioral factors that may affect cancer growth and help in detection and treatment.

Bladder Cancer

In the US, bladder cancer is expected to strike about 53,000 men and 18,000 women this year. The increased risk among men is mainly due to environmental factors, including smoking (more men smoke) and job-related exposure to toxins—especially in the processing industries, such as textile, metal, rubber and printing, which often use heavy metals and other carcinogens. When such carcinogens are inhaled, they pass into the urine where they can lead to cancer in the bladder. The inhalation of carcinogens while smoking cigarettes also increases bladder cancer risk, as does exposure to secondhand smoke.

While men have greater average exposure to such carcinogens, their risk also is higher because they urinate less often, on average, than women (seven times daily rather than eight), exposing the bladder to potential carcinogens longer.

Self-defense for men and women: Don't smoke. If you have symptoms of bladder cancer, such as blood in your urine, see your doctor. If you're at increased risk for bladder cancer due to your job, ask your doctor about one of several new tumor marker tests that can help identify bladder cancer early. Drinking water (about 50 ounces daily) also has been shown to reduce bladder cancer risk.

Colorectal Cancer

This year, colorectal cancer is expected to strike about 76,000 men and about 71,000 women in the US. Studies show that hormone replacement therapy significantly lowers menopausal women's risk for colorectal cancer—so younger women's higher estrogen levels also may have a protective effect.

A person's average bowel transit time—the time it takes food to pass through the digestive tract—also seems to play a role over several decades. Women, being smaller on average, have shorter intestines, reducing transit time. A diet high in fruits and vegetables cuts transit time. Women average three-and-one-half to four daily servings of fruits and veggies, while men average two to two-and-one-half.

Self-defense for men and women: Starting at age 50, get checked regularly for precancerous polyps with a *colonoscopy* (examination of the colon using a lighted, flexible tube) or, in some cases, flexible *sigmoidoscopy* (a similar procedure that examines the lower one-third of the colon). Follow your doctor's advice on the frequency of these tests.

Esophageal Cancer

One of the primary risk factors for esophageal cancer is chronic acid reflux—also known as *gastroesophageal reflux disease* (GERD). With GERD, the esophagus is repeatedly exposed to acidic stomach contents, which can cause cellular changes in the esophageal lining that may lead to cancer.

In the US, esophageal cancer is expected to affect about 13,000 men and about 3,500 women this year.

The main reason: Men are much more likely than women to have GERD—and related risk factors, such as drinking alcohol excessively, which increases stomach acid production…and having big bellies, which increase pressure on the stomach contents.

Self-defense for men and women: Drink in moderation (up to one drink daily if you're a woman…up to two drinks daily if you're a man) and lose weight, if necessary. If you have chronic acid reflux (common symptoms include burning in the throat, chronic cough or chronic hoarseness), seek medical treatment, such as prescription medication, to reduce symptoms.

Liver Cancer

This year, liver cancer is expected to affect about 16,000 men and 6,000 women in the US. Men are more likely than women to develop and die from liver cancer, largely because men are at greater risk for cirrhosis—the main risk factor for this type of malignancy. Men also have higher rates of hepatitis B and hepatitis C, both of which can cause cirrhosis. Twice as many men as women drink alcohol excessively, which also increases cirrhosis risk.

Self-defense for men and women: Drink moderately (as described earlier)…avoid hepatitis by protecting yourself against infected blood and body fluids by practicing safe sex and making sure that any nail salons you visit use sterilized manicure tools…and know hepatitis B and C symptoms (brief, flulike illness, nausea, vomiting and diarrhea, loss of appetite, abdominal pain and jaundice) so you can get treatment if you become infected.

Lung Cancer

Lung cancer—the deadliest of all malignancies—is expected to strike about 116,000 men and approximately 103,000 women in the US this year.

Statistics show that women are more likely to be among the 10% of lung cancer patients who never smoked. Although exposure to secondhand smoke and other carcinogens (such as asbestos and radon) play a role in lung cancer, women's risk for this disease may be influenced by estrogen, which some studies indicate can fuel lung tumor growth. Hormone replacement therapy, for example, has been shown to increase risk of dying from lung cancer, particularly among female smokers. Even so, women have better survival rates than men for all types and stages of lung cancer.

Groundbreaking research: The role of estrogen is being investigated in studies under way at the University of Pittsburgh and the University of California, Los Angeles. Specifically, researchers are studying whether women with lung cancer fare better when given the estrogen-blocking drug *fulvestrant* (Faslodex) in addition to the lung cancer drug *erlotinib* (Tarceva).

Self-defense for men and women: Do not smoke, and avoid second-hand smoke, radon and asbestos whenever possible.

Melanoma

Melanoma, the most dangerous form of skin cancer, is more common among women than men under age 40…occurs equally in both sexes between ages 40 and 50…and strikes significantly more men than women after age 50.

Some research theorizes that estrogen may account for the difference in melanoma rates in men and women. In total, about 30,000 women and 39,000 men in the US are predicted to develop melanoma this year.

Important new study finding: Researchers at New York University Langone Medical Center found that women under age 40 diagnosed with melanoma were much more likely to have a variation in a potentially cancer-promoting gene called MDM2. Besides offering an explanation for melanoma's prevalence in younger women, the discovery suggests that screening for this variation with a blood test may help identify women at risk and increase early detection of melanoma while it is most treatable.

Self-defense for men and women: Undergo yearly skin exams by a dermatologist, and perform self-exams in front of a mirror to identify changes in size, shape or color of existing moles and to check for new moles, spots or freckles that look unusual.

Otis Brawley, MD, practicing medical oncologist in Atlanta, chief medical officer of the American Cancer Society (*www.cancer.org*) and professor of hematology and medical oncology at the Emory University School of Medicine, also in Atlanta.

Candlelit Carcinogens?

Burning widely used paraffin candles indoors increases harmful pollutants, including some carcinogens.

Solution: Candles made from beeswax or soy don't produce the same pollutants as petroleum-based paraffin.

American Chemical Society

Don't Stand in Front Of the Microwave

Virtually everything with a cord or battery emits electromagnetic radiation—but some devices emit much more than others. The official exposure limit for electromagnetic radiation, set by the Federal Communications Commission, is based on old research that considered tissue heating to be the danger threshold.

New research: Radiation levels up to 1,000 times lower than the FCC's guidelines have been shown to affect our health.

Magda Havas, PhD, one of the leading experts in this field, explains what to do...

Cell Phones

A study published in *The American Journal of Epidemiology* reported that cell-phone users who spent more than 22 hours a month on their cell phones were 58% more likely to develop tumors of the *parotid* (salivary) *gland* than those who didn't use cell phones as often. Another study found that the risk for *gliomas* (a type of brain tumor) and *acoustic tumors* (where the ear meets the brain) doubled on the same side of the head after a decade of cell-phone use.

Studies funded by the telecommunications industry consistently have shown that cell phones are safe.

Main flaws: These studies typically lasted six years or less, not long enough for tumors to develop. In addition, most of the studies defined "heavy use" as using a cell phone just a few times a week—far less than the hours that many people spend on their cell phones every day.

Self-defense: Use cell phones only for emergencies or to retrieve messages. Return calls on a regular phone. *When you do use a cell phone...*

• **Regularly switch the phone from one side of your head to the other** to minimize one-side radiation exposure.

• **Turn off your cell phone when you're not expecting a call.** Even when you're not talking, cell phones send and receive signals to communicate with towers and satellites.

• **Never let the cell phone touch your ear or other body parts.** When talking, hold it at least one inch away from your head. Text-messaging is better than talking because the phone is farther away from your head. Bluetooth (wireless technology) uses radiation, but generally, levels are lower than those from your cell phone. Turn off cell phones in shirt or pants pockets.

• **Use a pneumatic (plastic air-tube) earpiece to reduce the brain's exposure to radiation.** Mercola (877-985-2695, *http://products.mercola.com*) sells these headsets, which have a hollow tube near the head rather than a wire running to the ear.

• **Don't use a phone in the car.** Using a cell phone or any wireless device while driving (or while in a train, bus or plane) uses more power because the phone must continually be reconnecting with antennas. Also, the signal is reflected by the metal around you, so your exposure inside is higher than it is outside.

Cordless Phones

Cordless phones, the kind with a base station and remote handsets that you can use anywhere in your house, use very similar frequencies to those used by cell phones. They pose the same risks.

Cordless phones with the designation Digitally Enhanced Cordless Telecommunications (DECT) technology are the worst, because they constantly emit radiation whether you're using the phone or not. They're more dangerous than having a cell-phone antenna inside your home.

Self-defense: Replace all cordless phones with corded phones.

WiFi

The majority of new computers, printers and similar devices now are equipped with WiFi (wireless) capabilities. Wireless signals are a strong source of electromagnetic radiation. As long as you are using a device that is receiving and sending information to and from the Internet without wires (this includes BlackBerries and iPhones), then you are being exposed to radiation.

Self-defense: Use cables to connect your Internet service to computers, not a wireless router. Similarly, it's safer to hardwire your printer to the computer than to use a WiFi connection. Hardwiring means that you won't be able to easily use a single computer throughout the house or to "beam" a signal to your printer from another room. Some people find this inconvenient, but the added safety is worth it. You can have additional Internet cables installed in multiple rooms.

If you do use a wireless router: Place it as close as possible to the devices that it controls. At greater distances, the router is forced to amplify its signal. Turn off the router when you're not using the computer.

If you don't use a wireless router: Find out how to disable the WiFi settings in your computer and printer. In the "on" position, these settings prompt the devices to emit electromagnetic energy in order to find the nearest available router.

Microwave Ovens

Medical technicians leave the room when X-rays are taken. People should be just as cautious with microwave ovens. Reason: Just about every microwave oven that I have tested, including the newest models, leaks radiation. In my home, I could detect electromagnetic radiation from the microwave 20 feet away.

Self-test: Put your cell phone inside the oven, and close the door (do not turn on the microwave). Call the cell-phone number. If you hear the phone ring, the cell-phone signal was able to pass through the walls of the oven—meaning that microwaves are able to pass out.

Self-defense: Leave the kitchen when the microwave is on.

Dirty Electricity

Household electricity normally is delivered at 60 cycles per second. Along with this stable current, however, come higher frequencies—spikes in power that cause surges of radiation from appliances and even unused electrical outlets.

This so-called "dirty electricity" has been linked to fatigue, headaches, difficulty concentrating and even cardiac symptoms in people who are sensitive (known as *electrohypersensitivity*).

Self-defense: Surge protectors, commonly used to protect computers and other electronic equipment, will "clean" household current to some extent.

Better: Graham-Stetzer Filters. These devices filter electrical "noise." You just plug them into wall outlets. They're designed to clean up entire circuits in the house. The average North American home needs about 20 filters. When you plug the filters in, you can use a microsurge meter to measure the levels of dirty electricity and try to get the levels below 40 GS units. The filters and meters are available at some hardware stores and online at *www.stetzerelectric.com* and *www.lessemf.com*.

Cost: About $35 for a filter, $125 for a meter.

Plasma Televisions

Plasma TVs generate high levels of dirty electricity. Using one filter won't solve the problem—people with plasma TVs might have to use three or more filters to clean up the power, compared with just one filter for an LCD TV.

Self-defense: LCDs produce nearly as good a picture and produce less dirty electricity than plasma TVs.

Magda Havas, PhD, associate professor of environmental and resource studies at Trent University in Peterborough, Ontario, Canada. She is a leading expert on radio-frequency radiation, electromagnetic fields, dirty electricity and ground current.

Vitamin E Reduces Lung Cancer Risk

Researchers from University of Texas MD Anderson Cancer Center looked at the association between lung cancer risk and four forms of vitamin E—alpha-, gamma-, beta- and delta-tocopherol. Patients with and without lung cancer answered a food-frequency questionnaire to determine intake.

Results: Those who consumed more of the four vitamin E tocopherols daily had a 55% reduction in lung cancer risk compared with those with the lowest average intake. Independently, alpha-tocopherol produced the best results. Those who consumed more than 7.73 mg daily had a 53% reduction in lung cancer risk compared with those who had less than 4.13 mg daily. The other forms of vitamin E did not independently affect lung cancer risk.

Vitamin E strengthens the immune system, has potent anti-inflammatory effects and acts as an antioxidant, stopping free radicals from damaging cells. To get the most protective form of vitamin E—alpha-tocopherol—consume almonds and other nuts, sunflower seeds, vegetable oils (one of the best is wheat germ oil) and leafy green vegetables. Aim for at least one serving of each of these foods daily. Or take 400 international units (IU) daily of vitamin E.

Mark A. Stengler, NMD, naturopathic medical doctor in private practice, La Jolla, California, and author of the *Bottom Line/Natural Healing* newsletter. *www.drstengler.com.*

Hot Tea Danger

In a study of 871 men and women, those who drank very hot tea (158°F or higher) several times a day were eight times more likely to develop cancer of the esophagus (the muscular tube that leads from the throat to the stomach) than those who drank warm or lukewarm tea. (The boiling point of water is 212°F.)

Theory: Very hot liquids can damage cells in the lining of the esophagus, potentially leading to cancer.

Self-defense: Before drinking tea or any other hot beverage, wait at least four minutes for the beverage to cool after being poured.

Reza Malekzadeh, MD, professor and director, Digestive Disease Research Center, Tehran University of Medical Sciences, Iran.

Meat, Dairy and Pancreatic Cancer

Men and women who ate the most fat, particularly from red meat and dairy sources, had a 53% and 23% higher rate, respectively, of pancreatic cancer than those who ate the least, according to a National Cancer Institute study. Those who ate the most saturated fat had a 36% higher rate of the cancer than those who consumed low levels.

Best: Limit the amount of total fat you consume to less than 30% of your total diet, particularly saturated fat from animal and dairy products.

Mark A. Stengler, NMD, naturopathic medical doctor in private practice, La Jolla, California, and author of the *Bottom Line/Natural Healing* newsletter. *www.drstengler.com.*

Five Ways to Prevent Colorectal Cancer

There are 147,000 new cases of colon and rectal cancer every year, and 50,000 people die from these cancers—making colorectal cancer the third biggest cancer killer of men (after lung and prostate) and women (after lung and breast).

But a recent study shows there are five ways to reduce your risk for the disease...

Study Details

Researchers at the George Institute for International Health in Australia analyzed data from 103 studies on risk factors for colon cancer. *Five risk factors stood out...*

●**Alcohol.** Those drinking the most—on average, about a drink a day—had a 60% higher risk than light drinkers (a few times a week, or less) or nondrinkers. "I was surprised by the strength of this association between alcohol consumption and colorectal cancer," says Rachel Huxley, DPhil, the study leader.

After alcohol, there were a number of other risk factors that were "remarkably consistent" at increasing or decreasing risk by about 20%, she says...

●**Meat.** A high intake of red and processed meat was linked to a 20% increased risk.

●**Sedentary lifestyle.** People who had the most physical activity—either recreational or on the job—had a 20% lower risk than those who had the least.

●**Overweight.** Excess pounds were linked to a 20% higher risk of the disease.

●**Smoking.** Smokers had a 20% higher risk of colorectal cancer. "Smoking had not been previously considered a cause of colon cancer" and "should be added to the list of tobacco-associated" cancers, says Dr. Huxley, who is now an associate professor at the University of Minnesota.

Dr. Huxley speculates that all these factors cause "a chronic, low-level inflammation" in the intestines that can eventually trigger colon cancer.

Beef, Butter, Booze and Body Fat

"Colorectal cancer is a disease of lifestyle," says Dr. Huxley. "If you change your behaviors—drink in moderation, maintain a healthy weight, eat a well-balanced diet without an excess of red meat, exercise regularly and quit smoking—you can substantially reduce your risk of the disease."

"And that's not just true of people with a family history of colorectal cancer," she adds. "It's true for everyone. And you'll get the bonus of lowering your risk for other types of cancers, and for heart disease."

"The recipe for reducing your risk of colorectal cancer is to cut beef, butter, booze and body fat," says Keith Block, MD, medical director of the Block Center for Integrative Cancer Treatment in Chicago, director of Integrative Medical Education at the University of Illinois College of Medicine and author of *Life Over Cancer* (Bantam). "And it's time to add cigarettes to that list."

His advice...

●**If you drink, limit alcohol to rare occasions.** "I used to tell people that drinking a little wine or beer is fine," he says. "Then data showed that even a little drinking increased the risk for breast cancer. Clearly, for cancer prevention, it's best to shift away from alcohol altogether."

●**Maintain normal weight.** "A low-grade inflammatory condition can also promote the risk or progression of colon cancer," says Dr. Block. "And extra weight—particularly belly fat—leads to a pro-inflammatory environment.

"I don't need to tell you how difficult it is to lose weight and keep it off. But to reduce your body's fat stores, I recommend the basics—a low-calorie, high-fiber diet that emphasizes whole-grains, vegetables and fruits, plus moderate aerobic exercise for 30 to 60 minutes a day."

●**Cut back on red and processed meat.** "For a source of animal protein, you are better off with cold-water fish, such as salmon or mackerel, which are high in inflammation-reducing omega-3 fatty acids," says Dr. Block.

Also important: The study also linked diabetes to a 20% increased risk for colon cancer. "High levels of blood sugar substantially increase the risk for colon cancer," says Dr. Block. (And death from the disease if you get it—in one study, people with diabetes with colon cancer survived only six years, compared with 11.3 years for people without the disease.)

To help control blood sugar levels, he recommends consuming whole grains at every meal, and eating small amounts of food throughout the day (three meals, with two or three snacks).

● **Exercise regularly.** "If walking were a drug, pharmaceutical companies would be in a frenzy to patent it," says Dr. Block. "A sedentary lifestyle is a bad idea."

● **Stop smoking.** "Research demonstrates that for every 15 cigarettes you smoke, at least one genetic mutation occurs" says Dr. Block. "Over time, those thousands of mutations are drivers for malignancy. If you want to prevent cancer, you must stop smoking."

Rachel Huxley, MA, DPhil, associate professor, School of Public Health, University of Minnesota, Minneapolis.

Keith Block, MD, medical director of the Block Center for Integrative Cancer Treatment in Chicago, director of Integrative Medical Education at the University of Illinois College of Medicine and author of *Life Over Cancer* (Bantam). *www. blockmd.com.*

Exercise: Rx for Cancer

The oncologists have finally taken a lesson from the fitness instructors.

"Oncologists should recommend exercise to their patients, because of the accumulating scientific evidence that exercise can improve both the quality of life and the prognosis for cancer patients," says Melinda Irwin, PhD, of Yale University, at a recent annual meeting of the American Association for Cancer Research. As one standout example of that evidence, Dr. Irwin cited a study showing that regular physical activity can reduce the death rate by 67% in breast cancer patients—a reduction, she says, that matches "standard medical treatments" for the disease.

However, continues Dr. Irwin, only half of cancer patients say that their oncologists even mention exercise.

It's well worth their mentioning it—and you hearing about it. Because if you're in the midst of a cancer treatment such as chemotherapy or radiation and want to reduce side effects such as fatigue...or if you're a cancer survivor who wants to prevent the recurrence of cancer...or if you've never set foot in an oncologist's office, but want to prevent

cancer from happening in the first place—recent studies show there's probably no stronger Rx than exercise.

Newest Research

Dozens of new studies show that exercise can help you walk (or run or bike or swim) away from cancer.

● **Preventing cancer.** In a 17-year study of more than 2,600 men, Finnish researchers found that men who exercised an average of 30 minutes a day had a 37% lower risk of developing and dying from any cancer. The findings were in the *British Journal of Sports Medicine.*

● **Preventing prostate cancer.** Researchers at the Duke University Medical Center studied 190 men who had a prostate biopsy (removal of tissue to test for cancer). Those who had been exercising regularly had a 35% lower risk of having the disease. And among those who had prostate cancer, exercise was linked to a 14% lower risk of developing an aggressive, faster-growing form of the disease. The findings were in the *Journal of Urology.*

In another study, researchers at the National Cancer Institute found that four or more hours of exercise a week decreased the risk of prostate cancer in African-American men by 41%. (Black men have a 30 to 50% higher risk for prostate cancer, and often develop a more aggressive form of the disease, with a death rate twice as high as white men.)

● **Preventing endometrial cancer.** Researchers at the National Cancer Institute analyzed health data from more than 109,000 women and found that those who exercised five or more times a week had a 23% lower risk of developing endometrial cancer, compared with those who rarely exercised. When they focused their analysis on overweight women, they found those who exercised lowered their risk by 39%.

● **Preventing breast cancer.** In a study of more than 110,000 postmenopausal women, those who engaged in more than seven hours per week of moderate or vigorous exercise for the previous 10 years had a 16% lower risk of developing breast cancer, compared with inactive women. The findings were in *BMC Cancer*.

●**Preventing the recurrence of breast cancer.** Researchers in Canada analyzed health data from more than 1,200 breast cancer survivors and found that those who exercised the most had a 56% lower risk of dying from breast cancer (or any other cause), compared with those who exercised the least. The findings were in the *International Journal of Cancer*.

And in a Chinese study on more than 1,800 breast cancer survivors, those who engaged in any type of regular exercise—such as taking a brisk, 45-minute walk three days a week—reported less emotional distress, better body image, better relationships and a greater ability to engage in the daily activities of work or school.

●**Surviving colon cancer.** Researchers at the Harvard School of Public Health studied 668 men with colon cancer—and found that those who exercised the most had a 53% lower risk of dying from the disease, compared with men who exercised the least. The findings were in *Annals of Internal Medicine*.

●**Help for leukemia fatigue.** Researchers at the UNC Lineberger Comprehensive Cancer Center at the University of North Carolina at Chapel Hill found that regular exercise (a customized program that could include stretching, aerobic exercise, strength training, and "core" exercises such as Pilates) can dramatically relieve fatigue and depression in people with leukemia, with fatigue decreasing by 64% and depression by 40%.

"This result is important because of the numerous side effects related to cancer treatment for leukemia, which requires confinement to a hospital room for four to six weeks to avoid the risk of infection," says Claudio Battaglini, PhD, the study leader.

"We have demonstrated that these patients not only can complete an exercise program in the hospital, but that they receive both physical and psychological benefits that could assist in their recovery." The findings were published in *Integrative Cancer Therapies*.

●**Cancer survivors—exercise, and survive longer.** Researchers in England found that cancer survivors who engaged in at least three, 20-minute sessions of vigorous exercise a week were 53% less likely to die, compared with people who didn't exercise. The findings were in *Cancer Causes and Control*.

Whole Body Fitness Program

"It used to be that oncologists told cancer patients to go home and rest—they were treated as if they were fragile, like china," says Keith Block, MD, Medical Director of the Block Center for Integrative Cancer Treatment in Chicago, Director of Integrative Medical Education at the University of Illinois College of Medicine, and author of *Life Over Cancer* (Bantam). "But the most recent research shows the more exercise you get, the better your odds of surviving cancer and reducing the debilitating side effects of cancer treatment."

Dr. Block's treatment for his cancer patients includes a "whole-body fitness program" that consists of...

●Muscle strengthening (through resistance training, using either weights or resistance bands such as Thera-bands),

●Muscle lengthening (through stretching or yoga),

●Cardiovascular endurance (through an aerobic exercise such as walking) and

●Cardiovascular recovery (also called "interval training," or short, intense bursts of aerobic exercise).

"Individualize your exercise program to your needs and capabilities," says Dr. Block. For those who have been sedentary, he says the ideal fitness program consists of regular, short bouts of low-to-moderate exercise that increases in intensity and duration as your fitness improves.

Start slow, increase gradually. That opinion is seconded by Julie Goodale, a personal trainer and certified cancer exercise trainer in New York.

"In spite of feeling exhausted from cancer treatments or being really out of shape, find an activity you enjoy and try exercising at an appropriate level," says Goodale.

But a fairly common mistake at this point is ramping up your workout too quickly, she says. "And if you increase too much, too quickly, you're risking injury, because your muscles might not be strong enough."

Better: "Stick with your workout for a week or two before increasing," she advises. "When you're ready to begin increasing, do it gradually, giving your muscles a chance to adjust to the new level.

"You can increase the duration, intention or frequency of your workout—but only increase one element at a time. If you started out with a short amount of time, try increasing the duration first. For example, you walked slowly for 20 minutes—next time you walk, increase the time by 10%, to 22 minutes. After you adjust to that, keep the time the same, but increase the intensity, walking a little faster. After that, add another day of walking into your week—if you started out walking three days, walk four. The same gradual approach holds true for strength training."

To recover from cancer, try interval training. "During cancer treatment, you will undergo events that are emotionally and physically draining, such as surgery and chemotherapy," says Dr. Block. "One of the few ways to improve your recovery capacity is by placing yourself in an exercise-induced stressful situation, over and over, and then training your body to tackle the stress and return to its healthy baseline—for instance, returning your heart rate to normal after strenuous physical activity."

That type of repetitive strenuous activity is called "interval training"—and you can do it for 15 to 30 seconds, 40 or 50 times a day, gradually building up to one minute, two minutes or three-minute sessions of high-intensity exercise, says Dr. Block.

Interval exercises can include running up and down stairs, running in place or jumping jacks—any exercise that quickly boosts your heart rate.

"With interval training, it's amazing how the body is very quickly trained to bounce back—and impressive to see cancer patients shift rapidly into a stronger state," says Dr. Block.

Melinda Irwin, PhD, associate professor, Yale School of Public Health.

Claudio Battaglini, PhD, assistant professor, Department of Exercise and Sport Science, University of North Carolina.

Julie Goodale, personal trainer and certified cancer exercise trainer in New York. *www.life-cise.com.*

Keith Block, MD, medical director of the Block Center for Integrative Cancer Treatment in Chicago, and author of *Life Over Cancer* (Bantam). *www.blockmd.com.*

Muscle Health Linked to Cancer Survival

In a study of 250 obese people with lung or gastrointestinal cancer, those with normal muscle mass lived an average of 10 months longer than those who had sarcopenia (depleted muscle mass).

Theory: Muscle mass may play a role in the body's immune response to cancer.

If you have cancer: Get screened by your doctor for sarcopenia and discuss moderate strength training.

Carla Prado, PhD, researcher, department of oncology, University of Alberta, Cross Cancer Institute, Canada.

Lifting Weights Relieves Lymphedema

Throughout your body are hundreds of *lymph nodes*—small, bean-shaped structures, rich in lymphatic fluid, where the immune system's *lymphocytes* (white blood cells) encounter viruses and other foreign particles and are programmed to repel the invaders.

One or more lymph nodes are usually removed during breast cancer surgery. Too often, the result is *lymphedema*—a buildup of lymphatic fluid in the arm, causing painful swelling in the arm and hand.

To prevent postsurgical lymphedema, women are usually told not to overuse the at-risk arm. Don't carry bags full of groceries, don't tote a heavy purse, don't pick up a child, don't lift a heavy suitcase—in fact, don't ever lift anything over 15 pounds!

Not stressing the arm, they are told, is *protecting* the arm. *Turns out that advice is wrong...*

Less Severe Symptoms

Researchers at the University of Pennsylvania School of Medicine studied 141 breast cancer survivors with lymphedema, dividing them into two groups. One group didn't change their exercise habits. But the other group started weight lifting—13 weeks of twice-weekly, 90-minute classes with a fitness instructor, followed by 39 weeks of unsupervised twice-weekly weight lifting.

During the year of working out, the women wore a custom-fitted compression garment on the affected arm while weight lifting... were asked weekly about any change in their symptoms...and their arms were measured monthly, to detect any change in swelling.

Results: Over the year, lymphedema worsened in 19 of the 70 nonlifters (29%), compared with only nine of the 70 weight lifters (13%). The weight lifters also reported less severe symptoms. Plus, after the year was over, the weight lifters had a sixfold greater improvement in body image and relationships—they felt much better about their bodies and appearance, and were more satisfied with their sex lives.

The findings were in the *New England Journal of Medicine*.

"Our study shows that participating in a safe, structured weight-lifting routine can help women with lymphedema take control of their symptoms and reap the many rewards that resistance training has on overall health," says Kathryn Schmitz, PhD, MPH, the study leader.

"Breast cancer survivors *can* safely participate in slowly progressive weight lifting—

and they can gain the benefits of weight lifting without any increase in their lymphedema symptoms," she says. "In fact, this type of exercise may actually help them feel better."

Put Aside Your Fear

If you're a breast cancer survivor who wants to start lifting weights (also called *strength training* or *resistance training*), here are recommendations from Vik Khanna, a clinical exercise specialist certified by the American College of Sports Medicine (ACSM), and chief "exercise" officer at Galileo Health Partners near Baltimore, Maryland.

- **First, talk to your doctor and/or oncologist.** "Make sure you're cleared for physical activity—that you're healthy enough to lift weights," says Khanna.

- **Next, put aside your fear.** "A woman might be concerned because all the medical advice to date has been to rest the at-risk or affected arm," says Khanna. "But this study destroys that medical mythology. It shows that engaging in physical activity is overwhelmingly beneficial. A woman can confidentially say to herself, 'The evidence is in my favor—weight lifting is going to help me.'"

- **Strength train in a facility, under the guidance of a qualified trainer.** The women in the study were trained and guided by fitness professionals at a YMCA.

Working with a fitness professional at a fitness facility is an excellent way to start weight lifting, says Khanna—and the Y is a good choice, because it's family friendly and usually has good trainers.

Resource: To find a nationwide list of the approximately 150 YMCAs that offer training to cancer survivors (LIVESTRONG at the YMCA, in collaboration with the Lance Armstrong Foundation), visit the Web site *www.livestrong.org*, and under "Grants and Programs" click "National Partnerships," and then click "LIVESTRONG at the YMCA."

Smart idea: If there's no Y nearby, and you're using another fitness facility, it's important to make sure your trainer is qualified, says Khanna. He recommends talking to the supervisor of the trainers in the facility, and asking whether any personal trainer on the staff has received formal instruction in working with a cancer survivor, and has done so safely and successfully.

You could also look for a trainer certified by the ACSM to work with cancer survivors—a "Certified Cancer Exercise Trainer." To locate one, visit the ACSM Web site (*www.acsm.org*) and use the ProFinder tool under "General Public."

Or, if you live near a university-based or hospital-based cancer center, call and ask if they can recommend a fitness professional in the community to help you with a strength-training program.

"You want the best-educated, most highly credentialed person you can find," says Khanna. "The trainer should make sure you do the exercise properly; talk to you about how you feel before, during and after exercise; monitor the health of your arm and encourage you to see the doctor if something seems amiss." The trainer doesn't need to be a medical professional, he adds, but he/she does need to understand the medical implications of what you're doing.

● **Strength train on your own.** Perhaps you don't feel you're ready to be seen in public. Perhaps a gym is too costly. Perhaps transportation is a problem. Or perhaps after a few weeks of strength training in a gym, you're ready to strength train on your own. For whatever reason, you want to strength train at home.

"For many people, starting at home is best done with basic equipment, such as resistance bands, tubes or pairs of dumbbells, starting at 3 to 5 pounds" says Khanna. "You can equip a very functional home gym for $50 to $100. And many of these products come with an illustrated guide that shows you how to do enough exercises to create a whole-body workout.

"Sit down and create a strength-training session that you can do three times a week—starting each time with the large muscles of the legs, hips and lower back, and progressing to the small muscles of the chest, shoulders, arms and upper back."

Resources: To purchase basic, at-home strength-training equipment, Khanna uses two Web sites: *www.performbetter.com* and *www.power-systems.com*. You can also buy these supplies at sporting-good retailers, such as Dick's or Sports Authority.

● **Use a whole-body approach.** The women who participated in the study at the University of Pennsylvania didn't just exercise the affected arm, points out Khanna.

"They learned strength-training exercises for their lower body, their arms, their torso and their core," he says. The whole-body workout is important, he says, because muscles work in balance, and because strength training the entire body offers many health benefits—including preserving and strengthening bone, and reducing the risk of falls.

● **Start slowly.** The study used a cautious approach to weight lifting. First, the researchers established what is called a "1 rep maximum" for each exercise (the most weight a person can lift safely and correctly in a particular exercise). Then, the program started at a somewhat lower level of resistance that allowed participants to do 10 repetitions, for 2 or 3 sets. (Each movement in an exercise is a rep; a group of successfully completed reps is a set.) When the participants could safely and correctly do two to three sets of 10 reps, the trainers helped them increase the weight of the exercise.

"That's exactly the way you want to do it," says Khanna.

"By adding weight in small increments, you stay within your physical and psychological comfort zone, and you create a steady path of improvement."

Weight lifting example: On a strength-training machine, you can safely and correctly do a 1 rep maximum in the bicep curl with 30 pounds. You then use 20 pounds, until you can successfully do 2 sets of 10 reps. At that point, you increase the weight in increments of 2.5 to 5 pounds. You do 2 sets of 10 reps with the new weight before you again increase the weight.

Resistance band example: You start with "extra-light" resistance bands and then move to light, medium, heavy, etcetera.

● **Don't set a limit to your strength.** "People usually underestimate how quickly they'll gain strength," says Khanna.

"But don't be afraid to get stronger—strong muscles are an intrinsic good, and they have no downside. If you're using strength training for cancer recovery, go as far as your body and spirit will take you."

Kathryn Schmitz, PhD, MPH, associate professor of epidemiology, University of Pennsylvania School of Medicine.

Vik Khanna, clinical exercise specialist and chief "exercise" officer at Galileo Health Partners, Baltimore, Maryland, *www.galileohealth.net.*

Acupuncture Cools Hot Flashes Caused by Cancer Drugs

As if breast cancer weren't bad enough. After the chemotherapy and radiation, women usually take anti-estrogen drugs (such as Tamoxifen) for five years, which often trigger severe hot flashes and night sweats. (So severe, that many women are forced to stop taking the cancer-suppressing drug!)

The standard medical treatment for these hot flashes is *venlafaxine* (Effexor), an antidepressant drug. It works (though doctors don't know why), but it comes with its own set of possible side effects, such as nausea, dry mouth, dizziness and anxiety.

Good news: A new study shows that a nondrug treatment works just as well as Effexor. *Acupuncture...*

Benefits, Not Side Effects

A team of researchers led by doctors at the Henry Ford Health System in Detroit, Michigan, studied 59 breast cancer survivors with hot flashes, dividing them into two groups. One group received 12 weeks of treatment with acupuncture—the technique from Traditional Chinese Medicine (TCM) that inserts tiny needles into "acupuncture points" on the body, stimulating and balancing what TCM practitioners call *qi*, or life-force. The other group received a daily dose of Effexor for 12 weeks.

After 12 weeks, both groups had the same benefit—a 50% reduction in hot flashes and depression. But many in the drug group also had side effects from Effexor.

And when the drug and acupuncture treatments were stopped after 12 weeks, the drug group started having lots of hot flashes again—but the acupuncture group didn't. In fact, they didn't experience any sizable increase in the number and severity of hot flashes for the next three months.

And, unlike the drug group, many of the women receiving acupuncture also said they had more energy, greater clarity of thought and more well-being. Twenty-five percent also reported a boost in sex drive.

The findings were in the *Journal of Clinical Oncology.*

"Acupuncture offers a safe, effective and durable treatment option for hot flashes—something that affects the majority of breast cancer survivors," says Eleanor Walker, MD, the study leader. "And compared with drug therapy, acupuncture actually has benefits, as opposed to more side effects."

And in another recent study on acupuncture and hot flashes, doctors in Norway found that 10 weeks of acupuncture reduced hot flashes by 50% and night sweats by 60%. There was also a 44% reduction in the Kupperman Index—a measurement of common menopause symptoms, such as insomnia, anxiety, depression, headaches and muscle pain.

Find an Acupuncturist

"Acupuncture supports the whole system—not only helping to lessen hot flashes, but balancing the entire body and creating better health," says Elizabeth Trattner, OMD, an acupuncturist and doctor of oriental medicine in Bay Harbor Islands, Florida.

To find a qualified acupuncturist near you, she recommends visiting the Web site of the National Certification Commission for Acupuncture and Oriental Medicine (*www.nc caom.org*) and clicking "Find a Practitioner" on the home page. She also counsels finding a practitioner who has treated other people with breast cancer.

(For more information on the best way to find and choose an acupuncturist, see page 23 in "Aches & Pains from Head to Toe." Also see appendix page 354 for information on acupuncture as a healing modality.)

Eleanor Walker, MD, division director of breast services, Department of Radiation Oncology, Henry Ford Hospital, Detroit, Michigan.

Elizabeth Trattner, OMD, acupuncturist and doctor of oriental medicine in Bay Harbor Islands, Florida. *www.eliza bethtrattner.com.*

The Cancer Recovery Diet

When you are facing cancer, it is more important than ever to follow a nutritious diet that strengthens your immune system and helps your body detoxify. This often is challenging, however, because some cancer treatments interfere with the body's ability to take in or use nutrients. *Cancer patients undergoing chemotherapy and/or radiation often experience...*

• Damage to salivary glands resulting in a dry mouth, difficulty swallowing and unpleasant changes in taste.

• Nausea and vomiting.

• Impaired absorption of nutrients and calories due to changes in the normal intestinal bacteria.

These factors and the resulting loss of appetite deplete the body's stores of nutrients and can lead to excessive weight loss that impedes your recovery, strains your immune system and adds to fatigue.

The following nutrition plan designed by Mitchell Gaynor, MD, clinical professor of medicine at Weill Cornell Medical College of Cornell University, is for cancer patients undergoing treatment—as well as for those who finished treatment within the past year—to help rebuild nutrient reserves. All supplements below are sold at health-food stores and/or online.

Important: Discuss your diet and supplement use with your oncologist—this helps the doctor determine the best treatment and follow-up regimen for you. *What to do...*

• **Eat plenty of protein.** Protein helps repair body tissues and prevent unwanted weight loss. It also helps minimize the memory and concentration problems ("chemo brain") common among patients on chemotherapy. The recommended dietary allowance (RDA) for women is 38 grams (g) of protein per day and for men it is 46 g—but for cancer patients, Dr. Gaynor recommends at least 70 g per day.

Example: With breakfast, include one egg (7 g) and eight ounces of unsweetened soy milk (8 g)...with lunch, a cup of lentil soup (10 g) and eight ounces of low-fat yogurt (12 g)...as a snack, two ounces of almonds (12 g)...with dinner, three ounces of chicken or fish (21 g) or one cup of soybeans (29 g).

Helpful: Consider a healthful protein supplement— such as Biochem Sports Greens & Whey, which provides 20 g of protein per one-ounce serving.

• **Have eight ounces of low-fat yogurt or kefir daily.** Check labels and choose unsweetened brands with live active cultures of lactobacillus acidophilus and bifidobacterium. Chemotherapy and radiation destroy beneficial bacteria in the gut. Restoring them with probiotics helps alleviate nausea, optimizes immune system function and reduces production of cancer-promoting chemicals.

Alternative: Try a probiotic supplement that contains at least one billion colony forming units (CFUs) per gram. Choose coated capsules to protect the probiotics from stomach acids. Take on an empty stomach upon awakening and also one hour before lunch and dinner.

Good brand: Natren Healthy Trinity (866-462-8736, *www.natren.com*).

● **Boost fiber.** This combats constipation, a common side effect of chemotherapy. Aim for six to 10 servings of whole grains daily.

Examples: One slice of whole-grain bread…one-half cup of cooked brown rice, rolled barley, millet or buckwheat…one-half cup of old-fashioned oatmeal.

● **Also eat seven to 10 servings of fruits and vegetables daily,** which provide fiber and cancer-fighting phytonutrients (plant chemicals). If you have lost your taste for vegetables, have juice instead—it is easier to swallow. Carrots, celery, watercress and beets make delicious juices. Juicers are sold at kitchenware stores ($50 and up).

● **Focus on anti-inflammatory foods.** The same enzyme (called COX-2) that causes inflammation also may increase levels of compounds that allow cancer cells to grow. Lowering the body's inflammatory response may be protective.

Best: Eat cold-water fish (salmon, sardines, herring, mackerel, cod) at least three times per week—these are rich in anti-inflammatory omega-3 fatty acids. Dr. Gaynor recommends avoiding tuna, swordfish and shark, which may contain mercury and other metals.

Alternative: Take 2.5 g of a fish oil daily with food.

Also helpful: Use curry powder liberally to spice up vegetables, meats and poultry—it is a natural anti-inflammatory.

● **Eat foods rich in calcium, magnesium and vitamin D.** These bone-building nutrients are especially important for cancer patients who take steroid medication to control nausea, because steroids can weaken bones. Increase your intake of foods that provide calcium (low-fat dairy, fortified cereals, leafy green vegetables)…magnesium (nuts, beans, quinoa)…and vitamin D (fish, fortified dairy). Also supplement daily with 1,500 mg of calcium citrate…400 mg of magnesium…and 1,000 international units (IU) of vitamin D-3.

● **Minimize intake of sugar and white flour.** Eating these foods temporarily increases your levels of insulin-like growth factor (IGF), which has hormonelike effects. Although the long-term consequences are unclear, some research suggests a link between high IGF levels and cancer, especially of the breast and colon.

● **Drink plenty of fluids.** Dehydration contributes to decreased salivation…promotes inflammation…and stresses the kidneys and liver, making it harder for these organs to detoxify the body. Drink at least six eight-ounce glasses of water, broth or tea per day.

Beneficial: Green tea contains compounds that may inhibit *angiogenesis* (creation of blood vessels that feed cancer cells).

● **Opt for organic.** Conventionally grown produce often has pesticide and herbicide residues that stress the liver. Choose free-range chicken and beef from grass-fed cows to minimize exposure to antibiotics and hormones in the feed of nonorganic animals. Remove the skin from poultry and fish before cooking, even if organic—skin tends to store a high concentration of toxins.

Helpful: A dietitian who specializes in oncology nutrition can help monitor your nutrient intake and recommend alternatives if certain foods are difficult to eat.

Referrals: American Dietetic Association, 800-877-1600, *www.eatright.org*.

Mitchell Gaynor, MD, clinical professor of medicine at Weill Cornell Medical College of Cornell University and founder and president of Gaynor Integrative Oncology, both in New York City. *www.gaynoroncology.com*.

The Vegetarian Advantage

It's official—the vegetarian diet has gone mainstream.

The American Dietetic Association recently issued an updated "position paper" on the diet, declaring that "appropriately planned vegetarian diets, including total vegetarian or vegan diets, are healthful, nutritionally adequate and may provide health benefits in the prevention and treatment of certain diseases."

Those diseases include heart disease, diabetes, obesity—and cancer. "Vegetarians tend to have lower overall cancer rates," according to the paper. Why?

"Vegetarian diets tend to be lower in saturated fat and cholesterol and have higher levels of dietary fiber, magnesium and potassium, vitamins C and E, folate, carotenoids, flavonoids and other phytochemicals," the paper continued. "These nutritional differences may explain some of the health advantages of those following a varied, balanced vegetarian diet."

And over the last year, the anticancer advantages of emphasizing plant foods and minimizing (or even eliminating) meat have become clearer and clearer...

Newest Research

●**All cancers.** Researchers at the University of Oxford in Britain analyzed 12 years of health data from more than 61,000 British men and women. Vegetarians had a 22% lower risk of cancer than people who ate meat. The findings were in the *British Journal of Cancer.*

●**Colon cancer.** Korean researchers studied more than 1,000 people and found that those with the highest intake of folate (a B vitamin found abundantly in green, leafy vegetables, chickpeas and lentils) had a 66% lower risk of colon cancer, compared with those with the lowest intake. "Adequate intake of folate appears to assume the role of a protective agent against cancer," says Joel

Mason, MD, of the Jean Mayer USDA Human Nutrition Research Center on Aging at Tufts University, in a paper on folate and cancer in *Nutrition Reviews.*

In another study, researchers at the National Cancer Institute found that people who consistently ate a diet high in fruits, vegetables and fiber and low in fat, had a 50% lower risk of developing colon polyps, benign growths, some types of which, increase the likelihood of developing colon cancer later on.

●**Breast cancer.** In a study of more than 65,000 postmenopausal women, researchers found that those who ate a Mediterranean-style diet rich in fruits, vegetables and olive oil had a 15% lower risk of developing breast cancer than those who ate a so-called Western diet rich in meat, eggs, butter and processed foods. The findings were in the *American Journal of Epidemiology.*

●**Prostate cancer.** Researchers at the National Cancer Institute analyzed nine years of health data from more than 175,000 men. Those who ate the most red meat (beef and pork) and red processed meat (bacon, red-meat sausage and hot dogs) had a 12% higher risk of developing prostate cancer, compared with men who ate the least—and a 33% higher risk of developing advanced prostate cancer.

●**Lymph cancers.** Researchers from the Mayo Clinic analyzed 20 years of health data from more than 35,000 people. Those who ate seven servings a day or more of fruits and vegetables had a 31% lower risk of developing cancers of the lymph system, such as non-Hodgkin lymphoma, compared with those eating three or fewer servings a day. The findings were in the *International Journal of Cancer.*

Best: Yellow and orange vegetables, and cruciferous vegetables (such as broccoli) were linked with the greatest reduction in cancer risk.

●**Endometrial and uterine cancer.** Researchers at the Cancer Institute of New Jersey found that women with a higher intake of antioxidant vitamins found in plant foods —such as beta-carotene, vitamin C and vitamin E—had a lower incidence of endometrial and uterine cancer.

• **Pancreatic cancer.** Researchers at the National Cancer Institute analyzed six years of health data from more than 500,000 people. Those eating the highest amount of saturated fat—found primarily in red meat and dairy products—had a 36% higher risk for pancreatic cancer. Study results were published in the *Journal of the National Cancer Institute.*

Starting a Vegetarian Diet

How do you switch to a vegetarian diet? The following are suggestions from Suzanne Havala Hobbs, DrPh, MS, RD, a registered and licensed dietician, clinical assistant professor at the University of North Carolina, author of numerous books, including *Living Vegetarian for Dummies* (Wiley)—and a vegetarian herself.

• **Educate yourself.** "As you make the transition, it's a great idea to spend several weeks reading everything you can about vegetarianism," she says. She recommends…

Books: The New Becoming Vegetarian by Vesanto Melina and Brenda Davis (Healthy Living Publications), *Simply Vegan* by Debra Wasserman (Vegetarian Resource Group) and her book *Living Vegetarian for Dummies* (Wiley).

Organizations and Web sites: Vegetarian Resource Group (VRG), the biggest vegetarian organization in the world, at *www. vrg.org.*

The North American Vegetarian Society (NAVS), at *www.navs-online.org.*

Try this: "NAVS puts on the annual Vegetarian Summerfest in Johnstown, Pennsylvania, and the 5-day event is a wonderful way to learn how to put a vegetarian diet into practice," says Dr. Hobbs. For more information, visit the Web site *www.vegetariansum merfest.org.*

• **Reduce your meat intake.** "While you're doing background reading about vegetarian diets, there are easy ways to reduce your meat intake," says Dr. Hobbs.

Add two or three meatless main meals to your diet each week. "Begin with easy and familiar entrées," she says.

Examples: spaghetti with tomato sauce, vegetarian pizza, bean burritos, vegetable lasagna and pasta primavera.

• **Try vegetarian convenience foods.** "Most supermarkets carry these products," says Dr. Hobbs. "Substitute them for their meat counterparts."

Examples: veggie burger patties, veggie breakfast meats, frozen vegetarian diners and veggie hot dogs.

When you eat meat, make it a side dish or condiment. "Keep meat portions small, and extend the meat by mixing it with rice, vegetables, pasta or other plant products," she says.

Example: "Rather than eat a chicken breast or entrée, cut it up and mix it into a big vegetable stir-fry that feeds four to six people."

• **Make the switch.** After a few months of educating yourself and reducing your meat intake, you're ready for a meatless lifestyle, says Dr. Hobbs. *To make the final transition…*

• **Plan a cutoff date after which you'll eat only meatless meals.** "Mark that date on your calendar," she advises.

• **Stop buying meat.** "A week or two before the cutoff date, stop buying meat and products containing meat, such as soup with ham or bacon and baked beans with pork.

• **Practice.** Congratulations! You're a vegetarian. You have adopted one of the most effective anticancer diets. *To stay that way…*

• **Socialize without meat.** "Invite friends and family to your home for vegetarian meals," says Dr. Hobbs.

• **Plan ahead.** Is staying vegetarian a problem during holidays, vacations and other breaks in your routine? If so, use the educational material you gathered during your transition phase to strategize how to stay vegetarian during those times. *Example:* "When on vacation, eat at ethnic restaurants known for their many good meatless dishes," she says. *However:* For safety's sake, vegans (vegetarians who don't eat any animal products, including dairy) should take a nutritional supplement that includes vitamin B-12, which is found only in animal products.

Joel Mason, MD, Jean Mayer USDA Human Nutrition Research Center on Aging, Tufts University.

Suzanne Havala Hobbs, DrPh, MS, RD, registered and licensed dietician, clinical assistant professor at the University of North Carolina and author of numerous books, including *Living Vegetarian for Dummies* (Wiley).

Eating Fish Helps Prostate Cancer Survival

A 22-year Harvard School of Public Health study of 20,167 men found that fish intake did not reduce the incidence of prostate cancer but did improve survival rates among men who had prostate cancer. Men with prostate cancer who ate fish five or more times weekly had a 48% lower risk of dying from the disease than those who ate fish less than once a week.

Several animal studies have shown that omega-3 fatty acids found in fish inhibit prostate cancer growth. One component of omega-3 fatty acids, known as *eicosapentaenoic acid* (EPA), and one of its metabolites have been shown to suppress the proliferation of prostate cancer cells.

Recommendation: Consuming five weekly servings of fish, especially those with the least mercury and other contaminants, such as sardines, trout and wild Alaskan salmon. Or take a fish oil supplement that supplies a combined daily total of 1,000 mg of EPA and *docosahexaenoic acid* (DHA).

Mark A. Stengler, NMD, naturopathic medical doctor in private practice, La Jolla, California, and author of the *Bottom Line/Natural Healing* newsletter. *www.drstengler.com.*

Protection from Stomach Cancer— Broccoli Sprouts

In a Johns Hopkins University School of Medicine study, adults who were infected with the *Helicobacter pylori* (H. pylori) bacteria ate either two-and-a-half ounces of broccoli sprouts or the same amount of alfalfa sprouts daily for two months.

Result: After eight weeks, stool and breath tests indicated that those who ate the broccoli sprouts had significantly lower levels of biomarkers of the H. pylori infection. There was no change in the alfalfa sprouts group.

That broccoli sprouts appear to reduce the levels of H. pylori in humans is good news, since this bacteria can lead to ulcers and digestive cancers. Broccoli sprouts are rich in sulforaphane, a biochemical that triggers the production of gastrointestinal enzymes and can protect against potentially cancer-causing chemicals and inflammation. Broccoli sprouts also support the body in the detoxification of carcinogenic substances. Add broccoli sprouts to your salad or on sandwiches. Aim to eat up to two-and-a-half ounces a day, the amount used in the study.

Mark A. Stengler, NMD, naturopathic medical doctor in private practice, La Jolla, California, and author of the *Bottom Line/Natural Healing* newsletter. *www.drstengler.com.*

Can Garlic Repel Cancer?

Is garlic a viable cancer fighter? A recent meta-analysis of 19 published studies found no strong link between garlic intake and reduced risk for a wide number of cancers. The research team, led by Oran Kwon, MD, at Ewha Women's University in Seoul, South Korea, did acknowledge credible evidence linking garlic intake to reduced risk for colon, prostate and ovarian cancer, but qualified the data as "very limited."

According to Andrew Rubman, ND, an issue with meta-analyses—studies that evaluate data from numerous others to reach a conclusion—is that researchers are able to pick and choose among previous studies to skew their findings in a particular direction. It is possible, he says, that the studies showing no discernable effects of garlic used products that were relatively weak or garlic processed at high temperatures, which would diminish its healthful properties.

Dr. Rubman continues to support garlic as one among many cancer-prevention tools when it is part of a healthy diet. He says that preliminary human studies, evaluated by Natural Standard (*www.naturalstandard. com*), a clinical database that evaluates evidence-based natural therapies, suggest that regular consumption of garlic, particularly unprocessed, may reduce the risk of developing several types of cancer, including gastric and colorectal. "More studies are necessary to better evaluate preventative or curative capacity," Dr. Rubman adds.

Dr. Rubman notes that it is best to crush raw garlic to release its healthful enzymes and then let it rest for 10 minutes or so to "bloom." Most people start a dish by heating garlic in oil, which is fine, but Dr. Rubman advises adding garlic at the end of the cooking process as well to ensure that you'll get the full health value, since some of its cancer-fighting properties are reduced—even destroyed—by heat. Another possible solution is to take capsules of cold-pressed extraction of garlic (he recommends those made by a Japanese company called Kyolic, *www.kyo lic.com*). However, with such excellent garlic available in markets today, Dr. Rubman says he sees no reason not to consume it fresh in your favorite dishes.

Andrew Rubman, ND, medical director, Southbury Clinic for Traditional Medicines, Southbury, Connecticut. *www. naturopath.org*.

Scheduled for Radiation Treatment? Drink a Glass of Wine

"Nearly all cancer patients who get radiation treatment experience some form of painful skin damage, from mild sunburn all the way to blisters," says Paul Okunieff, MD, adjunct professor of radiation oncology at the James P. Wilmot Cancer Center of the University of Rochester, in New York.

To prevent the damage, an oncologist will typically prescribe *ethyol* (Amifostine), a cell-protecting drug.

But a single dose costs about $400. The drug also can have severe side effects, including low blood pressure, allergic reactions, weakness, drowsiness, fever and vomiting. And studies show that it may actually protect breast cancer cells from radiation treatment. No wonder that one-third of patients prescribed Amifostine stop taking it.

Now, a team of Italian cancer doctors has discovered what they say may be an "equally effective, but less expensive, and less toxic natural substance" to protect radiated skin.

A daily glass of wine...

Less Skin Damage

The doctors analyzed the wine-drinking habits of 348 women treated with radiation therapy after breast cancer surgery.

They found that only 14% of those who drank a glass of wine on the day of their radiation treatment had acute skin damage—compared with 32% of patients drinking one-half glass of wine, and 38% of those who didn't drink wine.

They also found that 35% of patients who drank two glasses of wine on the day of treatment had skin damage—showing that when it comes to the protective effects of wine, more isn't merrier.

Why it works: The study was conducted in Italy, so the researchers speculate that the women were drinking red wine. And certain compounds in red wine—particularly the antioxidants and the tannins (which give red wine its dry effect)—have been shown to protect cellular DNA from damage, the underlying cause of radiation's side effects, explains Gabriella Macchia, MD, a study researcher and physician in the Radiotherapy Unit, Department of Oncology at Catholic University in Campobasso, Italy.

But however the wine worked, "our findings clearly indicate that wine has a radio-protective effect," wrote Dr. Macchia and her colleagues, in the *International Journal of Radiation Oncology, Biology and Physiology*.

One Glass of Wine a Day

"If a woman undergoing radiation for breast cancer is a wine drinker, she should maintain that habit, drinking one glass of wine a day—ideally, ½ glass at lunch and dinner," says Dr. Macchia.

If you're not a drinker, Dr. Macchia advises maximizing your intake of antioxidants by eating more whole foods, such as fruits, vegetables, whole grains and legumes.

She also says that drinking one glass a day of red grape juice may be just as effective as drinking red wine—because studies show that red grape juice has the same heart-helping benefits as red wine (such as reducing the risk of blood clots, lowering "bad" LDL cholesterol and lowering high blood pressure).

Dr. Macchia says more study on the "protective effect of wine" is needed, including finding out if wine might protect against radiation-caused skin damage in the treatment of other types of cancer.

Gabriella Macchia, MD, Radiotherapy Unit, Department of Oncology, Catholic University in Campobasso, Italy.

Paul Okunieff, MD, adjunct professor of radiation oncology, James P. Wilmont Cancer Center, University of Rochester, New York.

Cultured Milk Products May Reduce Bladder Cancer Risk

The large intestine is the center of the body's immune system, the protective core that works hard to keep the body safe from harmful microbes that cause disease. Researchers in Sweden have discovered that eating more probiotic foods—in this case, fermented milk products such as yogurt and "sour milk" (a product similar to buttermilk but made by fermentation with different bacteria)—are beneficial not only for the gut but for the nearby bladder.

The study, published in the *American Journal of Clinical Nutrition*, assessed the diets of 82,000 men and women over nine years. Participants who had eaten yogurt were more likely to remain cancer-free than those that hadn't. Specifically, researchers found that those individuals who had reported eating two or more servings of sour milk and yogurt per day had a 38% lower risk of bladder cancer.

Maintaining a Healthy Microbial Balance

Maintenance of a healthy microbial colony in the large intestine is particularly essential to maintaining bladder health, notes Andrew L. Rubman, ND. Beneficial bacteria help defend it and the intestinal tract from carcinogens and other dangerous microbes in the food you eat.

Although this study examined sour milk and yogurt in particular, Dr. Rubman notes that other fermented dairy products such as kefir, sour cream and buttermilk likewise contain protective bacteria (*lactobacillus* and/or *bifidobacterium*). In fact, he noted, nondairy fermented foods confer much of the same benefit. Options include tangy Korean *kimchi* (a spicy cabbage side dish), pickled cucumbers, tempeh, miso and tamari (a soy product).

Over time, eating fermented foods like these will not only improve your gut function, but your immune health overall.

Andrew L. Rubman, ND, medical director, Southbury Clinic for Traditional Medicines, Southbury, Connecticut. *www.southburyclinic.com.*

Slow Down Prostate Cancer with Green Tea

This year, nearly 200,000 American men will be diagnosed with prostate cancer, and more than 27,000 will die from the disease—making prostate cancer the most diagnosed cancer among men, and the second biggest cancer killer. In fact, death rates for advanced-stage prostate cancer haven't gone down in the last decade, in spite of new treatments.

But a recent study shows that more men with prostate cancer might survive—if they drink green tea or take a supplement of green tea extract.

A Good Addition

Researchers at Louisiana State University Health Sciences Center studied 26 men with prostate cancer who were scheduled to have their prostates surgically removed (radical prostatectomy).

For one month before the operation, the men took a daily dose of a green tea extract called Polyphenol E, a supplement standardized for high doses of catechins, the cell-protecting, disease-fighting antioxidants in green tea. It contains 1.3 grams of total catechins, including 800 milligrams (mg) of *epigallo-catechin-3-gallate*, or EGCG (the most active ingredient in green tea), and lower amounts of *epicatechin*, *epigallocatechin* and *epicatechin-3-gallate*. (Polyphenol E is not yet on the market.)

The extract didn't stop cancer in its tracks—but it definitely slowed it…

After one month, the men had an average decrease of 9.9% in *vascular endothelial growth factor* (VEGF)—a protein that helps provide blood supply to tumors, spurring their growth and spread.

They also had an 18.9% decrease in *hepatocyte growth factor* (HGF)—a protein linked to cancer *metastases* (cancer spreading beyond its original site to other parts of the body) and to shorter survival time. (In some men, the decreases in VEGF and HGF were as high as 30%.)

The men also had a 10.4% decrease in prostate specific antigen (PSA), a prostate-manufactured protein that typically increases during prostate cancer.

Additionally, there was a significant decrease in *insulin-like growth factor* (IGF) and *IGF binding protein-3* (IGFBP-3)—two compounds that speed the growth of cancer cells and shield them from dying.

The findings were published in *Cancer Prevention Research*.

This study supported the findings of an earlier, year-long Italian study, which showed that taking an EGCG supplement reduced the risk of prostate cancer in men with *high-grade prostatic intraepithelial neoplasia* (HGPIN), abnormal cellular changes that turn into prostate cancer 30% of the time. Only one man in the EGCG group developed prostate cancer, compared with nine in the group not taking EGCG.

"There is reasonably good evidence that many cancers are preventable, and our study using a plant-derived substance supports the idea that plant compounds found in a healthy diet can play a role in preventing cancer development and cancer progression," says Jim Cardelli, PhD, the study leader. "Green tea may be a good addition to traditional therapies for prostate cancer, such as chemotherapy or radiation."

Standout scientific evidence: In other recent research on green tea and cancer—scientists in Japan found that people drinking five or more cups of green tea a day were 42% less likely to develop leukemia and other blood cancers, compared with people drinking less than one cup a day…and researchers at the University of Texas MD Anderson Cancer Center found that people with pre-cancerous signs of oral cancer who took green tea extract were 22% less likely to develop oral cancer, compared with people who didn't take the extract.

The Best Green Tea

To guarantee a sufficient intake of EGCG at the level that has been found beneficial to prevent or slow prostate cancer, try one or more of the following strategies, says Patrick M. Fratellone, MD, executive medical director of Fratellone Medical Associates in New York City and an attending physician at St. Luke's Hospital, Roosevelt Hospital and Beth Israel Hospital in New York City.

● **Drink green tea.** The amount of EGCG in the supplement given to the men was the equivalent of drinking 12 cups of green tea a day. A preventive level may be four to six cups.

Best: For maximum intake of EGCG, try whole-leaf loose tea rather than a teabag, using 1 teaspoon per cup, says Dr. Fratellone.

Steep the tea for 5 to 10 minutes before drinking, and do not reuse.

● **Take a supplement of green tea extract.** For prevention, 400 mg a day of a supplement standardized to 90% EGCG. For cancer support, 800 mg a day.

Add one or more drops of green tea liquid extract to green tea or another beverage. As with the supplement, look for a product that is standardized to a high level of EGCG.

Example: HerbaGreen from Herbasway, at 90% polyphenols, 50% from EGCG.

Caution: If you have prostate cancer, take an EGCG supplement only with the approval and supervision of your oncologist, says Dr. Fratellone.

And, he adds, there are several precautions for anyone drinking large amounts of green tea or taking a green tea extract. Talk to your doctor if...you take an antiplatelet drug (blood thinner) such as *warfarin* (Coumadin) because green tea also thins the blood...you use a bronchodilator for asthma or chronic obstructive pulmonary disease because green tea can increase its potency...or

you take an antacid because green tea can decrease the effect.

Jim Cardelli, PhD, professor of microbiology and immunology, LSU Health Sciences Center, Shreveport.

Patrick M. Fratellone, MD, executive medical director of Fratellone Medical Associates in New York City. *www.fratel lonemedical.com.*

Pomegranate Juice— Potent Prostate Protection

P is for pomegranate juice and its potential to fight prostate cancer. Researchers from the University of California at Los Angeles tracked *prostate-specific antigen* (PSA) levels in men who had undergone prostate cancer treatment, and found that those who drank a daily eight ounces of POM Wonderful (a widely available brand) had significantly slower cancer progression.

According to Christopher Amling, MD, a spokesman for the American Urological Association, this study followed 48 men whose cancer had been treated with either surgery or radiation, monitoring the success of the treatment by tracking degree of change in PSA (known as *PSA doubling time*). The pomegranate juice group fared far better than those who didn't drink it, regardless of whether their initial treatment was radiation or surgery. In fact, in about one-third of men, PSA levels not only didn't rise as fast, but actually decreased.

Dr. Amling says that researchers believe that the polyphenol antioxidants in pomegranate juice may slow cancer growth, noting that they have not isolated the specific active ingredients responsible. Since the juice contains dozens of plant-based chemicals, the combination may have a synergistic effect that could be more potent than any individual nutrient on its own.

Does this mean that pomegranate juice can prevent prostate cancer? That's a claim no responsible researcher is willing to make. But it certainly seems to offer some protection for those with the disease. "Pomegranate juice looks promising as a nontoxic strategy for slowing the progression of prostate cancer, but its true benefit will be unknown until phase III trials are complete," Dr. Amling said.

Christopher Amling, MD, spokesman for the American Urological Association.

The Perfect Anticancer Drug

Vitamin D knows how to handle cancer. It can stop *differentiation*—new cells becoming cancer cells. It can promote *apoptosis*—the death of cancer cells. It can prevent *metastasis*—the spread of cancer cells. And vitamin D can block *angiogenesis*—cancer cells developing a new blood supply.

"In short, vitamin D seems like the perfect anticancer drug," says John Cannell, MD, executive director of the Vitamin D Council (*www.vitaminDcouncil.org*).

And that's exactly what new studies are showing...

Newest Research

• **Doubling survival rates in colon cancer.** Researchers at the Dana-Farber Cancer Institute in Boston analyzed nearly two decades of data on blood levels of vitamin D in women newly diagnosed with colon cancer. They found the women with the highest blood levels of vitamin D at diagnosis had 50% less risk of dying from the disease, compared with women with the lowest levels.

• **Reducing the risk of breast cancer.** Swedish researchers studied more than 2,500 women and found that those with the highest blood levels of vitamin D were 48% less likely to develop breast cancer. "Low blood levels of vitamin D have been linked to higher risk for many different cancers, including breast, colon and prostate," says Keith Block, MD, medical director of the Block Center for Integrative Cancer Treatment in Chicago, director of Integrative Medical Education at

the University of Illinois College of Medicine and author of *Life Over Cancer* (Bantam).

• **Reducing risk of non-Hodgkin lymphoma.** Doctors at the Cancer Research Center of Hawaii studied more than 215,000 people, and found that African-American women with the highest dietary intake of vitamin D were 50% less likely to develop this type of cancer.

• **Slowing prostate cancer.** Sunlight triggers the formation of vitamin D in the skin—and English researchers found that men with prostate cancer who spent the most time outdoors had a 51% lower risk of developing an advanced form of the disease.

• **Reducing the risk of esophageal cancer and oral cancer.** A study in *Annals of Oncology* found that people with the highest dietary intake of vitamin D had 42% less risk for developing esophageal cancer and 24% less risk for developing oral cancer, compared with those with the lowest intake. Heavy smokers with the lowest intake of vitamin D had eight times the risk for oral cancer and 10 times the risk of esophageal cancer, compared with heavy smokers with the highest intake.

• **Slowing the spread of melanoma.** Researchers in Germany found that cancer spread more slowly in melanoma patients with the highest blood levels of vitamin D. The findings were in *Anticancer Research*.

• **Reducing the risk of endometrial cancer.** Researchers in Sweden studied nearly 30,000 women and found that those who used vitamin D–producing tanning beds three or more times a year were 40% less likely to develop endometrial cancer.

• **Preventing the painful side effect of a common cancer drug.** Joint pain is a common side effect from aromatase inhibitors such as *letrozole* (Femara), which block the production of the hormone estrogen. High levels of estrogen increase the risk for recurrence in many women with breast cancer. Doctors at the University of Kansas Medical Center studied 60 breast cancer survivors about to take letrozole, measuring their vitamin D levels. Sixty-three percent of the women were deficient—and all of them received vitamin D supplements (50,000 IU a week). After four months on the drug and the supplement, women with the highest blood levels of vitamin D were more likely to be free of joint pain than women with the lowest.

Boost Your Blood Level

"Vitamin D is clearly linked with preventing cancer and combating an existing cancer," says Dr. Block. However, as studies show, many people with and without cancer are deficient in the nutrient—including 50% of seniors and an estimated 70% of cancer patients. To combat this widespread deficiency, he recommends that everyone actively boost their levels. *His approach…*

•**Get tested regularly for vitamin D levels.** To understand the vitamin D test, you need to know a bit more about this unique nutrient, says Dr. Block.

Technically, vitamin D isn't a vitamin—it's a hormone.

When sunlight strikes the skin, the body makes *cholecalciferol* (the naturally occurring form of vitamin D)…which the liver turns into *calcidiol* (25-hydroxyvitamin D)…which the kidneys turn into *calcitriol* (1,25-dihydroxyvitamin D), a hormone.

The test for vitamin D measures 25-hydroxyvitamin D in nanograms per milliliter (ng/mL) or nanomoles per liter (nmol/l) of blood. (To convert nmol/l to ng/ml—the more common measurement—multiply by 2.5.)

The medical community is slowly acknowledging that blood levels once considered normal may be too low to ensure optimal health and healing.

Dr. Block recommends a "bare minimum" of 50 ng/mL. He says the optimum is between 60 and 90. And at his clinic, he "repletes" deficient cancer patients so that their levels are between 80 and 90.

He recommends healthy people receive two vitamins D tests a year, and cancer patients receive four tests a year. *After you've received the results, the next step is to…*

•**Supplement with vitamin D.** There are many individual factors that determine how much vitamin D to take, says Dr. Block. They include age (seniors are less able to make and use vitamin D)…where you live (people in northern climes make less during the winter)…skin color (darker-skinned people make less)…and genetic irregularities that can block the ability to make or use vitamin D (tests are being developed to detect these).

Work with your primary care physician or oncologist to determine the right level of vitamin D supplementation for you.

However, as a general recommendation, Dr. Block advises taking a minimum of 2,000 IU a day of vitamin D-3, the natural and more usable form of the compound.

•**Spend some time in the sun.** If you live above the 35th parallel north (bisecting California, and paralleling the northern borders of Arizona, New Mexico, Texas, Oklahoma, Arkansas, Mississippi, Tennessee and North Carolina), you're unlikely to make enough vitamin D during the winter to keep levels normal, says Dr. Block.

The best strategy for optimizing levels for those above the 35th parallel—during the late spring, summer and early fall, sunbathe 10 to 15 minutes without sunscreen, three to four times a week, with a minimum of clothing. "This is safe and sensible sun exposure," says Dr. Block.

John Cannell, MD, executive director of the Vitamin D Council. *www.vitaminDcouncil.org.*

Keith Block, MD, medical director of the Block Center for Integrative Cancer Treatment in Chicago, director of Integrative Medical Education at the University of Illinois College of Medicine and author of *Life Over Cancer* (Bantam). *www. blockmd.com.*

Chapter 5

DEPRESSION & OTHER EMOTIONAL OBSTACLES

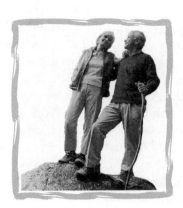

What Really Cures Depression

One in four Americans—more than 70 million people—will become clinically depressed at some point in their lives. That is, their everyday experience will match the official criteria for major depression in the *Diagnostic and Statistical Manual of Mental Disorders, Fourth Edition* (DSM-IV), published by the American Psychiatric Association—they'll have at least five of the following nine symptoms (and definitely have either symptom number 1 or 2), nearly every day for two weeks or more...

1. Persistent sadness, anxiety or "empty" mood

2. Loss of interest or pleasure in all (or nearly all) activities

3. A large increase or decrease in appetite/weight

4. Insomnia or hypersomnia (greatly increased sleep)

5. Slowing of physical movements, or severe agitation

6. Intense fatigue

7. Excessive feelings of guilt or worthlessness

8. Difficulty concentrating or making decisions

9. Frequent thoughts of death or committing suicide.

Depending on the intensity of those symptoms, major depression is labeled *mild, moderate* or *severe*.

Severe depression debilitates your life—you can hardly sit up in bed, let alone get out of it. In mild and moderate depression, you have a lot of psychological pain, but you're able to function. Four out of five people with depression have the mild to moderate variety.

But whether their depression is mild, moderate or severe, just about everybody who is diagnosed with the condition receives a prescription for an antidepressant drug, with

150 million antidepressant prescriptions written in the US each year.

There's only one problem with those antidepressants.

For the majority of people, they don't work.

That's the conclusion of a recent study in the *Journal of the American Medical Association*, which showed that antidepressants provide little or no benefit for people with mild or moderate depression...

Negligible Effects

Researchers at the University of Pennsylvania analyzed data from six studies involving more than 700 depressed people. Antidepressants were anticlimactic.

"True drug effects—an advantage of antidepressant medications over placebo—were nonexistent to negligible among depressed patients with mild, moderate or even severe baseline symptoms, whereas they were large for patients with very severe symptoms," says Jay C. Fournier, the study leader.

But, says Fournier and his colleagues, the majority of depressed patients don't have the severe symptoms for which antidepressants actually work.

He also noted that most of the previous studies that have "proved" antidepressants work involved *only* patients with severe depression—a fact that doctors and patients frequently overlook. (And drug companies never mention.)

Lifestyle Changes

"What this and other studies show is that the majority of people on antidepressants—the four out of five depressed people with mild or moderate depression—are essentially taking an expensive placebo with nasty side effects, such as weight gain and lowered libido" says Stephen Ilardi, PhD, associate professor of clinical psychology at the University of Kansas, and author of *The Depression Cure: The 6-Step Program to Beat Depression without Drugs* (Da Capo).

"It's unrealistic to think that simply taking a pill is going to provide a viable long-term solution to a major form of mental illness," Dr. Ilardi adds.

What *can* provide a long-term solution? *Lifestyle changes*, says Dr. Ilardi. In fact, he thinks that the epidemic of depression—with rates 10 times higher than they were two generations ago—may be caused by modern lifestyle, just like the epidemics of heart disease, type 2 diabetes and obesity. Some of the same lifestyle factors that cause those diseases are also toxic to the brain, causing depression.

Those toxic lifestyle factors include a diet low in brain-nourishing omega-3 fatty acids...a lack of exposure to sunlight...a society where personal relationships are frayed and isolation is the norm...too little sleep...and a psychological attitude that values mental rumination over action.

"There is an enormous body of scientific evidence showing that changing one or more of these lifestyle factors can change the brain in positive ways that help relieve depression," says Dr. Ilardi.

Dr. Ilardi calls his practical approach for changing those lifestyle factors Therapeutic Lifestyle Change, or TLC. In a study he conducted on depressed people who had failed to get well on antidepressant medications, 75% improved on the TLC program.

Here are some of Dr. Ilardi's lifestyle recommendations—for preventing depression, reversing depression or preventing a relapse. (He also recommends that you get your doctor's okay before beginning the regimen.)

● **Nourish your brain.** The brain is 60% fat—and omega-3 fatty acids, found mainly in fish, wild game, nuts, seeds and leafy vegetables—are critical building blocks for brain structure and function, says Dr. Ilardi. Our hunter-gatherer ancestors ate five to ten times more omega-3 fat than we do—and the lack of omega-3s in our diet puts us at increased risk for depression.

Recommended: A daily fish oil supplement containing high doses of two omega-3 fatty acids—1,000 mg of EPA (*eicosapentaenoic acid*) and 500 mg of DHA (*docosahexaenoic acid*).

Product: An economical supplement is Mega EFA from Neutraceutical Sciences Institute, available online at *www.vitacost.com.*

● **Don't think, do.** "Depression is closely linked to a toxic thought process psychologists call *rumination*—the habit of dwelling on negative thoughts, turning them over and over in your mind," says Dr. Ilardi. "Unfortunately, many depressed people spend literally hours ruminating every day."

Recommended: "You can only put an end to ruminating when you're caught up in something else—something absorbing," says Dr. Ilardi. "In most cases, it just takes a few minutes of immersion in a good alternative activity before the spell is broken."

Some ideas for alternative activities—engage in conversation...pursue shared activities, such as volunteering...listen to music... listen to books on CD...watch DVDs.

"Brainstorm and make your own list," says Dr. Ilardi. It could include gardening...playing an instrument...cooking...shopping...playing with a dog.

● **Exercise.** "Modern life is notoriously sedentary, and most Americans are woefully out of shape," says Dr. Ilardi. "This is unfortunate, because exercise is a remarkably potent antidepressant." There are more than 100 studies showing the antidepressant effects of exercise, he noted. In one, exercise (30 minutes of brisk walking, three times a week) was just as effective in relieving depression as the antidepressant Zoloft—and those taking Zoloft rather than exercising were three times more likely to become depressed again.

Recommended: "Walking is an ideal antidepressant exercise—our bodies are designed to do it, and it's something just about everyone can do," says Dr. Ilardi. And it takes only ninety minutes a week to provide an antidepressant effect." Other antidepressant activities include jogging, swimming, cycling, tennis and jumping rope.

● **Savor sunlight.** "Without enough light exposure, the body clock eventually gets out of sync," Dr. Ilardi says. "When that happens, it throws off important circadian rhythms that regulate energy, sleep, appetite and hormone levels. The disruption of these important biological rhythms can, in turn, trigger clinical depression."

Recommended: A half hour of sunlight a day is enough to reset your body clock. Consider a brisk thirty-minute walk outdoors every morning.

You could also talk to your doctor about morning use of a "light box," a device that provides a concentrated dose of 10,000 lux (the same light you would receive walking on a beach about 40 minutes after sunrise). Use it for 30 minutes a day, immediately after waking up.

Resource: The Center for Environmental Therapeutics has an online store that sells a light box that has been used in clinical studies on light therapy for depression—the Day-Light, from Uplift Technologies. Order at *www.cet.org* or call 800-387-0896.

● **Find social support.** "When it comes to depression, relationships matter," says Dr. Ilardi. "People who lack a supportive social network—family, friends, neighbors—face an increased risk of becoming depressed, and of remaining depressed once an episode strikes. Fortunately, we can do a great deal to improve the quality and depth of our connections with others, and this can have a huge payoff in terms of fighting depression and reducing the risk of recurrence."

Recommended: Let your friends know you're depressed, says Dr. Ilardi. "I believe our friends have a right to know what we're going through, especially when we're facing a treacherous enemy like depression. Honest disclosure about our struggle is essential to maintaining—or reestablishing the health of any friendship."

● Spend regular time together with family and friends in shared activity, such as walking, working out, grabbing a meal, playing games, going to a concert, attending a play, watching a film and so on.

● Cultivate friends at a distance through social networks, video chats and in Internet chat rooms and forums…volunteer…attend local worship services…join a social organization or club, such as the Rotary…find a self-help group…join a sports league.

● **Deepen sleep.** "Sleep and mood are intimately connected," says Dr. Ilardi. "Disrupted sleep is one of the most potent triggers of depression, and there's evidence that most episodes of mood disorder are preceded by at least several weeks of subpar slumber."

Recommended: There are several habits of healthy sleep, says Dr. Ilardi. *You should…*

● Use the bed only for sleeping.

● If possible, keep the same bedtime every night.

● Get up at the same time every day.

● Avoid napping.

● Avoid bright light at night.

● Avoid caffeine and other stimulants after 12:00 p.m. (Caffeine persists in the body—if you drink a strong cup of coffee with 200 mg of caffeine at noon, you'll still have 25 mg of caffeine in your body at midnight.)

● Turn down your thermostat at night. A mild drop in temperature helps increase sleep drive.

● Avoid taking your problems to bed with you. Instead, find a task that is both engrossing and relaxing, such as inhaling and exhaling slowly and deeply from your diaphragm, the large muscle that sits right below the lungs.

● Don't try to fall asleep. The harder you try, the more elusive it becomes.

Jay C. Fournier, MA, Department of Psychology, University of Pennsylvania.

Stephen Ilardi, PhD, associate professor of clinical psychology at the University of Kansas and author of *The Depression Cure: The 6-Step Program to Beat Depression without Drugs* (Da Capo). *www.thedepressioncurebook.com.*

To Achieve Long-Term Happiness, Challenge Yourself

You might think that the secret to everyday and long-term happiness is avoiding emotional, mental and physical stress as much as possible.

Surprising: A new study shows that the momentary stress and lack of pleasure from mastering any challenging activity—such as learning to play a new instrument or speak a new language—can lead to more daily and long-term happiness.

Competence Creates Happiness

For two days, 132 study participants kept a log, reporting how they spent each hour, the enjoyment and stress experienced during that hour, and their level of enjoyment at the end of the day.

When the participants did something difficult that led to an increase in their competence—such as learning to play tennis, learning to play the guitar, mastering advanced math or becoming skilled at using a new software program—they reported less enjoyment and more stress and less happiness in the moment.

But they reported more happiness at the end of the day!

Set Goals and Persist

"'No pain, no gain' is the rule when it comes to increasing happiness from increasing our competence at something," says Ryan Howell, PhD, the study leader and assistant professor of psychology at San Francisco State University.

"People often give up their goals because it's stressful to achieve. But we found there is benefit at the end of the day from undergoing the stress of learning to do something well.

"And what was particularly striking is that you don't even have to reach your goal to see the daily benefits to your happiness and well-being—you just have to make progress toward your goal."

His recommendations…

● **Understand that real happiness requires some unhappiness.** "People are often surprised to learn their pursuit of happiness isn't always enjoyable," says Dr. Howell. "But understanding that stress and a lack of pleasure are key to competence, and that competence is a key to happiness, can help us persist in mastering activities that give us true and lasting satisfaction."

● **Understand that momentary pleasure doesn't guarantee long-term happiness.** "People tend to think they're going to derive a huge amount of joy from a snippet of pleasure—the kind of pleasurable life portrayed in TV commercials, when someone seems ecstatically happy as they eat a taco or drink a beer," says Dr. Howell. "But that kind of pleasure isn't permanent. A life of flourishing happiness is based on meaning-driven activities with significant goals—and they take hard work."

● **Persist.** "Set your goals and keep at them, even when you feel like stopping—you'll be glad you did!"

Ryan Howell, PhD, assistant professor of psychology at San Francisco State University. *www.bss.sfsu.edu/rhowell/.*

Which Psychotherapy Is Right for You?

Research has shown that emotional problems can be just as disabling—and deadly—as physical illnesses. Depression, for example, can worsen a variety of serious health ailments such as heart disease, diabetes, arthritis and asthma.

Latest development: A US law was recently passed that requires health insurers to provide equal coverage for the treatment of physical and emotional problems beginning in 2010. This change will allow more people to afford psychotherapy.

How Psychotherapy Works

Psychotherapy involves communication between a therapist and the person seeking help, usually in a series of weekly individual sessions ($75 to $200 each, depending on the part of the country where you live) that typically last 45 to 50 minutes each.

Important: You are most likely to get good results from psychotherapy if you work with a competent therapist who makes you feel understood and accepted. A recommendation from a physician, trusted friend, relative or member of the clergy is often helpful.

In many states, anyone can call himself/herself a therapist, but only licensed practitioners are sure to have appropriate training and qualifications. Clinical psychologists (who hold an advanced degree, such as a doctor of philosophy, PhD, in psychology or a doctor of psychology, PsyD)…social workers (who hold a master's degree in social work with an emphasis in clinical approaches)…and psychiatrists (medical doctors who can prescribe medication)—among many other practitioners—all can be licensed to practice psychotherapy.

To verify that a therapist is licensed by the professional body that governs his specialty, contact your state's health department.

Most therapists specialize in a particular type of therapy or a combination of therapies.

Best types of therapy include…

Cognitive Behavioral Therapy (CBT)

Main premise: Psychological problems are tied to irrational beliefs and thoughts—for example, a depressed person thinking that everything in his life is bad. When the irrational beliefs are replaced with more realistic ones, symptoms typically improve.

What it's good for: Depression, anxiety, obsessive-compulsive disorder, eating disorders and post-traumatic stress disorder.

Typical duration: Six to 20 sessions.

Psychodynamic Therapy

Main premise: Difficulties in the present are rooted in feelings and actions from your earlier life.

What it's good for: Difficulty forming or maintaining relationships and interpersonal conflict at work or with friends or family members.

Typical duration: Because patterns that are identified in psychodynamic therapy can be subtle and elusive, it may last for six months to two years or more.

Interpersonal Therapy (IPT)

Main premise: Psychological problems result from difficulties in connecting and communicating with other people.

What it's good for: A person who lacks satisfying relationships or is adjusting to life changes (divorce or job loss, for example).

Typical duration: IPT generally adheres to a timetable, such as 12 to 16 weekly sessions, established at the onset of therapy.

Therapy Settings

Even though most psychotherapy occurs in individual sessions with the patient and a therapist, there are other settings in which the therapies described earlier may be used alone or in combination.

Among the most common…

• **Group therapy.** A group of five to 10 people meet and give one another feedback—most often, in the presence of a therapist.

What it's good for: A specific problem that participants share—such as anger, a phobia, panic attacks, social anxiety or grief.

Typical duration: Groups that focus on problems that are shared by its members (such as those described above) are likely to be limited to 12 to 20 sessions. Other groups, which tackle long-standing issues, such as emotional isolation or excessive dependency, can go on indefinitely. Members may stay for several months or years and then be replaced by new members. Sessions generally last 60 to 90 minutes for both types of groups.

Important: Insurance often does not cover group therapy, which typically costs 50 to 75% of the cost of individual therapy.

• **Family therapy.** This approach is based on the belief that a person's emotional difficulties are related to the way his entire family interacts. Usually, all available family members—the more the better—gather to clarify the roles each plays and the relationships among them.

What it's good for: Any issue in which the resources of an entire family can be tapped to address the problems of a member, including an adult child, a grandparent or a divorced spouse. Family therapy also can help families deal with the serious illness or death of a member.

Typical duration: Twelve to 20 weekly sessions. The cost of family therapy, which is covered by some insurance plans, is determined by the length of the session (typically 90 to 120 minutes each).

• **Couples therapy.** By meeting with both partners at the same time, the therapist can hear each partner's complaints and watch them interact. This allows the therapist to help the couple identify problematic patterns—such as repeated criticism or refusal to change—and make suggestions.

What it's good for: Marital crises (such as infidelity) or frequent fighting, particularly when the same issues come up repeatedly.

Typical duration: Weekly sessions for 20 weeks to a year.

Important: Insurance often does not cover couples therapy. Sessions typically run 60 to 90 minutes with fees set accordingly.

Jonathan Jackson, PhD, clinical professor of psychology at Adelphi University and director of Adelphi's Center for Psychological Services at the Derner Institute of Advanced Psychological Studies, both in Garden City, New York.

Eliminate the Excuses That Hold You Back

When things don't go our way, our subconscious minds offer up excuses. We try to pin our failures and bad habits on factors outside our control—our genes...our upbringing...our busy schedules...our bad luck. We're never really to blame.

Escaping blame might make us feel better for a moment, but soon we start to accept our excuses as truths about who we are, what we are capable of and how the world works. Once this happens, excuses become mental viruses, limiting what we can accomplish.

Seven ways to eliminate excuses...

1. Remove all labels. When we define ourselves with a word or two, we place limits on what we can achieve. Labeling ourselves "fat" gives us an excuse for not losing weight...labeling ourselves "big spenders" gives us an excuse for not saving.

Stop accepting labels that you place on yourself and that are placed on you by others—even if you have lived with these labels your whole life.

Strategy: When a label is placed on you—by yourself or someone else—repeat the affirmation "I am capable of accomplishing anything I place my attention upon."

Example: My daughter labeled herself "unathletic" when she was a child and used this as an excuse to avoid physical activities. Years later, she made a conscious decision to remove this label and now enjoys exercise.

2. Converse with your subconscious mind. Excuses such as "That's just the way I am" or "That's how I was raised" are rooted in the assumption that we cannot alter subconscious behaviors. But we can change subconscious behaviors—if we become more conscious of them.

Strategy: Treat the part of you that encourages the behavior that you would like to change as if it were a separate entity. Imagine that it has a physical form. Have conversations with it. Explain to it that you know

it's accustomed to being in control, but now you have taken charge.

Example: When the little creature inside me that loves sugar encourages me to drink soda or eat dessert, I tell it that I'm now in charge and that I've decided to reduce my sugar intake.

3. Practice mindfulness. I used to think I had a poor memory. I would forget everything from my appointments to where I left my car keys. Forgetfulness really was just an excuse I used to justify my not keeping track of my schedule and my possessions.

Strategy: Keep your conscious mind focused on where you are and what you're doing at this moment, and your forgetfulness will disappear.

Example: When I enter my house, I remind myself to notice my car keys in my hand. I feel the keys' shape in my palm and listen to the jingling sound they make. I pay attention as I place the keys in the spot that I have selected for them.

4. Commit to overcoming inertia. Our excuses tell us that it's okay if we fail to achieve what we set out to do today. We'll do it tomorrow...maybe. Our excuses tell us it's okay to stay with what's safe. Trying something different could be difficult and risky. Left unchecked, these excuses will prevent us from ever reaching our goals.

Strategy: Have conversations with yourself about the person you intend to become and what you're willing to do to bring this about. Next, write out a contract with yourself summarizing what you've agreed to do and the schedule on which you've agreed to do it. Review this contract every day.

Example: Before I start writing a book, I write a contract with myself detailing how much work I'm going to do each day and when I'm going to do it. The written agreement helps me recollect that I am in the process of redefining myself.

5. Harness the power of affirmations. What we think helps shape what we become. When we think in excuses, we believe our

excuses and stop believing that we can succeed. Use your thoughts to shape your life in
more useful ways instead.

Strategy: When you catch yourself making an excuse, replace it with an affirmation—a positive statement about what you
are...what is available to you...or what you
will become.

Affirmations include *Whatever I need is already here, and it is all for my highest good*
and *I deserve health, happiness and success.*

Example: If you want more love in your
life, cut yourself off when you start to think
of excuses such as *I'm not attractive enough
to find a partner* and replace them with affirmations such as *I deserve to find love.*

6. Live in a supportive universe. If you
see the world as an unfriendly place, you will
have a handy excuse for any failure—something always will seem to stand in your way.
Instead, view the universe as helpful.

Strategy: Remind yourself frequently that
the universe is trying to help you achieve
your goals. Soon people and events will stop
conspiring against you and start conspiring
to assist you.

Example: In an unfriendly universe, if
your car breaks down, the 100 drivers who
don't stop to help are proof that the world
is out to get you. If your car breaks down
in a supportive universe, the 101st driver
who does stop is evidence that the universe
is on your side. This attitude will keep you
in a state of contentment and peace instead
of anxiety. It also enables you to attract the
right people into your life.

7. Don't complain, and don't explain.
Complaints and explanations are key allies of
excuse makers. When we complain, we place
blame on someone or something else for our
problems. When we explain ourselves, we
often get drawn into arguments about our
actions and beliefs, then use excuses to defend our positions.

Strategy: Explain your decisions only
when they directly affect other people. Decisions about your own life are not anyone

else's business. They need to be explained
only to yourself.

Example: Some of my goals sound
strange to others. In the past, I often found
myself making excuses when I tried to explain them—and those excuses affected how
I viewed the goals. Now I share my goals
with only a few people whom I trust deeply.

Wayne Dyer, PhD, an internationally renowned author and speaker in the field of self-development. *www.
drwaynedyer.com.*

The Downside of Positive Thinking

I am a loveable person...
I will succeed...
I say yes to life!
I'm good at this...
I am at peace...

Those phrases are affirmations—positive
statements about yourself and your inten-
tions that you repeatedly think, say or write,
to polish your self-image and propel you into
effective action.

You can find positive affirmations on blogs,
Web sites and billboards...in greeting cards,
self-help books and magazines. They play repeatedly on the soundtracks of self-help CDs.

"The belief that we should think 'posi-
tively' permeates our culture," says Joanne V.
Wood, PhD, a professor of psychology at the
University of Waterloo in Canada.

There's only one problem with that belief—a new study shows that if you're already
feeling bad about yourself, affirmations can
make you feel a whole lot worse.

Affirmations Can Backfire

In the study, a team of researchers led by Dr.
Wood asked a group of people to fill out a
questionnaire that rated self-esteem. Those
with the lowest and highest self-esteem were
then asked to participate in the next phase of
the study, during which they were assigned
one of two tasks.

1. Repeat the statement "I'm a loveable person" for four minutes (positive self-statement).

2. Write down thoughts and feelings for four minutes.

After the participants completed the task, the researchers took another measure of their self-esteem. And it hadn't necessarily changed for the better.

"People with low self-esteem felt worse about themselves after repeating the positive self-statement, compared with those with low self-esteem who wrote down their thoughts and feelings," says Dr. Wood. "In contrast, people with high self-esteem did feel better after repeating the positive self-statement—but only a little bit better than those with high self-esteem who wrote down their thoughts and feelings.

"In other words, for people with low self-esteem, repeating an affirmation backfired—it made them feel worse immediately afterward, rather than better."

What happens: "If you have low self-esteem and you affirm that you're actually feeling good about yourself, you're going to stimulate the opposite thought," says psychologist Kirk Strosahl, PhD, cofounder of acceptance and commitment therapy (ACT), and author of *The Mindfulness and Acceptance Workbook for Depression* (New Harbinger). "That's a demonstration of how thinking actually works—when you try to affirm one side, you automatically activate the other side. Substituting the positive for the negative amplifies the negative."

Avoid the Outlandish

"Since conducting the study, which was reported widely in the media, I've heard from many people around the world who have tried positive self-statements that haven't worked for them," says Dr. Wood.

"For example, a nurse in the Netherlands wrote me, 'I've read a lot of books about positive thinking. Every time I tried hard to practice the theories, but I felt much more anxiety and insecurity. I've felt very bad about myself. What did I do wrong?'"

Is there any way to do affirmations right? *Yes, says Dr. Wood...*

● **Be specific and moderate.** Dr. Wood believes that a positive self-statement might be useful if it is specific rather than overly general, and moderate rather than extreme.

"Repeating a statement that doesn't contradict one's self-view could help," she says. "Rather than a sweeping phrase such as 'I am a loveable person,' remind yourself of a specific attribute that you are confident about, such as 'I am a good listener.' My research indicates such specific self-statements can boost mood.

"However, avoid overly general and outlandish phrases, such as 'I accept all aspects of myself completely.'"

Kirk Strosahl, PhD, cofounder of acceptance and commitment therapy (ACT) and author of *The Mindfulness and Acceptance Workbook for Depression* (New Harbinger).

Joanne V. Wood, PhD, professor of psychology at the University of Waterloo, Canada.

Feeling Down? Sit Up!

Want to feel more confident and sure of yourself? It could be as easy as sitting up a little straighter in your chair.

New research shows that improving your sitting posture can also improve your self-confidence...instantly!

Posture Affects Confidence

Researchers in the Psychology Department at Ohio State University studied 71 students, telling them (falsely, for the sake of the study) that they were participating in two studies—one from the Art School, on factors that contribute to a person's acting ability; and one from the Business School, on factors that contribute to professional job performance and satisfaction.

Each student was seated at a computer terminal and instructed to either "sit up straight and push out your chest" or "sit slouched forward with your face looking at your knees."

Then they were told to write down either three positive or three negative traits about themselves that they thought would relate to professional job performance.

Lastly, they took a survey, rating themselves on how well they would perform as a future professional employee.

"The results were striking," says Richard Petty, PhD, professor of psychology at Ohio State University and a study author.

"Students who wrote positive thoughts about themselves rated themselves more highly when in the upright rather than the slouched posture—because the upright posture gave them more confidence in their positive thoughts," says Dr. Petty.

"Most of us were taught that sitting up straight gives a good impression to other people," he added. "But it turns out that posture can also affect how you think about yourself. If you sit up straight, you convince yourself of the rightness of your own thinking. And sitting up straight is something you can train yourself to do."

Head Up, Chin Level, Chest Open

That's also the opinion of Michele Benza, a Pilates teacher and founder of Michele Benza Image Consulting and Posture, in San Francisco.

"If you have bad posture—if you carry your head down and your shoulders forward—you communicate a lack of self-confidence to yourself and to others," she says. "But if your entire body is erect—if your head is up, your chin parallel to the floor, your chest open and your shoulders back and relaxed—you're telling yourself and the world that you are enthusiastic about who you are and what you are doing."

Here are some of the recommendations for a better sitting posture that Benza gives to all her image consultant clients on their first visit. "Practice them on a regular basis and they will become easy," she says.

● **Good sitting posture.** Sit directly on your "sitz bones" (*ischial tuberosities*)—the pressure points you feel at the junction of your thigh and butt when you sit on a hard,

flat surface. Don't scoot forward and slouch backward, so that you're practically sitting on your upper butt or lower back.

● Keep your head straight forward, with your ears in line with your shoulders, and your shoulders square with your hips.

● Keep your chin parallel to the floor.

● Keep your shoulders back and relaxed.

● Keep your chest open.

● Over all, elongate—your neck, your chest and your waist. "Grow taller," says Benza. "Imagine a string pulling you up from the crown of the head toward the ceiling and the sky."

Michele Benza, Pilates teacher and founder of Michele Benza Image Consulting and Posture, San Francisco. *www.michelebenza.com.*

Richard Petty, PhD, professor of psychology, Ohio State University, Columbus.

The Healing Power Of Writing

Grief involves a complex mix of emotions. Along with sadness and loneliness come strange sensations of unreality and frightening feelings of helplessness. You may be angry at the unfairness of the situation or relieved that the loved one's suffering is over—then feel guilty for having such thoughts. When even sweet memories bring pain, the quagmire of conflicting feelings can keep you stuck in despair, unable to understand or resolve your emotions.

For many people, writing provides a means to identify these wrenching emotions, to grow personally and to find a new path to acceptance and peace. Grief expert Fran Dorf conducts Write to Heal workshops nationwide to help people cope with loss. *Her insights...*

Fran's Story

After my son Michael died, I, a professional writer, couldn't bring myself to write a word.

People told me, "Maybe it would help to write." But writing seemed illogical. How do you write a scream? What words convey weeping, rage, terror, paralysis, self-recrimination, failure, the physical pain of grief?

One day, two years after my son's death, I bought a composition notebook. I stared at that first blank page. Then, over and over again, I wrote the same two words—"Help me."

A few days later, I picked up the notebook again. This time I wrote, "Grief is a faucet that I can't turn off." I kept writing, "Grief is..." and filling in different metaphors. Soon, I was writing all the time again.

It took three years, but what grew out of that journal was my novel, *Saving Elijah*. Looking back, I realize that I used my writing to rebuild the structure of my life—not only to restart my career, but to reconnect with the world.

The Power of the Pen

Through writing, the human soul can reveal itself and find expression. But grief journaling isn't necessarily shared with family and friends or mailed to a publisher. Rather, it is a kind of self-therapy that helps you identify, integrate and ultimately even transform your most frightening and difficult feelings.

Vital: Do not worry about your grammar or spelling...do not censor, edit or appraise yourself...do not fret if you've never considered yourself a good writer...do not imagine what others would think if they read your words. This frees you to really feel the feelings—and that is what's important when you write to heal.

You need only a pen and a notebook. These work better than a computer because you can carry your journal everywhere and write whenever the urge strikes. *Exercises to get started...*

● **Begin with, "I remember..."** Write this at the top of the first page of your journal, then list a simple one-sentence memory of your loved one.

Example: "I remember when my husband and I went sailing in Florida." Then write "I

remember" again, this time choosing a different memory. Continue this way for 10 minutes, allowing your mind to wander to all corners—to bad memories as well as good ones—without passing judgment on the memory's meaning or relative importance. Try to identify the various feelings these recollections conjure up. Putting a name to an emotion is the first step in coming to terms with it.

● **Flesh out the details.** Choose one memory from your list and elaborate on it. What was the weather like? What were you wearing? What did you do, see, smell, hear, think and feel? Give the story a beginning, a middle and an end.

Next: Retell the story in the third person, as if it happened to someone else and you were merely observing. Creating a narrative helps you gain distance from and begin to cope with the raw emotion of difficult memories.

● **Try a written meditation.** Take a half-dozen objects connected with the person you've lost and lay them on a table. Contemplate them for a while, and then meditate on one that "speaks" to you. Divide a page of your journal into four squares. In one square, describe the object...in another, write how the object makes you feel...in the third square, write what the object reminds you of...and in the last square, speak in the voice of the object. This can help you separate thoughts from feelings...and uncover hidden emotions, such as rage or fear.

● **Compose a dialogue with God.** Imagine a scene in which you meet God (or whatever name you use for a supreme being or higher power). Give the details of the setting and describe what your supreme being looks like—not necessarily in flowing robes, but in a form meaningful to you and your life. You ask, "Why me?"...and God answers, "Why not you?" What do you say next, and what reply do you receive?

Another option: Write a letter to the person you lost...or write a letter that you think your loved one might write to you, as if from the afterlife. Let yourself express the anguish, anger or guilt you are harboring. Then open your mind and heart to whatever philosophical insights may be revealed to you.

Going through grief is rather like writing a novel. No two people do it exactly the same way...there is no straight progression that carries you through from start to conclusion...and you cannot tell in advance just what the journey will bring. But journaling can help you do the hard work—so that you wind up in a place of hope, strength and renewal.

Fran Dorf, therapist, poet, essayist and author of the novels *Saving Elijah* (Putnam) and *Flight* (Vivisphere). Find more exercises and/or subscribe to her blog, Bruised Muse, at *www.frandorf.com*.

How to Calm an Angry Person

When someone is angry, our instinctive reaction typically is to get defensive (if the person is angry at us) or to give advice (if he/she is angry at someone else). These responses are not useful—they do not resolve the situation and even may inflame the angry person further.

More effective...

When You Are Not the Target

The best way to calm someone who is angry at someone else is to let him vent. Don't interrupt or tell him why he shouldn't be angry or that he should let it go. Don't talk about the time you got mad about the same thing—this implies that your reaction is more important than his.

When he has talked himself out, acknowledge his feelings—whether or not you agree with his views.

Example: "Wow, you're really angry with your boss. I can see how upset you are."

After listening and acknowledging, ask if there is any way you can help. In many cases, the other person will say that you have helped just by listening. You also might be able to assist with brainstorming and problem-solving. But if you try to solve the problem before hearing the person out or without his approval, he most likely will feel angrier.

When the Anger Is Directed at You

When someone lashes out at you, the primitive part of your brain is activated. This creates the impulse to defend yourself from attack by telling the other person he is wrong or irrational or by getting angry yourself.

Instead, before responding, pause for a few moments and silently ask yourself four questions...

1. Is this situation important?

2. Is my reaction appropriate?

3. Is the situation modifiable?

4. If so, is taking action worth it?

To remember the four questions when you are under stress, use the partial acronym I AM WORTH IT. **I** stands for Important...**AM** stands for Appropriate and Modifiable... **WORTH IT**, of course, stands for the last question.

If the answer to all four questions is "yes," then assert yourself by telling the person...

- Exactly what he is doing.

- How it makes you feel.

- What, specifically, you would like him to do differently.

Keep your voice fairly quiet and your tone neutral. Describe behavior, not motives or personal characteristics.

Example from Redford Williams, MD: My wife used this technique when I came home in a bad mood at the end of a tough day. Virginia was preparing dinner. On the kitchen counter was a big stack of mail-order catalogs that she had promised to look through a few days earlier. I snapped, "What are these damn catalogs doing here?"

Virginia didn't say a word for about 20 seconds. Then she replied calmly, "Redford, you just walked into the kitchen and said, 'What are these damn catalogs doing here?' (She told me what I had done.) I came home early to make dinner, and now, I am feeling hurt, unappreciated and, frankly, angry at you. (She told me how it made her feel.) Would it be possible for you to come home at the end of the day and not have the first words out of your mouth be something critical?" (What she would like me to do.)

I turned around, walked out of the kitchen, came back in and said, "Mmm, smells good. What's for supper?"

When I first arrived home, Virginia could have fueled an argument by snapping back, "What's the matter with you, coming home and criticizing me?" Instead, during those 20 seconds of silence, she asked herself the four questions. Then she made a specific observation and a request for change.

If you need to respond to an angry outburst in a setting where expressing personal feelings is not appropriate—for example, at work—use a results-oriented word, such as "helpful."

Example: "Bill, you just told me that my marketing idea for the new product is the stupidest thing you ever heard. I need to let you know that calling my suggestion stupid isn't helpful. If you could give me some of the reasons you think it won't work, I'd appreciate it."

If your answer to any of the four I AM WORTH IT questions gets a "no"—focus on controlling your reaction. Don't say anything to the person. Instead, if the situation isn't important or can't be changed, say to yourself, "Hey, it's not that important," or "There's nothing I can do to change this guy." If requesting change isn't appropriate or worth it, you can distract yourself by thinking about something pleasant or doing something else...or by taking a few deep breaths and thinking the word *calm* as you inhale and *down* as you exhale. This is not the same as passively giving in. You are evaluating the situation and making a rational decision.

Redford Williams, MD, director of the Behavioral Medicine Research Center at Duke University Medical Center in Durham, North Carolina and author of numerous books, including *In Control* (Rodale). *www.williamslifeskills.com*.

To Overcome Shyness, Talk to Yourself

You're painfully shy—a condition psychologists call *social anxiety* or *social phobia*.

Maybe you have a hard time starting or maintaining a conversation...or going to a party...or having friends over for dinner...or meeting new people...or expressing a personal opinion...or sending back food in a restaurant. Maybe you're always afraid of making a mistake in public...or speaking in a meeting...or shopping in a busy store.

Maybe you're so shy, you can't even bring yourself to call a therapist to set up an appointment to help you with the problem.

Maybe you don't have to.

A new study shows that using a self-help book to overcome social anxiety can be an effective alternative to professional help...

Therapy Without the Therapist

Researchers at the University of North Carolina at Chapel Hill and the Mayo Clinic studied 21 people with social anxiety, dividing them into two groups.

One group was given a step-by-step self-help workbook to overcome shyness. (They also met with a therapist for 30 minutes every other week or so to review the book's assignments, but they didn't receive therapy during those sessions.)

The other group was "wait-listed." They were told they would receive therapy when a therapist was available.

After two months, the group using the self-help book was in much better psychological shape. They had 30 to 35% less social anxiety...their social anxiety was 33% less severe...they had 13% less general anxiety... and they had 59% less depression.

There was little or no change in any of those parameters in the wait-listed group.

Then, the researchers gave the self-help book to those who had been wait-listed.

Three months later they too had significant psychological improvements—with 34 to 55% less social anxiety...33% less severe social anxiety…19% less general anxiety… and 49% less depression.

The findings were in the *Journal of Behavior Therapy and Experimental Psychiatry*.

"Using the book didn't provide the same type of robust gains that would typically be achieved by seeing a therapist, but it did provide significant improvement," says Jonathan Abramowitz, PhD, the study leader. "The participants weren't getting up and dancing on tables—but they could do more activities than they had been able to do, and they felt more comfortable going out in public."

Important: Dr. Abramowitz points out that the people in the study had mild or moderate social anxiety, rather than severe variety. In mild to moderate social anxiety, you endure social experiences with a lot of discomfort, and you often avoid them. In severe social anxiety, you're not even able to leave your house.

The Book That Changed Their Lives

The book used in the study was *The Shyness & Social Anxiety Workbook: Proven Step-by-Step Techniques for Overcoming Your Fear* (New Harbinger), by Martin Antony, PhD, and Richard Swinson, MD.

The book is based on cognitive-behavioral therapy (CBT) for social anxiety, which studies have repeatedly shown is effective in relieving the problem.

"CBT is a technique that teaches individuals to be more aware of their negative thoughts and to replace them with less negative thoughts," Dr. Antony explained. "People learn to treat their beliefs as guesses about the way things may be, rather than as facts. They are taught to examine the evidence supporting their anxious beliefs, and to consider the possibility that an alternative belief is true." This is the cognitive dimension of CBT.

CBT for social anxiety also involves exposure, he says—gradually and repeatedly confronting feared situations until they no longer trigger fear. This is the behavioral dimension of CBT.

The content of *The Shyness & Social Anxiety Workbook* mirrors the type of treatment you'd receive from a cognitive-behavioral therapist. *The chapters help you…*

- Educate yourself on your condition,
- Conduct a self-assessment (for example, what triggers your social anxiety and the physical ways you respond),
- Choose the best strategies to overcome your social anxiety,
- Make and implement a plan using the chosen strategies,
- Learn effective communication and
- Maintain improvements and plan for the future.

In the study, the participants read and implemented the book at the pace of one or two chapters per week, over eight weeks.

"I recommend reading the entire book fairly quickly and then going back to the beginning and reading more closely," says Dr. Antony. "Next, spend a week or two on each chapter—which will pretty much duplicate the type of process you would experience in therapy."

Bottom line: "Your best option for social anxiety is to seek out a therapist who practices CBT," says Dr. Abramowitz. "But if there's not a therapist available, or you're too anxious to go and talk to someone, using this particular self-help book might help."

"Some people use the book to accompany therapy," Dr. Antony says. "Some use the book for information and then seek out therapy. And some people only use the book, and do all the exercises—and the book changes their lives."

Jonathan Abramowitz, PhD, professor and associate chair of psychology, University of North Carolina.

Martin Antony, PhD, and Richard Swinson, MD, coauthors of *The Shyness & Social Anxiety Workbook: Proven Step-by-Step Techniques for Overcoming Your Fear* (New Harbinger). *www.martinantony.com.*

Calm Down with Chamomile

Gad! That may be the worried exclamation you uttered after being diagnosed with *generalized anxiety disorder* (GAD).

The diagnosis is made when you've been worrying nearly constantly, day after day, month after month, for six months or more… you worry about nearly everything, from big issues to small details…and your worry rides tandem with physical problems, such as headaches and insomnia.

If a primary care physician made the diagnosis of GAD, it's likely he also prescribed an anxiety-reducing drug—either a *benzodiazepine*, such as Xanax, Valium or Ativan; or an antidepressant, such as Paxil, Lexapro or Zoloft. *But those drugs are, well, worrisome…*

Benzodiazepines are potentially addictive—anxiety can increase if you suddenly stop taking the drug after a few weeks, forcing you back on the medication to relieve your intensified woes.

Antidepressants can deliver additional troubles, including weight gain, a stalled sex drive and even suicidal tendencies you didn't have before taking the medication.

"These side effects can lead dissatisfied patients to discontinue treatment," says Jay D. Amsterdam, MD, professor in the Department of Psychiatry at the University of Pennsylvania.

What's worse, the drugs may not even work!

"It's not reasonable to claim that drugs are the most effective treatment for anxiety," says David Burns, MD, author of *When Panic Attacks: The New, Drug-Free Anxiety Therapy That Can Change Your Life* (Broadway). "This claim has been by made by the American Psychiatric Association and has been widely publicized by the pharmaceutical industry. But it's not consistent with the latest research, which raises serious questions about the safety and effectiveness of the benzodiazepines and the antidepressants."

That's why many people with GAD decide not to take medications—and instead use a natural or alternative therapy to self-treat anxiety, says Dr. Amsterdam.

And in a first-of-its kind study, Dr. Amsterdam and his colleagues showed that one of those treatments may work quite well—the classically calming herb, chamomile…

Greater Reduction in Symptoms

The researchers studied 57 people who had been diagnosed with mild to moderate GAD. They divided them evenly into two groups—one group took a daily supplement of chamomile extract; the other group took a placebo.

For the first week of the study, those taking chamomile received a daily capsule of 220 milligrams (mg) of an extract of German chamomile (a specific variety of the herb), standardized to contain 1.2% apigenin (the active ingredient). In the second week, the dose was increased to two, 220 mg capsules. Every week thereafter, the patients were evaluated for anxiety levels, using a test called the Hamilton Anxiety Scale (HAM-A). Those who had only a small weekly reduction in the HAM-A score received an increased dosage—660 mg during week three; 880 mg during week four; and 1,100 mg during weeks five through eight.

At the beginning and end of the study, the participants were given two other tests to measure anxiety and well-being—the Beck Anxiety Inventory (BAI), and the Psychological General Well-Being Index (PGWBI).

Results: After two months, those taking the chamomile had an average 53% reduction in their HAM-A, compared with 35% for the placebo group.

They also had a 42% reduction in BAI, compared with 21% for those taking the placebo.

And the chamomile group had a 28% increase in well-being, compared with 18% for the placebo group.

Altogether, there was a "significant and clinically meaningful" difference between the performance of chamomile and the placebo, says Dr. Amsterdam.

How does chamomile work to reduce anxiety? "It's exact mode of action is unknown," says Dr. Amsterdam. It may work by affecting a stress hormone (*noradrenaline*) and brain chemicals (*dopamine* and *serotonin*) that play a role in anxiety. It also binds to the same cell receptors as benzodiazepines.

But no matter how it works, the study proved chamomile can work—and that doctors should consider recommending it to patients with GAD. "The demonstration of chamomile's efficacy…in patients with milder GAD may provide a wider acceptability of [this anti-anxiety] treatment in the general medical community," concluded Dr. Amsterdam and his colleagues, in the *Journal of Clinical Pharmacology*.

Use High-Quality Chamomile

"Chamomile is an excellent way to reduce anxiety," says Amanda McQuade Crawford, a medical herbalist in Los Angeles and author of *The Natural Menopause Handbook: Herbs, Nutrition & Other Natural Therapies* (Crossing Press). She points out that in Italy—a nation of high-strung espresso drinkers—chamomile is the standard treatment for overwrought nerves. "The whole nation—from mothers with little babies to retirees—relies on the herb for day-to-day anxiety control."

And those mothers and babies have nothing to fear from chamomile. The herb is well known for its safety, posing virtually no risk, Crawford says. (Only one of the study participants taking chamomile discontinued the herb, complaining of stomach upset. One participant also discontinued the placebo, complaining of an allergic reaction.)

For mild to moderate GAD, Crawford recommends starting treatment with chamomile tea—as long as you use high-quality chamomile.

"Look for a tea from whole, dried flowers rather than broken bits of petal and powder," she says. To test for quality, crush the whole, dried chamomile between your fingers—it should release an applelike scent. A quality tea is greenish-golden in the teacup, rather than tan-brown, and has a mildly bitter, applelike flavor.

She recommends having a cup whenever you feel anxious, drinking anywhere from one to three cups a day. "You should feel calmer 15 to 20 minutes after drinking the tea."

If you decide to opt for a supplement of chamomile, look for the same type of standardized extract used in the study, and experiment with dosages to see what works for you.

However: Effective treatment for anxiety also depends on understanding the ways in which you create your own anxiety, says Crawford. She recommends proven anti-anxiety therapies such as cognitive-behavioral therapy (CBT) or mindfulness-based stress reduction (MBSR)—using chamomile as a helpful addition.

Jay D. Amsterdam, MD, professor, Department of Psychiatry, University of Pennsylvania, Philadelphia.

David D. Burns, MD, adjunct clinical professor of psychiatry emeritus, Department of Psychiatry and Behavioral Sciences, Stanford University School of Medicine. He is the author of *When Panic Attacks* (Broadway) and *Feeling Good* (Harper).

Amanda McQuade Crawford, medical herbalist in Los Angeles and author of *The Natural Menopause Handbook: Herbs, Nutrition & Other Natural Therapies* (Crossing Press). *www.amandamcquadecrawford.com.*

Chapter 6

DIABETES

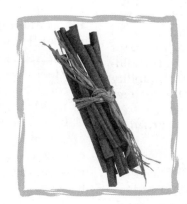

Lifestyle vs. Drugs for Preventing Diabetes— Lifestyle Wins!

More than a decade ago, researchers launched the Diabetes Prevention Program study (DPP) to discover the best way to prevent or delay type 2 diabetes. The study involved more than 3,200 individuals with prediabetes—people who were overweight and had higher-than-normal blood sugar (glucose), and were therefore at high risk for developing type 2 diabetes.

The researchers divided them into three groups. One group took the glucose-lowering drug *metformin* (Glucophage, Glucophage XR, Fortamet, Riomet). One group took a placebo. And one group went through a "Lifestyle Balance Program," learning new and healthy habits, such as exercising regularly and eating a low-fat diet.

After three years, the researchers tallied the new cases of diabetes to see which ap-

proach had worked best—and lifestyle was the winner. It reduced the rate of diabetes by 58%, compared with the placebo group. Metformin also worked, but not as well, reducing the rate by 31%.

After the DPP study was over, researchers offered the participants the opportunity to keep going with the lifestyle program or the drug—a continuation of the study, called the *Diabetes Prevention Program Outcome Study* (DPPOS). About nine out of 10 of the study participants opted to continue.

And now more than 10 years after the start of DPP, and more than seven years after the start of DPPOS, the newest results are in, published in the prestigious medical journal *The Lancet*…

Reducing Risk by Nearly 50%

And the winner is—lifestyle!

Compared with the placebo group, those in the lifestyle group had a 34% lower rate of developing diabetes.

And among those in the study who were aged 60 or older, lifestyle reduced the rate of developing diabetes by nearly 50%.

Those in the metformin group had an 18% lower rate.

Important: On average, the people in the lifestyle group regained 10 of the 15 pounds they lost during the three years of the DPP study. But 10 years of regular exercise and a healthier eating regimen was still protective against the development of diabetes. In other words, you don't have to lose a whole lot of weight to get a whole lot of benefit!

"Moderate weight loss through a lower-calorie, low-fat lifestyle, and regular exercise—usually walking—seems to be effective in lowering the risk for diabetes in people at very high risk for developing the disease, and that's certainly a positive finding," says Jill Crandall, MD, a study author, and director of the Diabetes Clinical Trials Unit at the Albert Einstein College of Medicine in New York City.

The Diabetes Prevention Program

"Changing your lifestyle to better health habits—including those aimed at reducing weight, improving diet and increasing exercise—can have long-term, sustained impact on preventing diabetes," agrees Neil H. White, MD, a study author at the Washington University School of Medicine in St. Louis.

Here are the some recommendations for lifestyle changes from the Diabetes Prevention Program...

• **Do 2½ hours of physical activity a week.** This will burn about 700 calories a week. Pick an easy activity you like, such as brisk walking. Spread the 2½ hours a week over 3 to 4 days (or more)—for example, ½ hour a day, on five days.

• **Three smart ways to eat less fat.** Incorporate the following straightforward lifestyle practices to reduce fat in your diet.

• Eat high-fat foods less often. *Example:* Don't eat French fries every day—have them only once a week.

• Eat smaller amounts of high-fat foods. *Example:* At the salad bar, don't use the ladle to pour on salad dressing—use a regular spoon from your place setting.

• Eat lower-fat foods instead of high-fat foods. *Examples:* choose pretzels instead of potato chips...use low-fat margarine instead of regular margarine...use salsa instead of sour cream on a baked potato.

• **Watch out for hidden fat.** Nearly 70% of the fat you eat isn't obvious, like a pat of butter—it's hidden in foods. *Example:* the hidden fat in a typical fast-food meal—a fried fish sandwich (5 teaspoons of fat), large French fries (6 teaspoons), apple pie (4 teaspoons) and milkshake (5 teaspoons)—equals 20 teaspoons of fat. That's close to eating a stick of butter!

• **Lower the fats in the meat you eat.** Meats are a major source of dietary fat. Buy lean cuts (round loin, sirloin, leg). Trim all the fat you see. Instead of frying—bake, roast, broil, barbecue or grill. Remove the skin from chicken and turkey. Drain off fat after cooking. Flavor meats with low-fat flavorings, such as Tabasco, catsup, lemon juice or Worcestershire sauce.

• **Healthy eating out.** Restaurant meals are often a major source of fat. If you're planning to eat dinner out, eat less fat and fewer calories at other meals during the day. Eat a little something before you got out, or drink a large, low-calorie beverage. Split a dessert.

Look for these low-fat choices on the menu...

• Pizza. Plain cheese pizza—and ask for half the cheese.

• Mexican. Grilled chicken or beef fajitas.

• Chinese. Stir-fried chicken or stir-fried vegetables.

• Italian. Spaghetti with meatless tomato sauce.

• Seafood. Broiled, baked or boiled—not fried.

• Steakhouses. Broiled chicken or fish, with a plain baked potato.

Resource: You can find guidelines for the entire Lifestyle Balance Program on the Web site of the Diabetes Prevention Program, *www.bsc.gwu.edu/dpp/index.htmlvdoc.* Click on "Manuals."

Jill Crandall, MD, director, Diabetes Clinical Trials Unit at the Albert Einstein College of Medicine in New York City.

Neil H. White, MD professor of pediatrics, Washington University School of Medicine, St. Louis.

Stay-Well Secrets for People with Diabetes or Prediabetes

We've all heard that diabetes is on the rise in the US, but few people realize the degree to which older adults are disproportionately affected.

Frightening statistic: Nearly one out of every three Americans over age 65 has diabetes, the highest rate among all age groups. Another one out of three older adults has a precursor to diabetes known as "prediabetes"—defined as a fasting blood sugar (glucose) level of 100 mg/dL to 125 mg/dL.

Many people downplay the seriousness of diabetes. That's a mistake. Because elevated glucose can damage blood vessels, nerves, the kidneys and eyes, people with diabetes are much more likely to die from heart disease and/or kidney disease than people without diabetes—and they are at increased risk for infections, including gum disease, as well as blindness and amputation. (Nerve damage and poor circulation can allow dangerous infections to go undetected.)

And diabetes can be sneaky—increased thirst, urination and/or hunger are the most common symptoms, but many people have no symptoms and are unaware that they are sick.

Despite these sobering facts, doctors rarely have time to give their patients all the information they need to cope with the complexities of diabetes. Fortunately, diabetes educators—health-care professionals, such as registered nurses, registered dietitians and medical social workers—can give patients practical advice on the best ways to control their condition.*

Good news: Most health insurers, including Medicare, cover the cost of diabetes patients' visits with a diabetes educator.

Here are some stay-well secrets to keep diabetes at bay…

Savvy Eating Habits

Most doctors advise people with diabetes or prediabetes to cut back on refined carbohydrates, such as cakes and cookies, and eat more fruits, vegetables and whole grains. This maximizes nutrition and promotes a healthy body weight (being overweight greatly increases diabetes risk). *Other steps to take…*

• **Drink one extra glass of water each day.** The extra fluid will help prevent dehydration, which can raise glucose levels.

• **Never skip meals—especially breakfast.** Don't assume that bypassing a meal and fasting for more than five to six hours will help lower glucose levels. It actually triggers the liver to release glucose into the bloodstream.

Better strategy: Eat three small meals daily and have snacks in between. Start with breakfast, such as a cup of low-fat yogurt and whole-wheat toast with peanut butter or a small bowl of whole-grain cereal and a handful of nuts.

Good snack options: A small apple or three graham crackers. Each of these snacks contains about 15 g of carbohydrates.

• **Practice the "plate method."** Divide a nine-inch plate in half. Fill half with vegetables, then split the other half into quarters—one for protein, such as salmon, lean meat, beans or tofu…and the other for starches, such as one-third cup of pasta or one-half cup

*To find a diabetes educator near you, consult the American Association of Diabetes Educators, 800-832-6874, *www.diabeteseducator.org.*

of peas or corn. Then have a small piece of fruit. This is an easy way to practice portion control—and get the nutrients you need.

Ask yourself if you are satisfied after you take each bite. If the answer is "yes," stop eating. This simple strategy helped one of my clients lose 50 pounds.

●**Be wary of "sugar-free" foods.** These products, including sugar-free cookies and diabetic candy, often are high in carbohydrates, which are the body's primary source of glucose. You may be better off eating the regular product, which is more satisfying. Compare the carbohydrate contents on product labels.

Get Creative with Exercise

If you have diabetes or prediabetes, you've probably been told to get more exercise. Walking is especially helpful. For those with diabetes, walking for at least two hours a week has been shown to reduce the risk for death by 30% over an eight-year period. For those with prediabetes, walking for 30 minutes five days a week reduces by about 60% the risk that your condition will progress to diabetes. *But if you'd like some other options, consider...***

●**Armchair workouts.** These exercises, which are performed while seated and are intended for people with physical limitations to standing, increase stamina, muscle tone, flexibility and coordination. For videos or DVDs, go to *www.armchairfitness.com* or call 800-453-6280.

Cost: $39.95 per video or DVD.

●**Strength training.** This type of exercise builds muscle, which burns more calories than fat even when you are not exercising.*** Use hand weights, exercise machines or the weight of your own body—for example, leg squats or bicep curls with no weights. Aim for two to three sessions of strength training weekly, on alternate days.

**Consult your doctor before starting a new exercise program.

***If you have high blood pressure, be sure to check with your doctor before starting a strength-training program—this type of exercise can raise blood pressure.

●**Stretching**—even while watching TV or talking on the phone. By building a stretching routine into your daily activities, you won't need to set aside a separate time to do it. If your body is flexible, it's easier to perform other kinds of physical activity. Stretching also promotes better circulation. Before stretching, do a brief warm-up, such as walking for five minutes and doing several arm windmills. Aim to do stretching exercises at least three times weekly, including before your other workouts.

Control Your Blood Glucose

If you are diagnosed with diabetes, blood glucose control is the immediate goal. Self-monitoring can be performed using newer devices that test blood glucose levels.

Good choices: LifeScan's OneTouch Ultra... Bayer's Contour...or Abbott Laboratories' FreeStyle.

The hemoglobin A1C test, which is ordered by your doctor and typically is done two to four times a year, determines how well glucose levels have been controlled over the previous two to three months.

If you have prediabetes: Don't settle for a fasting glucose test, which measures blood glucose after you have fasted overnight. It misses two-thirds of all cases of diabetes. The oral glucose tolerance test (OGTT), which involves testing glucose immediately before drinking a premixed glass of glucose and repeating the test two hours later, is more reliable. If you can't get an OGTT, ask for an A1C test and fasting glucose test.

If you have diabetes or prediabetes, you should have your blood pressure and cholesterol checked at every doctor visit and schedule regular eye exams and dental appointments. *In addition, don't overlook...*

●**Proper kidney testing.** Doctors most commonly recommend annual microalbumin and creatinine urine tests to check for kidney disease. You also may want to ask for a glomerular filtration rate test, which measures kidney function.

Do You Have Prediabetes?

If you are age 65 or older, you are at increased risk for prediabetes regardless of the characteristics described below. For this reason, you should ask your doctor about receiving a fasting glucose test.

If you are under age 65, answer the following questions. Speak to your doctor about receiving a fasting glucose test if you score 5 or higher.

Age	Points
20–27	0
28–35	1
36–44	2
45–64	4

Sex

Male	3
Female	0

Family History of Diabetes

No	0
Yes	1

Heart Rate (beats per minute)	Points
Less than 60	0
60–69	0
70–79	1
80–89	2
90–99	2
Greater than 100	4

To determine your heart rate, place the tips of the first two fingers lightly over one of the blood vessels in your neck or the pulse spot inside your wrist just below the base of your thumb. Count your pulse for 10 seconds and multiply that number by 6.

High Blood Pressure	Points
No	0
Yes	1

Body Mass Index (BMI)

Less than 25	0
25–29.9	2
30 or greater	3

Total Points

To determine your BMI, consult the National Heart, Lung and Blood Institute Web site, *www.nhlbisupport.com/bmi.*

Source: Annals of Family Medicine.

●**Meticulous foot care.** High glucose levels can reduce sensation in your feet, making it hard to know when you have a cut, blister or injury. In addition to seeing a podiatrist at least once a year and inspecting your own feet daily, be wary of everyday activities that can be dangerous for people with diabetes.

Stepping into hot bath water, for example, can cause a blister or skin damage that can become infected. To protect yourself, check the water temperature on your wrist or elbow before you step in. The temperature should be warm to the touch—not hot.

Stay Up to Date on Medications

Once diabetes medication has been prescribed, people with diabetes should review their drug regimen with their doctors at every visit. *Insulin is the most commonly used diabetes drug, but you may want to also ask your doctor about these relatively new medications...*

●**DPP-4 inhibitors.** These drugs include *sitagliptin* (Januvia), which lowers glucose levels by increasing the amount of insulin secreted by the pancreas. DPP-4 inhibitors are used alone or with another type of diabetes medication.

●**Symlin.** Administered with an injectable pen, *pramlintide* (Symlin) helps control blood glucose and reduces appetite, which may help with weight loss. It is used in addition to insulin.

If you have prediabetes or diabetes: Always consult a pharmacist or doctor before taking any over-the-counter products. Cold medicines with a high sugar content may raise your blood glucose, for example, and wart removal products may cause skin ulcers. Pay close attention to drug label warnings.

Theresa Garnero, advanced practice registered nurse (APRN), certified diabetes educator (CDE) and clinical nurse manager of the Center for Diabetes Services at the California Pacific Medical Center in San Francisco. She is author of *Your First Year with Diabetes: What to Do, Month by Month* (American Diabetes Association).

The Glycemic Index: A Reality Check

Nearly everyone has heard of the glycemic index. Little wonder—there are hundreds of books on the subject. But the glycemic index (GI) can make good nutrition too complicated, says Mark Stengler, NMD.

Background: The GI ranks foods by how much they elevate blood sugar levels. The index uses a scale of 0 to 100—with foods that result in the most rapid rise in blood sugar given the highest value. (Pure glucose serves as a reference point, with a GI of 100.) Eating too many high-GI ranked foods, such as pie or white bagels, causes a steep rise in blood sugar levels, increasing your risk of excess weight and diabetes. These foods also leave you feeling unsatisfied and often craving more sugars and starches.

Theory vs. reality: In theory, the GI is a good idea…in practice, it leaves a lot to be desired. Originally developed as a research tool, it has morphed into a weight loss technique for consumers. However, it often doesn't work in real-world settings. *Reasons…*

• **It measures individual foods.** GI rankings are based on individual foods, including bread, cereals, pastries, vegetables and fruits. But in reality, people eat combinations of foods, and a low-GI food (such as broiled chicken) may buffer the impact of a high-GI food (such as baked potato).

• **The health factor.** Low-GI foods aren't necessarily the most nutritious. You will find that broccoli and cauliflower are low on the GI, but so are ice cream and peanut M&Ms (peanuts have virtually no GI impact, so they buffer the sugar in M&Ms…just as the dairy protein in ice cream buffers the sugar in that food). Brown rice and carrots have high GI rankings, but they deliver healthier nutrients than low-GI potato chips, for example.

• **Inconsistent findings.** The average glycemic response (found in most of the GI diet books) doesn't always reflect individual responses. *Evidence:* In a study at Tufts University in Boston, participants' average response to white bread was 71, just one point off the GI reference of 70. However, *individual* responses ranged from 43 (moderately low) to 132 (very high). Furthermore, individual responses to the same food varied on different days—by as much as one-fifth… and if you ate a big dessert (high GI) at your previous meal, you'd probably have a higher GI response to carbohydrates at your next meal, no matter what you ate. We are biological individuals, not group statistics.

Advice: Using the GI to guide your diet can be as much of a hassle as counting calories or carbs—other techniques that people attempt and then abandon. Good nutrition can and should be simple. If you eat a diet rich in high-fiber vegetables and fruits, plus fish, chicken and legumes (such as beans and lentils), you'll be eating a healthful diet that happens to be a low-GI diet.

Mark A. Stengler, NMD, naturopathic medical doctor in private practice, La Jolla, California, and author of the *Bottom Line/Natural Healing* newsletter. *www.drstengler.com.*

Diabetes Medication Danger

Researchers at Wake Forest University have found that Avandia and Actos, two drugs that control type 2 diabetes, can almost double the risk for hip fractures in women.

Both medications—*rosiglitazone* (Avandia) and *pioglitazone* (Actos)—belong to a class of drugs known as *thiazolidinediones*. This is not the first time that these drugs have made headlines. In 2007, it was found that those who took rosiglitazone were at increased risk for heart attack. The FDA required warnings about heart attack and congestive heart failure to be added to rosiglitazone's label.

In the pharmaceutical industry, drugs are monitored through a practice known as post-marketing surveillance. Health-care professionals and the public voluntarily let the FDA know about any adverse effects experienced while using a drug. Manufacturers also are required to report any adverse events involving their drugs. Neither system is reliable. The disturbing findings about Avandia and Actos emphasize the need for more rigorous monitoring and reporting of side effects.

Many patients with diabetes can reduce or eliminate the need for medication with proper diet and exercise, along with certain natural supplements—including chromium…ginseng…and PolyGlycoplex (also known as PGX), a blend of fiber including glucomannan and Pycnogenol (extract from pine bark). If you must take medication to control your diabetes, talk to your physician about drugs other than Avandia and Actos. *Metformin* (Glucophage) has a long history as a reliable diabetes medication.

Mark A. Stengler, NMD, naturopathic medical doctor in private practice, La Jolla, California, and author of the *Bottom Line/Natural Healing* newsletter. *www.drstengler.com*

Defeat Diabetes Without Drugs

Type 2 diabetes is one of the many chronic diseases that often can be managed entirely without medication, particularly when it is diagnosed at an early stage.

Among people with insulin resistance, a precursor to diabetes, nearly all can reverse it with the same changes. Even with longstanding diabetes, many patients can discontinue most of their insulin/oral drugs when they make significant dietary and other lifestyle changes.

Catch It Early

About 24 million Americans have type 2 diabetes (once known as *adult-onset diabetes*), and at least 57 million have prediabetes, an intermediate condition in which levels of fasting glucose (blood sugar) are between 100 milligrams per deciliter (mg/dL) and 125 mg/dL.

What they have in common: An inability to effectively utilize insulin, the hormone

produced by the pancreas that allows glucose to move from the bloodstream into the body's cells.

Most people with diabetes are first diagnosed via a fasting blood sugar test. But by the time glucose levels are high, the disease already has progressed—and the cells that produce insulin may have suffered irreversible damage.

Better: The fasting serum insulin test.

Cost: About $50 (which may be covered by insurance). High levels of insulin indicate insulin resistance, a condition that precedes sharply elevated glucose.

Anyone with diabetes risk factors, including obesity, high blood pressure, elevated cholesterol or a waist circumference of more than 40 inches in men or 35 inches in women, should have the fasting serum insulin test.

Those who have diabetes or are at risk for diabetes should consider making the following lifestyle changes. People sometimes complain about the "restrictive" nature of the changes needed to control diabetes. It does take some effort, but far less than dealing with the complications of the disease—which may include blindness, nerve damage and amputation.

Near-Vegetarian Diet

One study found that 21 of 23 patients were able to discontinue oral diabetes drugs after switching to a mainly meatless diet—of those on insulin, 13 out of 17 were able to quit taking the insulin.

A plant-based diet is high in fiber, which slows digestion and the rate of glucose absorption into the blood. This causes the pancreas to secrete less insulin, and it makes cells more sensitive to insulin's effects. People who consume little or no meat also tend to have lower cholesterol and blood pressure—important for minimizing the cardiovascular complications of diabetes.

Carbohydrate Counting

Carbohydrate counting is among the most effective ways to control diabetes. *Main steps…*

• **Calculate net carbohydrate.** This is the amount of carbohydrate in a food minus fiber content. One cup of Kashi GoLean cereal, for example, has 30 grams (g) of total carbohydrates, but because this includes 10 g of fiber, the net carbohydrate is actually 20 g. You can find all of this information on food labels.

• **Identify carbohydrate choices.** One carbohydrate choice equals 15 g of net carbohydrates.

Example: A slice of whole-wheat bread is one carbohydrate choice (about 15 g of net carbs).

• **Eat 9 to 13 carbohydrate choices daily for optimal control.** Most people are advised to have three to five carb choices for breakfast.

Sample breakfast: One cup of old-fashioned oatmeal with milk or milk alternative, such as soy milk (two carbohydrate choices)...one cup of berries (one carb choice)... egg or tofu scramble with vegetables, such as mushrooms, bell peppers and onions (one carb choice)...one slice of toast with nut butter (one carb choice).

Have three to five carbohydrate choices at lunch and zero to three at supper. Eating lighter at night helps stabilize overnight and morning blood sugar levels.

Carbohydrate counting is confusing initially, but people quickly memorize the carbohydrate contents of the foods that they tend to eat most often.

Helpful: I advise patients to eat meals at the same time every day...and to eat about the same portion sizes to keep blood sugar levels stable.

Postmeal Exercise

Exercise helps people lose weight, which improves insulin sensitivity and reduces cardiovascular risk factors.

Even without weight loss, exercise is very effective for managing diabetes, particularly when you exercise after meals. Exercise after meals makes it easier for muscle cells to absorb glucose from the blood. Patients who check their blood sugar two hours after eating, then test it again after a brisk 20-minute walk, typically see a drop of at least 30 points.

Strength training also is helpful. People who lift weights or engage in other forms of resistance exercise (such as push-ups) two or three times a week have an increase in muscle tissue, which increases metabolism and insulin sensitivity.

Lower Stress

In an emergency, the body releases cortisol, the "fight-or-flight" hormone that increases blood glucose to produce a quick surge of energy. Unfortunately, the same thing happens in people with daily stress. Their cortisol—and glucose—remains at chronically high levels, making diabetes more difficult to control.

Stress management is critical if you have diabetes. Most people find that a daily walk keeps them calmer. In addition, hobbies are a good way to defuse tension and stress. Others learn to meditate or practice yoga. Whatever you find relaxing, make time for it at least a few times a day.

Stuart A. Seale, MD, medical director of Lifestyle Center of America, a diabetes center in Sedona, Arizona. He is coauthor, with Franklin House, MD, and Ian Blake Newman, of The 30-Day Diabetes Miracle (Perigee). www.diabetesmiracle.org.

Vitamin K KO's Diabetes

Vitamin K protects men against diabetes by reducing insulin resistance—a major factor in the development of type 2 diabetes.

Recent finding: Men who took 500 micrograms (mcg) of vitamin K daily for 36 months were significantly less likely to develop insulin resistance. The effect was not found in women.

Good food sources of vitamin K: Cooked kale, with more than 1,000 mcg per cup... cooked spinach, 760 mcg per cup...cooked collard greens, about 700 mcg per cup.

Sarah L. Booth, PhD, director, Vitamin K Research Laboratory at Tufts University's Jean Mayer USDA Human Nutrition Research Center on Aging, Boston.

Natural Help for the Diabetic Heart

If you have type 2 diabetes, you've already had a heart attack—whether you've had one or not!

"The guidelines for physicians from the American Heart Association are to treat a person with diabetes as if that individual has already had a heart attack," says cardiologist Seth Baum, MD, medical director of Integrative Heart Care in Boca Raton, Florida, and author of *The Total Guide to a Healthy Heart* (Kensington).

How Does Diabetes Hurt Your Heart?

As excess sugar careens through the bloodstream, it roughs up the linings of the arteries.

Insulin resistance (the subpar performance of the hormone that moves glucose out of the bloodstream and into muscle and fat cells) raises blood pressure, damaging arteries.

Diabetes also injures tiny blood vessels called *capillaries*, which hurts your kidneys, and nerves—damage that in turn stresses the heart.

The end result—an up to seven-fold increase in the risk of heart disease and stroke, the cardiovascular diseases (CVD) that kill four out of five people with diabetes.

But recent studies show there are several natural ways for people with diabetes to reverse the risk factors that cause heart disease…

First-Line Treatment

It's never too late to exercise—and a little goes a long way. Researchers at the University of British Columbia in Vancouver, Canada, studied 36 older people (average age 71) with type 2 diabetes, high blood pressure, and high cholesterol, dividing them into two groups.

One group walked on a treadmill or cycled on a stationary bicycle for 40 minutes, three days a week. The other group didn't.

To find out if the exercise was helping with CVD, the researchers measured the elasticity of the arteries—a fundamental indicator of arterial youth and health, with arterial stiffness increasing the risk of dying from CVD.

Results: After three months, the exercisers had a decrease in arterial stiffness of 15 to 20%.

"Aerobic exercise should be the first-line treatment to reduce arterial stiffness in older adults with type 2 diabetes, even if the patient has advanced cardiovascular risk factors such as high blood pressure and high cholesterol," conclude the researchers, in *Diabetes Care*.

Improve Risk Factors Quickly

Kenneth Madden, MD, the exercise study leader, and assistant professor of geriatric medicine at the University of British Columbia, says "You can improve every risk factor for diabetes and heart disease—and you can do it in a very short period of time."

• **Exercise at the right rate.** Dr. Madden recommends that older people with diabetes and cardiovascular disease see a doctor for a checkup before starting an exercise program.

Once you get the okay from your physician, he says to purchase and use a heart monitor during exercise, so you're sure that you're exercising at the level used by the participants in his study—60 to 75% of maximum heart rate.

Example: An estimate of your maximum heart rate is 220, minus your age. If you're 60, that would be 220 − 60 = 160. Exercising at between 60 to 75% of your maximum heart rate means maintaining a heart rate of between 96 and 120 beats per minute.

Finally, Dr. Madden advises you exercise the amount proven to improve arterial elasticity—a minimum of three sessions of aerobic exercise a week, of 40 minutes each.

• **Maximize magnesium.** Researchers in Mexico studied 79 people with diabetes and high blood pressure, dividing them into two groups. One group received a daily

450 milligrams (mg) magnesium supplement; one didn't.

Results: After four months, those on magnesium had an average drop of 20 points systolic (the higher number in the blood pressure reading) and 9 points diastolic (the lower number). Those on the placebo had corresponding drops of 5 points and 1 point.

"Magnesium supplementation should be considered as an additional or alternative treatment for high blood pressure in people with diabetes," says Fernando Guerrero-Romero, MD, the study leader.

What to do: "Magnesium acts as a natural vasodilator, relaxing arteries and lowering blood pressure," says Dr. Baum. "People with diabetes should incorporate a magnesium supplement into their regimen."

He suggests a daily supplement of 400 mg, about the level used in the study.

"People with diabetes and high blood pressure should also be encouraged to increase their dietary intake of magnesium, through eating more whole grains, leafy green vegetables, legumes, nuts and fish," says Dr. Guerrero-Romero.

• **Eat like a Neanderthal.** Researchers in Sweden tested two diets in 13 people with type 2 diabetes—the diet recommended by the American Diabetes Association (ADA), a generally healthful diet limiting calories, fat and refined carbohydrates; and a "Paleolithic" diet, consisting of lean meat, fish, fruits, vegetables, root vegetables, eggs and nuts—and no dairy products, refined carbohydrates or highly processed foods, whatsoever.

The basic diet: Eat more—lean meat, fish, shellfish, fruits, vegetables, eggs and nuts.

Eat less (or eliminate)—grains, dairy products, salt, refined fats and refined sugar.

Resource: You can order pre-packaged Paleolithic snacks and meals at *www.paleo brands.com*.

In terms of lowering risk factors for heart disease, the Paleolithic diet clubbed the ADA diet.

Results: After three months, it had done a better job of decreasing…

• High LDL "bad" cholesterol,

• High blood pressure,

• High triglycerides (a blood fat linked to heart disease) and

• Too-big waist size (excess stomach fat is linked to heart disease).

The diet was also more effective at increasing HDL "good" cholesterol.

And it was superior in decreasing glycated hemoglobin (A1C), a measure of long-term blood sugar control.

"Foods that were regularly eaten during the Paleolithic, or 'Old Stone Age,' may be optimal for prevention and treatment of type 2 diabetes, cardiovascular disease and insulin resistance," concludes Tommy Jönsson, MD, in *Cardiovascular Diabetology*.

What to do: "Eating a Paleolithic Diet is far easier than most people think," says Robb Wolf, owner of NorCal Strength and Conditioning in Chico, California, and author of *The Paleolithic Solution* (Victory Belt Publishing).

• **Have a cup of hibiscus tea.** Researchers in Iran studied 53 people with type 2 diabetes, dividing them into two groups. One group drank a cup of hibiscus tea twice a day; the other drank two cups a day of black tea. (The hibiscus tea was made from *Hibiscus sabdariffa*, which is also known as red sorrel, Jamaican sorrel, Indian sorrel, roselle and Florida cranberry.)

Results: After one month, those drinking hibiscus had…

• Higher HDL "good" cholesterol,

• Lower LDL "bad" cholesterol,

• Lower total cholesterol and

• Lower blood pressure.

The black tea group didn't have any significant changes in blood fats or blood pressure.

The findings were in *The Journal of Alternative and Complementary Medicine* and the *Journal of Human Hypertension*.

What to do: Consider drinking a cup or two of hibiscus tea a day, says Hassan Mozaffari-

Khosravi, PhD, an assistant professor of nutrition and the study leader.

Seth Baum, MD, medical director of Integrative Heart Care in Boca Raton, Florida, and author of *The Total Guide to a Healthy Heart* (Kensington). *www.vitalremedy.com.*

Kenneth Madden, MD, assistant professor of geriatric medicine at the University of British Columbia.

Fernando Guerrero-Romero, MD, director, Medical Research Unit, Clinical Epidemiology, Mexican Institute of Social Security.

Tommy Jönsson, MD, Department of Clinical Sciences, Lund University, Sweden.

Robb Wolf, owner of NorCal Strength and Conditioning, Chico, California, and author of *The Paleolithic Solution*, (Victory Belt Publishing).

Hassan Mozaffari-Khosravi, PhD, assistant professor of nutrition, Shahid Sadoughi University of Medical Sciences, Yazd, Iran.

Vitamin B-12—Better Than a Drug for Diabetic Neuropathy

Twenty-five percent of people with diabetes develop *diabetic neuropathy*—glucose-caused damage to nerves throughout the body, particularly in the hands, arms, feet and legs (peripheral neuropathy).

You experience tingling and prickling. Numbness. And pain—from annoying, to burning, to stabbing, to excruciating. Drugs hardly help.

"Many studies have been conducted on drugs for diabetic neuropathy, and no drug is really effective," says Anne L. Peters, MD, professor of medicine and director of the USC (University of Southern California) Clinical Diabetes Program, and author of *Conquering Diabetes* (Plume).

But a new study says a vitamin can help...

Less Pain and Burning

Researchers in Iran studied 100 people with diabetic neuropathy, dividing them into two groups. One group received *nortriptyline* (Pamelor, Aventyl), an antidepressant medication that has been used to treat neuropathy.

The other group received vitamin B-12, a nutrient known to nourish and protect nerves.

After several weeks of treatment, the B-12 group had...

- 78% greater reduction in pain,
- 71% greater reduction in tingling and prickling and
- 65% greater reduction in burning.

"Vitamin B-12 is more effective than nortriptyline for the treatment of painful diabetic neuropathy," conclude the researchers, in the *International Journal of Food Science and Nutrition.*

Latest development: A few months after the Iranian doctors conducted their study, research in the US involving 76 people with diabetes showed that the widely prescribed diabetes drug *metformin* may cause vitamin B-12 deficiency—and that 77% of those with the deficiency also suffered from peripheral neuropathy!

Anyone already diagnosed with peripheral neuropathy who uses metformin should be tested for low blood levels of B-12, says Mariejane Braza, MD, of the University of Texas Health Science Center and the study leader. If B-12 levels are low, she recommends supplementing with the vitamin, to reduce the risk of nerve damage.

Heal the Nerves

"If you take metformin, definitely take at least 500 micrograms (mcg) a day of vitamin B-12, in either a multivitamin or B-complex supplement," advises Jacob Teitelbaum, MD, author of *Pain-Free 1-2-3!* (McGraw-Hill). "It's the single, most effective nutrient for helping prevent and reverse diabetic neuropathy.

"On a good day, the best that medications can do for neuropathy is mask the pain," he continues. "But vitamin B-12 gradually heals the nerves."

Best: If you already have neuropathy, Dr. Teitelbaum recommends finding a holistic physician and asking for 15 intramuscular injections of 3,000 to 5,000 mcg of *methylcobalamin*, the best form of B-12 to treat peripheral neuropathy. "Receive those shots daily to weekly—at whatever speed is convenient to quickly optimize levels of B-12," says Dr. Teitelbaum.

Resource: To find a holistic physician, Dr. Teitelbaum recommends visiting the Web site of the American Board of Integrative Holistic Medicine, *www.holisticboard.org.*

If you can't find a holistic physician near you, he suggests taking a daily sublingual (dissolving under the tongue) dose of 5,000 mcg for four weeks. (Daily, because you only absorb a small portion of the sublingual vitamin B-12, compared with intramuscular injections.)

At the same time that you take B-12, also take a high-dose B-complex supplement (B-50). "The body is happiest when it gets all the B-vitamins together," says Dr. Teitelbaum.

He points out that it can take three to twelve months for nerves to heal, but that the neuropathy should progressively improve during that time.

Also helpful: Other nutrients that Dr. Teitelbaum recommends to help ease peripheral neuropathy include:

- **Alpha-lipoic acid (300 mg, twice a day)**
- **Acetyl-l-carnitine (500 mg, three times a day)**

Anne L. Peters, MD, professor of medicine and director of the USC Clinical Diabetes Program, author of *Conquering Diabetes* (Plume).

Mariejane Braza, MD, researcher, University of Texas Health Science Center and internist, Valley Baptist Medical Center, Harlingen, Texas.

Jacob Teitelbaum, MD, author of *Pain-Free 1-2-3!* (Mc-Graw-Hill) and *From Fatigued to Fantastic!* (Avery). *www.endfatigue.com.*

Protect Your Kidneys With Baking Soda

A part of your body that is beat up by the excess blood sugar of diabetes are the kidneys—the pair of bean-shaped, fist-sized organs that filter and clean blood.

"Of the 27 million cases of kidney disease in the US, more than half are caused by diabetes," says Katherine Tuttle, MD, clinical professor of medicine in the division of nephrology at the University of Washington School of Medicine.

When kidneys are weak and waste products loiter, your blood chemistry can become acid, a condition called *acidosis.* Acidosis erodes bones, hobbles the immune system, strains the heart, and even further injures the kidneys, pushing them faster toward total failure, or end-stage renal disease (ESRD)—the point at which you require either dialysis (regular cleaning of the blood by a machine) or a kidney transplant.

But a new study shows there may be an easy, inexpensive way to correct acidosis—baking soda...

Slowing Kidney Decline

For two years, researchers in England studied 134 people with advanced kidney disease and acidosis.

They found that adding a daily tablet of sodium bicarbonate (baking soda) to standard treatment dramatically slowed kidney decline.

Those taking baking soda had kidneys that were 69% more effective at cleaning the blood of *creatinine*, an acidic waste product, said the researchers, in the *Journal of the American Society of Nephrology.*

Only 9% of those taking baking soda had "rapid progression" of their kidney disease, compared with 45% of those who didn't take baking soda.

And only 6.5% of those taking the baking soda progressed to ESRD, compared with 33% of those who didn't.

And, the researchers note, taking baking soda didn't trigger higher blood pressure or more water retention—possible side effects from the sodium in sodium bicarbonate.

"A simple remedy like baking soda, when used appropriately, can be very effective," says Magdi Yaqoob, MD, the study leader, at the Royal London Hospital.

Is Baking Soda Right for You?

"While we would want to see several studies replicating these findings before routinely recommending baking soda to patients with kidney disease, these are remarkably positive results," says Dr. Tuttle. And, she adds, this type of therapy might be particularly positive for people with diabetes and kidney disease because they're very susceptible to acidosis.

Doctors already routinely treat acidosis in patients with kidney disease, she points out, but usually do so with medications such as sodium citrate, which converts to sodium bicarbonate in the body. She advises talking to your doctor to see if baking soda might be the right treatment for you.

"It's a therapy that is simple, easily available and cheap, compared with conventional medicines used to correct acidosis," she says. "You just have to learn exactly how much works in your case, and how to measure it carefully for the effective dosage. You also have to be tested regularly for possible side effects, such as high blood pressure and water retention."

Katherine Tuttle, MD, clinical professor of medicine in the division of nephrology at the University of Washington School of Medicine, Seattle.

Magdi Yaqoob, MD, professor of Renal Medicine, The Royal London Hospital, London, England.

Cinnamon—Cheap, Safe And Very Effective

Insulin is the hormone that controls blood sugar levels. Cinnamon is its twin.

"Cinnamon mimics the action of insulin," says Richard Anderson, PhD, a researcher at the Beltsville Human Nutrition Research Center in Maryland, and the coauthor of 22 scientific papers on cinnamon and diabetes. "Cinnamon stimulates insulin receptors on fat and muscle cells the same way insulin does, allowing excess sugar to move out of the blood and into the cells."

Several recent studies provide new proof of cinnamon's effectiveness in preventing and controlling diabetes...

Newest Research

● **Stopping diabetes before it starts.** In Britain, researchers studied healthy, young men, dividing them into two groups—one group received three grams of cinnamon a day and the other a placebo.

After two weeks, the men taking the cinnamon supplement had a much improved "glucose tolerance test"—the ability of the body to process and store glucose. They also had better "insulin sensitivity"—the ability of the insulin hormone to usher glucose out of the bloodstream and into cells.

● **Long-term management of diabetes.** The most accurate measurement of long-term blood sugar control is A1C, or *glycated hemoglobin*—the percentage of red blood cells that have been frosted by blood sugar. Seven percent or less means diabetes is under control—and a decrease of 0.5 to 1.0% is considered a significant improvement in the disease.

In a study by a doctor in Nevada, 109 people with type 2 diabetes were divided into two groups, with one receiving 1 gram of cinnamon a day and one receiving a placebo. After three months, those taking the cinnamon had a 0.83% decrease in A1C.

Those taking the placebo had a 0.37% decrease.

"We used standard, off-the-shelf cinnamon capsules that patients would find at their local stores or on the Internet," says Paul Crawford, MD, the study's author, in the *Journal of the American Board of Family Medicine*. And that cinnamon, he says, "gives diabetes care providers and diabetic patients an easily accessible, likely safe, and cheap alternative to help treat type 2 diabetes."

Important: He points out that the drop in A1C seen his study would decrease the risk of many diabetic complications—heart disease and stroke by 16%; eye problems (diabetic retinopathy) by 17 to 21%, and kidney disease (nephropathy) by 24 to 33%.

●**After a bad night's sleep, include cinnamon in your breakfast.** Several recent studies show that sleep deprivation—a nearly universal problem of modern life—increases the risk of diabetes.

Solution: Writing in the *Journal of Medicinal Food*, researchers in the Human Performance Laboratory at Baylor University recommend the use of cinnamon to reverse insulin resistance and glucose intolerance after sleep loss.

●**Oxidation under control.** Oxidation—a kind of biochemical rust—is one of the processes behind the development of diabetes. In a study by French researchers of 22 people with prediabetes, three months of supplementation with a cinnamon extract dramatically reduced oxidation—and the lower the level of oxidation, the better the blood sugar control.

"The inclusion of cinnamon compounds in the diet could reduce risk factors associated with diabetes," conclude the researcher, in the *Journal of the American College of Nutrition.*

Bottom line: cinnamon works. In a review study of the best research on cinnamon and diabetes to date, researchers in England concluded the spice has the power to fight high blood sugar. Their findings were in *Diabetes, Obesity and Metabolism.*

One Teaspoon Daily

"Try to get ¼ to 1 teaspoon of cinnamon daily," says Dr. Anderson. Sprinkle it in hot cereals, yogurt or applesauce. Use it to accent sweet potatoes, winter squash or yams. Try it with lamb, beef stew or chilies. It even goes great with grains such as couscous and barley, and legumes such as lentils and split peas.

Or you can use a cinnamon supplement.

Consider taking 1 to 3 grams per day, says Dr. Anderson, which is the dosage range used in many studies that show the herb's effectiveness.

Best: Cinnulin PF—a specially prepared water extract of cinnamon—is a supplement used in many studies showing the spice's effectiveness in supplement form. It is widely available in many brands, such as Swanson and Doctor's Best.

The dosage of Cinnulin PF used in studies is typically 250 mg, twice a day.

Richard Anderson, PhD, lead researcher at the Beltsville Human Nutrition Research Center, US Department of Agriculture, Maryland.

Paul Crawford, MD, assistant residency director, Nellis Family Medicine Residency, Mike O'Callaghan Federal Hospital, Las Vegas, Nevada.

How to Beat "Diabesity"— Fight Fat with Fat

Almost 90% of people with type 2 diabetes are overweight. In fact, these two problems are so closely related that one expert combined the words *diabetes* and *obesity*, calling the problem *diabesity*.

What happens: Insulin is the hormone that helps blood sugar (glucose) leave the bloodstream and enter cells. Now, imagine your cells are locks and insulin is the key, says Neal Barnard, MD, author of *Dr. Neal Barnards's Program for Reversing Diabetes* (Rodale). Extra fat clogs the locks, so insulin can't do its job.

Which is why losing even a little body fat can help prevent or delay diabetes, or help normalize glucose levels if you've already developed the disease.

And shedding extra body fat may be as easy as slightly increasing the fat in your diet, according to a surprising new study from researchers at Ohio State University.

The Power of CLA

The researchers studied 35 overweight, postmenopausal women (average age 60) with diabetes, dividing them into two groups.

One group took a daily supplement of conjugated linoleic acid, a saturated fat found in beef, lamb and dairy products. Studies have shown CLA can help burn body fat. (In one such study, people taking 3.4 grams a day of CLA lost an average of 4.5 pounds of fat and gained an average of 1.5 pounds of fat-burning muscle in three months—without cutting calories or increasing exercise.)

The other group took a supplement containing about two teaspoons of safflower oil, a vegetable oil rich in omega-6 polyunsaturated fats. (Omega-6 is a scientific term describing the specific chemical composition of a fat.)

After four months, the women taking CLA had lost a few pounds and an average of 3.2% of their body fat—without losing any muscle. (Losing muscle rather than fat is an unfortunate result of many diets.)

The women taking safflower oil didn't lose any weight. But they shed an average 6.3% of their belly fat and had a 1.6% increase in muscle.

Important: Excess belly fat is a risk factor for diabetes, possibly because it leads to a fattier pancreas and liver, two organs that play key roles in regulating glucose levels.

The women taking safflower oil also had an improvement in glucose control.

And they had a 20% increase in *adiponectin*, a hormone produced by fat cells that helps control glucose.

Salad Dressing Therapy

"The big surprise of this study was the effect of safflower oil on body fat and blood sugar—a result never seen before in scientific research," says Martha Belury, PhD, professor of human nutrition and the study leader.

Why safflower oil had that effect, she doesn't know. But that doesn't mean you can't benefit from it.

• **Safflower oil.** "If you're overweight and trying to improve blood sugar control, you should definitely begin to get two teaspoons a day of safflower oil in your diet," says Dr. Belury. "It's easy to do and it's inexpensive." You can also use another type of vegetable oil rich in omega-6 polyunsaturated fats, such as sunflower or corn.

• **Use the oil as a salad dressing, along with vinegar.** "I try to have a salad with oil and vinegar almost every day, because I know it's good for me," says Dr. Belury. Or cook with vegetable oil instead of butter.

• **CLA supplements.** Taking a CLA supplement is a personal decision, based on the cost of the supplement and the possible benefit, says Dr. Belury. "If I had 50 pounds to lose, and I could afford to take CLA, I would—because the supplement might help me lose that weight," she says.

Caution: Take the dosage recommended on the label—a larger dose won't speed or increase weight loss, says Dr. Belury. And take the supplement for at least three to six months, the time it takes for CLA to produce results.

Neal Barnard, MD, author of *Dr. Neal Barnard's Program for Reversing Diabetes*.

Martha Belury, PhD, professor, department of human nutrition at Ohio State University, Columbus.

Laugh Off Diabetes

Researchers recently looked at laughter's effect on people with diabetes. In this one-year study, 20 diabetes patients received medication for their diabetic condition, including *glipizide* (Glucotrol), but one group also watched humorous videos (which they selected) for 30 minutes daily. After one year, 26% of the "laughter group" patients had higher levels of HDL "good" cholesterol, compared with 3% of patients in the other group. The laughter group also had lower levels of inflammatory chemicals (such as C-reactive protein) linked with cardiovascular disease. Based on this research, people who have diabetes or are at risk for the disease may benefit from treating themselves to a good dose of laughter every day. If you follow this advice, choose any form of humor or comedy that appeals to you (such as movies, TV shows or books) and that produces joyful laughter.

Lee Berk, DrPH, MPH, preventive care specialist and psychoneuroimmunologist, Loma Linda University, Loma Linda, California.

Sleep Linked to Diabetes Risk

People who get too little or too much sleep are at greater risk of developing type 2 diabetes. The optimal amount of sleep is seven to eight hours each night. Compared with people who get that much sleep, those who get five hours per night or less have a 24% higher risk for diabetes. Those who sleep nine or more hours per night have a 48% higher risk.

Girardin Jean-Louis, PhD, associate professor of medicine and research director, Sleep Disorders Center, SUNY Downstate Medical Center at Brooklyn Center for Health Disparities, Brooklyn, New York.

The Martial Art That Defeats Diabetes

"People with diabetes often assume that for exercise to be beneficial, you have to be huffing and puffing, sweating and red-faced afterward," says Beverly Roberts, PhD, RN, a professor at University of Florida College of Nursing. "However, we found that a gentle activity such as tai chi can be just as beneficial in improving the health of people with diabetes."

Dr. Roberts is talking about a recent study that she and her colleagues conducted showing that regular practice of tai chi—an ancient martial art from China consisting of deep breathing and gentle, flowing movements—can help you lower blood sugar, manage diabetes more effectively, improve mood and boost energy levels.

Tai Chi for Glucose Control

A team of researchers from Korea and the US studied 62 people with type 2 diabetes—31 practiced tai chi twice a week, and 31 didn't.

After six months, those practicing tai chi had a greater drop in fasting blood sugar (a test that measures blood sugar after you haven't eaten for eight hours)...a bigger decrease in A1C (a measurement of long-term blood sugar levels)...more participation in diabetic self-care activities, such as daily measuring of glucose levels...happier social interactions...better mood...and more energy.

"For those with type 2 diabetes, tai chi could be an alternative exercise to increase glucose control, diabetic self-care activities and quality of life" conclude the researchers, in the *Journal of Alternative and Complementary Medicine*.

"Tai chi has similar effects as other aerobic exercises on diabetic control," says Dr. Roberts. "The difference is that tai chi is a low-impact exercise, which means that it's less stressful on the bones, joints and muscles than more strenuous exercise.

"Tai chi provides a great alternative for people who want the benefits of exercise on diabetic control, but may be physically unable to complete strenuous activities because of age, health condition or injury."

Standout Scientific Evidence

Many other recent scientific studies show that tai chi is good for diabetes...

• **Stronger immune system.** Researchers in Taiwan found that 12 weeks of tai chi improved the immune system of 30 people with type 2 diabetes (as well as lowering A1C levels). The findings were in the *British Journal of Sports Medicine*.

• **Healthier nerves.** Another team of Taiwanese researchers studied 32 people with type 2 diabetes and found that 12 weeks of tai chi improved the ability of peripheral nerves (in the arms, hands, legs and feet) to conduct nerve impulses, reporting their results in the *Journal of Rehabilitation Medicine*. That's important because many people with diabetes suffer from peripheral neuropathy—painful nerve damage in the arms, hands, legs and feet.

• **More mobility.** Researchers in Australia studied 38 people with type 2 diabetes and found that four months of tai chi practice improved their balance and walking speed. The findings were in *Diabetes Care*.

Helps in Several Ways

"These and other studies show that tai chi can have a significant effect on the management and treatment of diabetes," says Paul Lam, MD, of the University of South Wales School of Public Health, the author of five scientific studies on tai chi and diabetes.

"Tai chi can help with diabetes in several ways," he continues. "It can help you control blood sugar, reduce stress and minimize the complications of diabetes, such as high blood pressure, high cholesterol and the balance and mobility problems that accompany peripheral neuropathy."

Dr. Lam developed the tai chi program that was used in several studies on tai chi and diabetes—Tai Chi for Diabetes. It is available on DVD, and includes a complete tai chi routine, along with a warm-up, stretches, and qigong exercises (also from China) that increase the flow of chi (life force) in the parts of the body affected by diabetes.

Dr. Lam is also the coauthor of the book, *Tai Chi for Diabetes: Living Well with Diabetes* (Tai Chi Productions), which supplements the DVD.

Both the DVD and the book are available at *www.amazon.com*. You can also learn more about the Tai Chi for Diabetes program at Dr. Lam's Web site *www.taichifordiabetes.com*, where you can also order his DVD and book.

Also helpful: If you decide to take a tai chi class, look for an instructor who has practiced for at least three to four years, and who inspires you to the regular practice of tai chi, says Daniel Caulfield, a teacher of tai chi at Flow Martial and Meditative Arts, in Keene, New Hampshire. "The greatest benefit from tai chi comes from both taking a class with a qualified instructor and practicing at home at least 20 minutes a day."

(For a sampling of tai chi exercises, see appendix page 348.)

Beverly Roberts, PhD, RN, professor, University of Florida College of Nursing.

Paul Lam, MD, family physician, tai chi master, clinical teacher and lecturer, University of South Wales, Australia.

Daniel Caulfield, tai chi instructor at Flow Martial and Meditative Arts, Keene, New Hampshire. *www.flowmma.org.*

The Neighborhood Where No One Has Diabetes

Imagine a utopia for glucose—a neighborhood where normal, balanced blood sugar is a way of life, a neighborhood where...

• There are many opportunities to be physically active,

• Local sports clubs and other facilities offer many opportunities to get exercise,

• It is pleasant to walk,

• It is easy to walk,

• You often see other people walking,

• You often see other people exercising— jogging, bicycling or playing sports,

• There is a large selection of fresh fruits and vegetables available,

• The fresh fruits and vegetables are of high quality and

• A large selection of low-fat food products are available.

Well, scientists conducted a survey asking thousands of people if they lived in just such a neighborhood. *Their answers—published in the* Archives of Internal Medicine—*have produced new insights into the causes of diabetes...*

Reducing Risk by 38%

Researchers from the School of Public Health at Drexel University in Philadelphia analyzed the survey responses of 2,285 people, aged 45 to 84, who checked "yes" next to any of the above nine descriptions that fit their neighborhood, and checked "no" next to any of those that didn't fit.

In the five years after taking the survey, those who lived in healthy neighborhoods— neighborhoods where opportunities to exercise are abundant and fresh, low-fat food is available—were 38% less likely to develop diabetes.

Walk and Eat Well

Even if you live in a healthy neighborhood, you might not do what is best for your health, says Amy Auchincloss, PhD, the study leader. *She recommends...*

• **Personal action.** "Choose routine activities that involve physical exertion—activities that will help you be physically active, even when you don't feel like it," she says. "Walk rather than use a car if the traveling distance is less than two miles. Take the stairs instead of the elevator or escalator."

She also says to minimize your purchase of processed, prepared foods, opting instead for fresh.

"To prevent diabetes, eat more 'anti-diabetes' foods, which include whole grains, fruits and fresh vegetables—particularly dark green leafy vegetables," agrees Christopher Ervin, MD, a specialist in public health and former director of programs for the Georgia Diabetes Coalition. "And walk as often as possible—starting with 15 minutes a day, and gradually working your way up to one hour a day."

• **Social action.** "There are community groups and planning organizations that you can join to help advocate for making your city or town healthier," says Dr. Auchincloss.

"Many cities, for example, have public transportation advocacy organizations that also advocate for improving infrastructure for safe walking and bicycling." *Examples...*

• **Transportation Alternatives.** 127 W. 26 Street, Suite 1002, NY, NY, 10001. 212-629-8080, *www.transalt.org.*

• **Smart Growth Network.** The National Center for Appropriate Technology, Box 3838, Butte, MT 59701. 866-643-2767, *www.smartgrowth.org.*

Similarly, says Dr. Auchincloss, many organizations advocate for more fresh food in urban areas. *Two such organizations...*

• **The Food Trust.** One Penn Center, Suite 900, 1617 John F. Kennedy Blvd., Philadelphia, PA 19103. 215-575-0444, *www.thefood trust.org.*

• **The Prevention Institute.** 221 Oak Street, Oakland, CA 94607. 510-444-7738, *www.preventioninstitute.org.*

Amy Auchincloss, PhD, MPH, assistant professor and researcher, department of epidemiology and biostatistics, Drexel University School of Public Health, Philadelphia.

Christopher Ervin, MD, public health specialist and former director of programs for the Georgia Diabetes Coalition.

How to Balance Antioxidants and Blood Sugar

True to their name, antioxidants are nutrients that fight oxidation, the rustlike cellular injury that fuels the advance of many chronic diseases, including diabetes.

But recent studies show that taking a nutritional supplement containing antioxidants such as vitamins C, E and beta-carotene might actually harm people with diabetes. Or at least not help.

Newest Research

• **Blocking the benefits of exercise.** Researchers from Germany studied 39 healthy young men, dividing them into two groups. All the men exercised 85 minutes, five days a week, for four weeks. During those four weeks, one group of men took a daily supplement with vitamin C (1,000 milligrams [mg]) and vitamin E (400 IU), and one group didn't.

After four weeks, the men who didn't take the antioxidant supplement had a beneficial increase in insulin sensitivity—the ability of the hormone insulin to move glucose out of the bloodstream and into muscle and fat cells. But the men who took the antioxidant supplement had a decrease in insulin sensitivity—and therefore a possibly higher risk of developing diabetes. The researchers theorize that exercise-caused bursts of oxidation are good for the body, improving insulin sensitivity. But antioxidant supplements block that beneficial effect of exercise, and "may harm glucose metabolism," says Michael Ristow, MD, the study leader.

● **No protection from diabetes.** Researchers from the Harvard School of Public Health studied more than 8,000 women over age 40 with heart disease or risk factors for heart disease.

They divided the women into several groups. One group took a vitamin C supplement (500 mg a day), one took a vitamin E supplement (600 IU every other day) and one took a beta-carotene supplement (50 mg, every other day). Another three groups took placebos.

Overall, the study showed "no significant effects" of any of the three nutrients on the risk of developing diabetes, say the researchers in the *American Journal of Clinical Nutrition* (AJCN).

● **No protection from metabolic syndrome.** In that same issue of AJCN, researchers from France reported another set of anti-antioxidant findings.

They studied more than 5,000 people, dividing them into two groups. One group took an antioxidant supplement (containing vitamins C, E and beta-carotene, and the minerals zinc and selenium). The other group didn't.

After seven years, the researchers found the supplements provided no protection against metabolic syndrome—the gang of risk factors for diabetes that includes insulin resistance, extra belly fat, low "good" HDL cholesterol, high triglycerides (a blood fat) and high blood pressure.

These results "are consistent with recent reports of a lack of efficacy of antioxidant supplements," say the researchers.

Balancing Anti- and Pro-oxidants

"There is a delicate balance in our bodies between antioxidants and pro-oxidants," says Seth Baum, MD, medical director of Integrative Heart Care in Boca Raton, Florida, and author of *The Total Guide to a Healthy Heart* (Kensington). "On the one hand, pro-oxidants—the so-called free radicals we read so much about—are necessary to fight off in-

fections and heal injuries. On the other hand, antioxidants are necessary to keep excessive pro-oxidant activity in check.

"An intricate biochemical network maintains this balance. But taking high doses of antioxidants in a nutritional supplement may destabilize that network.

"However, antioxidants are important in maintaining and improving health—every doctor and scientist knows that."

Here is the advice Dr. Baum gives his patients to help them get the right amount of antioxidants...

● **Don't take a high-dose antioxidant supplement.** Instead, take a multivitamin-mineral supplement that includes 100% of the Daily Value (DV) of antioxidants (vitamins C, E and beta-carotene and the minerals zinc and selenium).

● **For complete confidence, take an antioxidant test.** For patients who want the most accurate picture of their antioxidant status, Dr. Baum recommends the Spectrox antioxidant test. "It provides the most accurate picture of your antioxidant activity—not just your blood level of antioxidants. If your antioxidant activity is low, your physician can recommend an antioxidant supplement—because you actually need to take it," he says.

Your doctor can find out more about the Sprectrox test at *www.spectracell.com.*

● **Eat more antioxidant-rich food.** Dr. Baum counsels all his patients to increase their antioxidant intake from food. "The way to achieve a healthy level of antioxidants isn't by taking a pill," he says. "It's by increasing your daily intake of antioxidant-rich vegetables and fruits, which deliver a natural balance of these nutrients. Eat a wide range of vegetables and fruits, of many colors—for example, leafy greens, blueberries, yellow corn, oranges and red peppers."

"For the maximum daily intake of antioxidants, try to eat three to five cups of fresh salad, three cups of cooked vegetables and four to five servings of fruit," advises Robin Jeep, coauthor of *The Super Antioxidant Diet and Nutrition Guide* (Hampton Roads).

Jeep points out that whole-grain, legumes and nuts and seeds are also loaded with antioxidants.

"Eating an abundance of natural whole plant foods loaded with antioxidants gives you the ability to reclaim your health," she says.

Red flag: If you have prediabetes or diabetes, both Jeep and Dr. Baum caution against eating too many high-sugar fruits, such as bananas, watermelons, pineapples, kiwis and mangos.

Michael Ristow, MD, professor, Department for Human Nutrition, University of Jena, Germany.

Seth Baum, MD, medical director of Integrative Heart Care in Boca Raton, Florida, and author of *The Total Guide to a Healthy Heart* (Kensington). *www.vitalremedy.com.*

Robin Jeep, chef, life coach and author of *The Super Antioxidant Diet and Nutrition Guide* (Hampton Roads).

Chamomile Tea Protects Against Diabetes Damage

Chamomile is one of the most popular herbal teas. People turn to chamomile tea to calm themselves at bedtime or to reduce cold and flu symptoms. Now recent studies show that this herb may also be helpful in preventing complications from type 2 diabetes.

Chamomile Quenches Free Radicals

According to Stanley Mirsky, MD, an associate clinical professor of medicine at the Mount Sinai School of Medicine in New York and coauthor of the *Diabetes Survival Guide*, chamomile is thought to be beneficial for people with diabetes because it is so rich in antioxidants that fight inflammation.

In Japan and the United Kingdom (same study, multiple international authors in different locations), researchers fed diabetic rats a chamomile extract prepared from the dried flowers of *Matricaria chamomilla* for 21 days. When compared with a similar group of diabetic rats who were fed the same diet

but without the chamomile, the chamomile-treated animals had a significant drop in blood sugar. There was also a decline in two enzymes that are associated with dangerous diabetic complications such as loss of vision, nerve damage and kidney damage.

Results of the study were published in the *Journal of Agricultural and Food Chemistry.* The researchers expressed hope that these preliminary findings might one day lead to a chamomile-based treatment for diabetes that would be cheaper and have fewer side effects than pharmaceutical treatments.

Even as this research continues, it may be helpful to add chamomile tea to your diet. For those who like it (and have no contraindications, as it is known to interact with certain medications), it may be a good substitute for sugary sodas or fruit juices, which can wreak havoc on blood sugar levels. Check with your doctor first.

Stanley Mirsky, MD, associate clinical professor of medicine, Mount Sinai School of Medicine, New York, and coauthor of the *Diabetes Survival Guide* (Ballantine).

Gourmet Cooking Secrets for People with Diabetes

Can people with diabetes eat healthfully and enjoy their meals at the same time? The answer is a resounding "yes," says Chris Smith, author of *The Diabetic Chef's Year-Round Cookbook* (American Diabetes Association). Smith uses fresh, seasonal ingredients to create healthy, interesting meals full of flavor for individuals with diabetes and everyone else at the table, while reducing the salt, sugar and fat that many have come to rely upon to add taste.

Healthy Eating...with Diabetes

Just like the rest of us, people with diabetes should eat nutritious meals that are low in fat (especially saturated and trans fat), moderate in salt and very sparing in sugar, while emphasizing whole grains, vegetables and fruit.

However, because people with diabetes are at a greater risk for life-threatening complications such as hypertension, heart disease and stroke, it's particularly important that they keep blood glucose control while maintaining normal levels of blood pressure and blood lipids (cholesterol). It can be challenging to do all that while still preparing flavorful and appealing food. Here The Diabetic Chef shares his secrets for preparing foods that are appropriate for people with diabetes and delicious enough for everyone.

Herbs and Spices Are Essential

Liven up your meals with garden-fresh herbs, many of which are available year-round. Fresh herbs are densely packed with flavor. You can use herbs in a variety of ways throughout the seasons.

●**Fine herbs,** such as thyme, oregano, dill, basil and chives, are usually available in the spring and summer. These should be added as a finish (at the end of the cooking process) to release their delicate flavors and aromatic qualities. "Use fresh basil with summer tomatoes and olive oil for pasta, or as a finish to a tomato sauce," says Smith. "Use chives as a delicate finish to soups, salads and sauces."

●**Hearty herbs** (rosemary, sage), available year-round, can be added earlier on in the cooking process. Use them with stews, soups and Crock-Pot dishes. They can withstand the heat of cooking without losing flavor and, in fact, the longer they're cooked, the more mellow and flavorful they are, says Smith.

●**Dried herbs must be rehydrated,** so use at the beginning of the cooking process (adding as you sauté onions for a sauce, for example). Your homemade tomato sauce with dried oregano and basil tastes better the next day as the flavor of the dried herbs fully blooms and combines with the other ingredients.

Herb typically describes the leaves of a plant, while spices are derived from any other part—including the root, seeds, bark or buds. Spices can be used to create a medley of flavors and can be evocative of different types of ethnic cuisines. "Spices bring great diversity to food," Smith says.

Other Tips for Healthful Eating

Overall, Smith points out that healthful eating is a matter of practicing what he calls "Nutritional MVP," which stands for moderation, variety and portion control.

From his cookbook, another suggestion is to learn how to do template cooking. Template cooking is taking one recipe and adapting it in different ways by using the same cooking method but substituting different ingredients, says Smith. "It gives you the freedom to be creative, which is the essence of good cooking." It also brings much-needed diversity to meals, so you are not forever serving the same old thing.

One example of a template recipe is the Simple Chicken Breast (see page 135). "There are only seven ingredients in this recipe but you can vary it with fresh, seasonal ingredients," says Smith. "For instance, in springtime you can exchange the olive oil for sesame oil and use lemon grass rather than garlic to create an Asian flavor. In summer, substitute fresh cilantro for the rosemary."

Try different cooking techniques to bring out the essence of foods.

●**Grill, broil, roast, sauté or steam food to enhance flavor without added fat or salt.** Slow-roast vegetables with a drizzle of olive oil in a 400-degree oven to bring out their true flavors. Many develop a natural sweetness when roasted. Season with garlic or add herbs to vary the taste. Rather than sautéing garlic or onions with butter or oil before adding them to soups or stews, try roasting in the oven.

●**Marinate foods in a few ingredients.** "The herbs, lemon and spice in the Simple Chicken Breast recipe create a vibrant flavor, and the extra-virgin olive oil allows the herbs and spices to reach their full bouquet," says Smith.

• **Sear meat** (brown on both sides in a pan for a few minutes before placing it in the oven) to enhance flavor without adding extra fat or salt. "Any kind and cut of meat can be seared," says Smith.

• **Pair dishes with colorful sides.** Instead of a plate full of brown items such as chicken and rice, liven up your plate with deeply colored fruits and vegetables that add variety and important *phytonutrients* (components of fruits and vegetables that are thought to promote health) to your diet.

• **Keep the pantry stocked with these healthy ingredients.**

Oils: extra-virgin olive oil, sesame oil, canola oil and grapeseed oil.

Vinegars: balsamic, champagne, rice and aged sherry vinegar.

Essential spices: cayenne pepper, chili powder, cinnamon, mustard, nutmeg, paprika and pepper.

Essential dry herbs: bay leaves, dill, basil, oregano, rosemary, thyme and sage.

Other essential products: chicken, vegetable and beef broth, dried beans, whole gluten-free grains such as quinoa and amaranth.

Essential fresh ingredients: lemons, limes, oranges, garlic, onions, shallots, carrots, tomatoes, potatoes, mushrooms, butter (salt free), sour cream (fat free), eggs, hard cheeses (Parmesan and Romano), mustard (grain, Dijon), capers and olives.

Template Recipe: Simple Chicken Breast Serves 4

4 chicken breast halves
1 tablespoon extra-virgin olive oil
1 tablespoon dried rosemary
1 tablespoon poultry seasoning
1 teaspoon salt-free lemon pepper
1 tablespoon minced garlic
½ teaspoon red pepper flakes
Cooking spray

1. In medium bowl, combine all ingredients and place chicken breasts in it. Cover and refrigerate 1 hour.

2. Preheat oven to 375°F.

3. Preheat sauté pan to medium-high heat. Spray pan with cooking spray. Add chicken breast to pan and sear to desired color, about 10 seconds, then turn over and sear other side.

4. When both sides are seared, remove chicken from pan and place in a baking dish or cookie sheet. Do not cover. Place in oven. Cook meat until internal temperature reads 165°F. When chicken is done, remove from oven and let rest for two to four minutes.

For more tips from Chef Smith go to: *www.TheDiabeticChef.com.*

Chris Smith, The Diabetic Chef, is an executive chef working in the healthcare field. Author of two cookbooks, *Cooking With the Diabetic Chef* and *The Diabetic Chef's Year-Round Cookbook* (both from American Diabetes Association), he lectures widely about cooking for people with diabetes.

Supplements That Help Manage Diabetes

Lifestyle change has always been the cornerstone treatment for people with type 2 diabetes. Beyond that, natural approaches are rarely discussed. Mark Stengler, NMD, recommends a number of plant-based remedies for those with diabetes, some of which date back hundreds, even thousands, of years…

According to Dr. Stengler, type 2 diabetes absolutely can be prevented and, in certain cases, even reversed with diet, exercise and appropriate dietary supplements.

To Prevent Diabetes…

• **Curb sugar cravings with Gymnema Sylvestre.** A staple of Ayurvedic medicine, this herb helps curb cravings for sugary foods that throw your blood glucose levels off balance.

Dr. Stengler believes gymnema sylvestre works best when used in combination with other glucose-balancing herbs, such as bitter melon and fenugreek. Ask your doctor.

• **Chromium can normalize sugar levels.** Your body requires adequate levels of chromium to properly control blood glucose levels. This essential trace mineral aids in the uptake of blood sugar into the body's cells, where it helps generate energy more efficiently. It can also reduce sweet cravings.

Dr. Stengler advises up to 1,000 micrograms of chromium a day (under your physician's supervision). He adds that this is a good mineral to take with gymnema.

• **Regulate blood sugar with fiber and fiber supplements.** Soluble fiber helps prevent or control prediabetes and diabetes by slowing the rate at which intestines release glucose into the bloodstream, thus modulating fluctuations in blood sugar levels. Rich sources of soluble fiber include plant foods, such as legumes, oat bran, rye, barley, broccoli, carrots, artichokes, peas, prunes, berries and bananas. In a small study in Taiwan, scientists found that supplementation with *glucomannan* (a soluble dietary fiber made from konjac flour) lowered elevated levels of blood lipids and glucose in people with diabetes.

Most Americans eat too much junk food and too little fiber. For his patients who fall into that category, Dr. Stengler typically prescribes one glucomannan capsule 30 minutes before lunch and dinner, and another before bedtime with a large glass of water.

Managing Symptoms...

• **Boost antioxidant levels with alpha-lipoic acid.** This powerful antioxidant kills free radicals that damage cells and cause pain, inflammation, burning, tingling and numbness in people who have peripheral neuropathy (nerve damage) caused by diabetes. Studies also suggest that alpha-lipoic acid (ALA) enables the body to utilize glucose more efficiently.

Dr. Stengler says to take alpha-lipoic acid daily under a physician's supervision.

• **Decrease blood glucose levels with chamomile tea.** Drinking chamomile tea, a rich source of antioxidants, may help prevent diabetes complications, such as blindness, nerve damage and kidney problems, according to recent research by UK and Japanese scientists.

Drink chamomile tea along with antioxidant-rich black, white and green teas, says Dr. Stengler.

• **Take omega-3 fatty acids to reduce inflammation.** These healthy fats improve the body's ability to respond to insulin, reduce inflammation, lower blood lipids and prevent excessive blood clotting. Good dietary sources of omega-3 fatty acids include cold-water fish, such as salmon or cod (eat two or three times a week), olive or canola oil, flaxseed and English walnuts.

Dr. Stengler's advice: Unless you know you are getting sufficient omega-3 fatty acids in your diet, it's good to take a daily fish oil supplement that contains about 1,000 mg of the omega-3 fatty acid *eicosapentaenoic acid* (EPA) and about 500 mg of the omega-3 fatty acid *docosahexaenoic acid* (DHA).

Caution: Because many dietary supplements lower blood sugar, and fish oil supplements may alter the way anticoagulant therapy functions, it is critical to work closely with your doctor before and while taking any of the above supplements. He/she will prescribe the right doses for you.

Diabetes Self-Care...

When addressing a difficult disease such as diabetes, all the nutrients and vitamins in the world will do no good if you do not also follow the basics of diabetes self-care: Maintain a healthy weight...get 20 to 30 minutes of exercise most days of the week...follow a diet that emphasizes lean proteins and healthy fats and limits simple carbohydrates...monitor blood glucose levels...and take diabetes, blood pressure and cholesterol medicine as prescribed by your physician. Dr. Stengler adds that even as simple a measure as taking a 10-minute walk after each meal can keep blood sugar under control. Start today.

Mark A. Stengler, NMD, naturopathic medical doctor in private practice, La Jolla, California, and author of the *Bottom Line/Natural Healing* newsletter. *www.drstengler.com.*

Chapter 7

DIGESTIVE DISORDERS

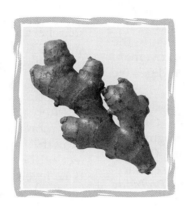

The Amazing Healing Power of Probiotics

The cells in your body are outnumbered—by the bacteria in your intestines!

"A total of one hundred trillion bacteria live in our digestive system—10 times more than the number of cells in our body," says Elizabeth Lipski, PhD, CNN, a clinical nutritionist in Ashville, North Carolina, and author of *Digestive Wellness* (McGraw-Hill).

Some of these bacteria can produce harmful toxins and carcinogens. But many of them are helpful—the so-called *probiotics*. And they're helpful in lots of different ways, says Dr. Lipski. *They...*

- Protect the intestinal lining, preventing colonization by bad bacteria and yeast;

- Stop the growth of bacteria that produce nitrates, a cause of cancer;

- Decrease the side effects of antibiotics, such as diarrhea;

- Stop the absorption of toxins from the gut;

- Manufacture B-complex vitamins;

- Help regulate *peristalsis,* the contraction of the intestinal walls that pushes waste matter through the digestive tract;

- Strengthen immunity;

- Help normalize cholesterol and triglycerides, blood fats that can cause heart disease and

- Break down and rebuild hormones.

"The overall composition of these helpful and harmful bacteria—our *intestinal flora*—usually remains fairly constant in healthy people," says Dr. Lipski. "However, the intestinal flora can become unbalanced—with the harmful bacteria no longer held in check—by aging, poor diet, disease, medications such as antibiotics or stress." In fact, she says, "digestive problems due to imbalanced flora have become widespread."

But, she adds, taking a probiotic supplement or eating foods rich in probiotics can help restore your helpful bacteria and counter those health problems.

Latest Research

Improving digestive well-being. Researchers in France studied 197 women with "minor digestive symptoms," dividing them into two groups. One group ate yogurt rich in the probiotic *bifidobacteria*; the other didn't.

After four weeks, 69% more women in the probiotic group reported an improvement in "GI well-being" and had fewer digestive symptoms.

Products: Yogurts and other food products rich in bifidobacteria include General Mills YoPlus yogurt, TCBY frozen yogurt and Attune Wellness bars, says Tracy Olgeaty Gensler, RD, a dietitian in Chevy Chase, Maryland, and author of *Probiotic and Prebiotic Recipes for Health* (Fair Winds).

• **Relieving irritable bowel syndrome.** Researchers in the US studied 44 people with irritable bowel syndrome—a constellation of digestive symptoms such as abdominal pain, cramping, bloating and diarrhea and/or constipation that affects 10 to 20% of Americans. Half received a daily probiotic supplement of *bacillus coagulans* and half didn't. After two months, those taking the supplement had much less abdominal pain and bloating.

Supplement: Sustenex, with GanedenBC, which is widely available. The dosage used in the study was one capsule a day.

You can find out more about the product at *www.sustenex.com*.

• **Easing ulcerative colitis.** This digestive disease—a severe inflammation of the lining of the colon and rectum—afflicts 500,000 Americans with symptoms such as diarrhea, bloody stools, abdominal pain and cramping, which come and go in flare-ups.

Researchers in India studied 77 people with "mild to moderate" ulcerative colitis, dividing them into two groups. One received a probiotic supplement twice daily for 12 weeks; one didn't.

After three months, 43% of the patients taking the probiotic were in remission. Only 11% of those taking the placebo saw improvement.

Supplement: VSL#3, a supplement with eight different strains of friendly bacteria. It is available at *www.vsl3.com*, or by calling 866-438-8753. Use it with your doctor's approval and supervision.

• **Better health after gastric bypass.** Researchers at Stanford University in California studied 44 patients who had gastric bypass weight-loss surgery. After the surgery, half the patients took a daily supplement of the probiotic *lactobacillus*, and half didn't.

After six months, the probiotic group had lost more weight, had less "bacterial overgrowth" in the stomach (a possible side effect of the surgery), and had higher vitamin B-12 levels (B-12 deficiency is another possible side effect).

Dosage: Lactobacillus supplements are widely available. In this study, the dosage was 2.4 billion organisms daily. (Supplement manufacturers use a number of different names to indicate the number of bacteria in a probiotic, such as *600 million organisms* or *1 billion microbes*, or simply a number after the name of the bacteria.)

• **Controlling gum disease.** Researchers in Japan studied 66 people, giving half of them a daily supplement of *lactobacillus salivarius*, a probiotic found in the mouth.

After two months, those taking the supplement had much lower levels of five types of oral bacteria that cause gum disease.

Probiotic supplements could beneficially affect gum disease, say the researchers, in the *Journal of Clinical Periodontology*.

Dosage: Supplements of lactobacillus salivarius are widely available. In this study, the daily dosage was 2 billion organisms.

• **Boosting immunity after a flu shot.** Researchers in France studied more than 300 people over 70 years of age. For four weeks before receiving a flu (influenza) shot, they drank either a dairy drink rich in the probiotic *lactobacillus casei* or a non-probiotic dairy drink.

In the five months after receiving the shot, those using the probiotic drink manufactured many more "influenza-specific antibodies"—the drink had powered up the immune system's ability to respond to the vaccine.

Product: DanActive yogurt, from Dannon.

• **Lowering cholesterol.** Researchers in Iran studied 14 people with high cholesterol, asking them to eat 10 ounces a day of either "ordinary" yogurt or probiotic yogurt with *lactobacillus acidophilus* and *bifidobacteria*.

After six weeks, those eating the probiotic yogurt had a "significant decrease" in total cholesterol, compared with those eating the ordinary yogurt.

Product: Yogurts containing these two bacteria include Stonyfield Farm low-fat and nonfat frozen yogurts, TCBY frozen yogurt, says Gensler.

Tracy Olgeaty Gensler, RD, dietitian in Chevy Chase, Maryland, and author of *Probiotic and Prebiotic Recipes for Health* (Fair Winds).

Elizabeth Lipski, PhD, CNN, clinical nutritionist in Ashville, North Carolina, and author of *Digestive Wellness* (McGraw-Hill). *www.lizlipski.com.*

Digestive Supplements For Optimum Health

A root cause of many chronic problems often turns out to be poor digestion and inadequate absorption of nutrients. And even most healthy people would feel much better if they improved their digestion. Mark Stengler, NMD, has created a protocol of supplements for better digestion.

Healthy Gut Protocol

In addition to clearing up all kinds of digestion problems, the following protocol gives the immune system a boost. You should experience improved energy, less gas and bloating, better concentration, less arthritis pain and fewer colds and infections.

Another benefit: This protocol helps people with chronic conditions cope with food sensitivities—reactions to foods containing sugar, dairy, wheat, corn or eggs that irritate and inflame the lining of the small intestine. Many holistic practitioners advise patients to identify these sensitivities with an elimination diet, in which one food at a time is avoided to determine if it is an offender. These diets can involve eliminating between 12 and 24 common foods—which can be time-consuming and stressful and deprive the body of valuable nutrients. This protocol enables you to eat many of the foods you want and get the nutrients you need.

Try all of the following supplements because each will have a different effect on digestion. Unless otherwise noted, they are safe for everyone, but discuss your intention to start this protocol with your doctor. Also, be sure to eat a healthful diet, avoiding alcohol, sugar, caffeine and hydrogenated fats (trans fatty acids found in packaged foods).

• **High-potency digestive enzymes.** These plant enzymes assist in the breakdown of all types of food. Because intolerance to dairy products and gluten (a protein in wheat and some other grains) is so common, Dr. Stengler recommends enzymes that contain *dipeptidyl peptidase* (DPP-IV), which help break down gluten and the milk protein casein. Try Integrative Therapeutics Similase GFCF (gluten-free/casein-free) (800-931-1709, *www.integrativeinc.com*). Take two capsules with or at the end of each meal.

Caution: These enzymes do not allow people with celiac disease to eat gluten, although they can help digest hidden gluten in foods. Avoid these enzymes if you have active gastritis or ulcers.

• **N-acetyl d-glucosamine (NAG).** This amino sugar helps to form the mucous coating on the intestine, which protects it from contact with digestive enzymes and acids and helps discriminate between normal and unhealthy particles. NAG seems to directly reduce food-sensitivity reactions. It also may promote a healthy balance of good flora throughout the intestines.

Recommended: NAG made by Allergy Research Group, which is available only through a health-care professional (800-545-9960, *www.allergyresearchgroup.com*). Take 500 mg twice daily before meals.

● **Glutamine.** This amino acid has been shown in several clinical studies to restore intestinal barrier function. It helps promote intestinal cell turnover, guards against intestinal infection and helps soothe inflammation of the digestive tract. Results often include less cramping and abdominal pain. Take 1,000 mg three times daily before meals.

● **Deglycyrrhizinated licorice (DGL).** This type of licorice root extract stimulates intestinal mucus production and has an anti-inflammatory and soothing effect on the lining of the digestive tract. Chew one 400-mg tablet three times daily before meals. One widely available, high-quality DGL is made by Natural Factors (800-322-8704, *www.naturalfactors.com*).

● **Probiotics.** These healthful bacteria help prevent overgrowth of yeast and other potentially harmful organisms in the intestines. They also help break down food and normalize gut immune reactions, reducing food sensitivities. Try probiotics made by Jarrow (800-726-0886, *www.jarrow.com*)...Bio-K+ (800-593-2465, *www.biokplus.com*)...or DDS Multiflora (800-422-3371, *www.uaslabs.com*). Follow instructions on the label.

What to do: Take these supplements for two months, and then evaluate how you feel. Most patients notice a marked improvement in their digestion, energy level and chronic conditions. If you continue to have digestion problems, see a holistic practitioner. If you're doing well, stay on the protocol for three months or more and assess how you feel. If you have a chronic condition and this protocol helps, you can stay on it indefinitely.

Mark A. Stengler, NMD, naturopathic medical doctor in private practice, La Jolla, California, and author of the *Bottom Line/Natural Healing* newsletter. *www.drstengler.com*.

IBS Breakthroughs

If you're among the estimated one in six American adults who suffers from chronic abdominal pain or discomfort due to irritable bowel syndrome (IBS), you know that effective, long-lasting treatment remains elusive.

Good news: The American College of Gastroenterology recently published a review of the most effective treatments, including dietary approaches, nondrug therapies and medications, that should finally give relief to people with IBS.

Do You Have IBS?

With IBS, the nerves that control the gastrointestinal tract are hypersensitive—that is, sensations that other people wouldn't notice, including those produced by the ordinary process of digestion, are amplified and often painful.

Research has shown that many times IBS begins after a severe bout of digestive upset caused by a bacterial or viral infection, such as "stomach flu" or "traveler's diarrhea"—perhaps because such infections temporarily or permanently affect nerves in the gastrointestinal tract.

What most people don't know: Researchers have found that people with a history of abuse (physical, emotional or sexual) are at heightened risk for IBS—probably due to stress on the intestinal nervous system.

Diagnosis of IBS can be tricky because symptoms, including abdominal pain, bloating and troublesome bowel patterns (frequent or persistent bouts of diarrhea, constipation or both, generally occurring at least three days a month), often wax and wane in severity. So-called "flares" (episodes of severe symptoms) may occur weeks, months—or even years—apart.

IBS symptoms that may be missed: Mucus in the stool or straining during, or a feeling of incomplete evacuation after, a bowel movement.

If you think you may have IBS: See your primary care doctor. IBS almost always can be identified with a standard history and physical exam.

When Food Is the Trigger

Lactose intolerance (the inability to digest dairy sugar) can lead to misdiagnosis because its classic symptoms—bloating and diarrhea—mimic those caused by IBS.

Advice: If your digestive problems seem to worsen when you consume dairy products, follow an elimination diet.

What to do: Go without all dairy products for seven to 10 days—and slowly reintroduce each type of dairy product, such as yogurt or cheese, to see how much you can tolerate before symptoms return.

IBS food triggers that often are overlooked—try the elimination diet (as described above) with each...

•**Soft drinks and other high-fructose drinks and foods.** *Fructose*—a sugar commonly added to carbonated soft drinks and sports drinks and naturally occurring in fruit juices and high-sugar fruits (such as dried fruits)—can cause bloating, gas and diarrhea in people with IBS.

•**Caffeine.** It stimulates the digestive tract and may cause cramps and more frequent bowel movements in people with IBS.

The Fiber Factor

For many people with IBS—especially those with recurrent constipation—adequate fiber intake (25 mg to 30 mg per day) helps relieve symptoms. If you are not consuming this much fiber, increase your intake of fruits and whole grains or take a fiber supplement containing psyllium (such as Metamucil or Konsyl).

Recommended fiber-rich foods: Raspberries, artichokes, green peas, almonds, oatmeal, oat bran and whole-grain bread.

Important: IBS patients who have recurrent diarrhea should limit fiber intake to about 10 g daily and avoid leafy greens and cruciferous vegetables (such as cauliflower) because high-fiber foods can worsen symptoms in these patients.

Best Alternative Approaches

If dietary changes (described above) do not relieve IBS symptoms, there is credible scientific evidence to support the use of two natural remedies for IBS...

•**Peppermint oil.** In enteric-coated capsule form, peppermint oil appears to relax smooth muscle in the gastrointestinal tract and therefore reduce IBS abdominal pain caused by muscle spasms. For dosage, follow label instructions.

•**Probiotics.** Probiotics augment the "friendly" bacteria in the large intestine. Probiotic dietary supplements containing the *Bifidobacterium* species are worth trying when bloating and diarrhea are prominent. Look for probiotic supplements providing at least 100 million colony-forming units per dose. Be patient—it may take up to three months to produce substantial benefits.

Best IBS Medications

If your IBS persists, there are medication options for...

•**Diarrhea.** Try an antidiarrheal medication, such as the over-the-counter (OTC) product *loperamide* (Imodium) or the prescription drug *diphenoxylate* and *atropine* (Lomotil). For diarrhea and abdominal pain, consider adding a low-dose of a tricyclic antidepressant, such as *imipramine* (Tofranil) or *amitriptyline* (Elavil). These antidepressants may affect how the brain interprets pain.

•**Pain and bloating.** A tricyclic antidepressant often reduces discomfort and other symptoms, including diarrhea, pain and bloating, to a tolerable level. If the drug causes side effects, such as dry mouth or dizziness, a selective serotonin reuptake inhibitor (SSRI), such as *citalopram* (Celexa) or *fluoxetine* (Prozac), can be used, but there is less proof that SSRIs are effective for IBS symptoms.

•**Constipation.** If you're consuming adequate levels of fiber (described earlier) but still have constipation, you may want to try an OTC laxative, such as *polyethylene glycol* (Miralax) or Milk of Magnesia for seven to 14 days. (See your doctor if symptoms persist after that trial period.) For more extended use, the prescription medication *lubiprostone* (Amitiza) has been shown to be effective for IBS with constipation.

Brian E. Lacy, MD, PhD, associate professor of medicine at Dartmouth Medical School and director of the gastrointestinal motility laboratory at Dartmouth–Hitchcock Medical Center in Lebanon, New Hampshire. He is author of *Making Sense of IBS* (Johns Hopkins).

Healthful Alternatives To Harmful Heartburn Drugs

What if you took a cholesterol-lowering drug and it increased cholesterol? What if you took a painkiller and it triggered pain? What if a drug meant to relieve a symptom caused or worsened the symptom instead?

Well, a new study shows that's exactly what can happen if you take a proton pump inhibitor (PPI), a heartburn medication that stops the production of stomach acid.

Fifteen million Americans have daily heartburn (also called acid indigestion, acid reflux disease, and gastrointestinal reflux disease or GERD)—painful, post-meal burning in your chest or throat when stomach acid leaks into the esophagus, the tube between the mouth and stomach. Another 60 million Americans have heartburn at least once a month.

And tens of millions of Americans take PPIs to control the problem.

Next to cholesterol-lowering statin drugs, PPIs are the most popular medications in the US, with sales totaling more than $11 billion a year—both prescription PPIs and over-the-counter PPIs such as *omeprazole* (Prilosec).

Are people taking so many PPIs because the drug causes the very problem it's meant to prevent? *Maybe...*

Heartburn Drug Causes Heartburn

Researchers from Copenhagen University in Denmark studied 120 healthy people, none

of whom had heartburn, dividing them into two groups.

One group took 40 milligrams a day of the PPI *esomeprazole* (Nexium) for eight weeks. Then they stopped and started a look-alike placebo. The other group took a placebo for twelve weeks. Many of those who took Nexium probably wished they hadn't started the drug—or stopped.

Within two weeks of stopping Nexium, 44% of those previously healthy people had developed GERD. They had burning...they had acid reflux...they had indigestion. Why did they develop heartburn after taking a heartburn drug?

Because of *rebound acid hypersecretion*, say the researchers.

After weeks of near-total suppression of the production of stomach acid by PPIs, acid production "rebounded" and went through the roof after the drug was stopped—causing heartburn.

"The observation that 40% of healthy volunteers—who had never been bothered by heartburn, acid regurgitation or dyspepsia—developed such symptoms in the weeks after cessation of PPIs is remarkable," says Christina Reimer, MD, the study leader.

And, say the researchers, since stopping the PPI can cause heartburn, people who take the drug may become dependent on the medication. They stop the drug...heartburn symptoms return...and they start taking it again to control the symptoms.

In other words, they're literally addicted to their heartburn drug!

Is that why up to 33% of the people who start PPIs stay on the drug—even though PPIs are typically prescribed for a few weeks? The researchers think so.

"Our results justify the speculation that PPI dependency could be one of the explanations for the rapidly and continuously increasing use of PPIs," they write, in *Gastroenterology*.

Think Twice Before Taking

You and your doctor definitely want to think twice before you decide to take PPIs, say researchers from the Mount Sinai School of Medicine in New York who reviewed recent scientific literature on PPIs. And not only because PPIs are potentially addictive. They're also potentially harmful.

"There are many unexpected side effects from this class of drugs," says Kenneth W. Altman, MD, PhD, the study leader.

They can...

• **Increase by 30% your risk of a hip fracture,** probably because PPIs decrease calcium absorption;

• **Increase by 89% your risk of developing "community-acquired" pneumonia (not acquired in the hospital),** probably because of the near-total absence of the stomach acid that typically kills swallowed bacteria;

• **Increase by 30% your risk of developing pneumonia in the hospital** (*Fact:* An estimated 40 to 70% of hospital patients are routinely given PPIs—even if they don't have heartburn);

• **Increase by 25% your risk of re-hospitalization after severe angina or heart attack,** and by 91% your risk of death after severe angina or a heart attack—if you were prescribed the blood thinner *clopidogrel bisulfate* (Plavix) and a PPI, a common prescription pattern;

• **Triple your risk of infection with diarrhea-causing *clostridium difficile*,** the leading cause of diarrhea in hospital patients and

• **Double your risk of a vitamin B-12 deficiency** (*Fact:* Low levels of B-12 are linked to many health problems, including nerve damage and memory loss).

What to Do

If possible, try to control your heartburn with diet and lifestyle changes before you take a PPI, say the researchers in *Otolaryngology —Head and Neck Surgery. The best way to do that...*

• **Figure out what foods are causing your symptoms.** "There are no universal dietary causes of heartburn," says Ronnie Fass, MD, a gastroenterologist and professor of medicine at the University of Arizona in Tucson. "Figure out exactly what worsens your symptoms—whether it's pizza or orange juice—and stay away from that food or beverage."

• **Lose weight.** Studies show that extra pounds double your risk of heartburn—and losing weight is one of the most effective ways to control the problem, says Dr. Fass.

• **Elevate the head of the bed.** Many people have heartburn symptoms during the night—but elevating the head of the bed by a few inches can reliably reduce nighttime heartburn.

What happens: A little extra gravity stops acid from flowing from the stomach into the esophagus.

"Use a 4 x 4 or 4 x 6 piece of wood under the legs at the head of the bed," says Elizabeth Lipski, PhD, CCN, a clinical nutritionist and author of *Digestive Wellness* (McGraw-Hill). "It's such a small change you won't even notice it, but it's enough extra gravity so that it works."

• **Talk to your doctor about stopping the drug.** If you decide you want to stop taking a PPI every day, talk to your doctor about *step-down therapy*—a two- to three-month treatment regimen that gradually lowers the dose of PPI and replaces it with another type of heartburn drug, such as the H2-blocker *ranitidine* (Zantac).

Red flag: PPIs are prescribed not only for heartburn but for a "wide variety of upper gastrointestinal symptoms" such as indigestion, says Kenneth McColl, MD. In fact, up to 70% of people who receive the drug don't have heartburn.

"The current finding that these drugs induce symptoms means that such liberal prescribing is likely to be creating the disease the drugs are designed to treat, and causing patients with no previous need for such therapy to require intermittent or long-term treatment," says Dr. McColl. "PPI therapy should be reserved for those with clear symptoms of heartburn or acid reflux."

Christina Reimer, MD, investigator, Department of Medical Gastroenterology, Copenhagen University, Denmark.

Kenneth W. Altman, associate professor, otolaryngology, Mount Sinai School of Medicine, New York.

Ronnie Fass, MD, gastroenterologist and professor of medicine at the University of Arizona, Tucson.

Elizabeth Lipski, PhD, CCN, clinical nutritionist and author of *Digestive Wellness* (McGraw Hill).

Kenneth McColl, MD, division of cardiovascular and medical sciences, University of Glasgow, Scotland.

Gas Be Gone!

The average person produces one to four pints of gas daily and expels it about 14 times a day. Sometimes gas gets trapped in the body, causing uncomfortable bloating. *What you should know…*

• **Flatulence occurs when bacteria ferment undigested carbohydrates in the colon.** The telltale noise is caused by vibration of the anal opening…odor depends on the foods eaten and types of bacteria present. Flatulence producers include asparagus, beans, bran, broccoli, brussels sprouts, cabbage, corn, onions, pasta, peas, potatoes, prunes and wheat. Dairy foods cause gas in people who lack the enzyme lactase needed to digest the milk sugar lactose. Called *lactose intolerance,* this gets more common with age.

Over-the-counter remedies: Charcoal tablets or *simethicone* (Gas-X) may help by breaking up big gas bubbles. Beano contains an enzyme that breaks down cellulose, a carbohydrate in legumes and cruciferous vegetables—take it just before eating. To help prevent gas, take a daily supplement that contains the probiotic *Bifidobacterium infantis,* such as the brand Align. For lactose intolerance, avoid dairy foods or try Lactaid supplements, which contain lactase.

• **Belching happens after you swallow air.**

Avoid: Fizzy drinks, gum, eating too fast, gulping, using a straw, smoking.

Another culprit: Anxiety makes people breathe rapidly and swallow more often.

Calming: Inhale for five seconds…hold five seconds…exhale for five seconds…hold five seconds…repeat.

See your doctor: If you are troubled by excess flatulence or belching, your doctor can check for underlying gastrointestinal problems.

Douglas A. Drossman, MD, professor in the division of gastroenterology and hepatology, and codirector of the Center for Functional Gastrointestinal and Motility Disorders at University of North Carolina, Chapel Hill, School of Medicine.

How to Stay Regular at 30,000 Feet

Being inactive for several hours and/or becoming dehydrated (which can occur during a plane flight) can slow the movement of stool through the colon, leading to constipation. To stay well-hydrated, drink plenty of water and other liquids, such as fruit and vegetable juices and clear soups. In addition, take an over-the-counter fiber supplement, such as Citrucel, to help prevent constipation. Take two capsules twice a day or one heaping tablespoon of the powdered form in eight ounces of liquid three times daily for three days before your trip. When taking a plane trip, bring some high-fiber food, such as prunes, to eat during the flight.

Charles D. Gerson, MD, codirector, Mind-Body Digestive Center, and clinical professor of medicine, Mount Sinai School of Medicine, both in New York City.

Apple Cider Vinegar For Acid Reflux

Apple cider vinegar (usually diluted in water) can be an effective natural treatment for preventing acid reflux. Acid reflux is caused by a weak or damaged esophageal sphincter (the valve between the stomach and esophagus). The sphincter is supposed to prevent the contents of the stomach from going upward. When it doesn't work properly, stomach acid flows into the esophagus. While there are no studies to prove why it works, vinegar may stimulate better digestive action and the closing of the esophageal sphincter.

Recommended: Mix one tablespoon of vinegar in eight ounces of water (not juice). Drink before meals or when experiencing reflux. In this small amount, vinegar is safe. Large amounts can adversely interact with certain drugs.

Mark A. Stengler, NMD, naturopathic medical doctor in private practice, La Jolla, California, and author of the *Bottom Line/Natural Healing* newsletter. *www.drstengler.com.*

The Common Fat That Triggers Ulcerative Colitis

You definitely don't want *ulcerative colitis*—an inflammatory bowel disease (IBD) that strikes the lining of the colon and rectum. (Crohn's, another IBD, can inflame any part of the intestinal lining.)

You don't want diarrhea that forces you to urgently seek out a bathroom...bloody stools...abdominal pain and cramping...and an increased risk of bowel cancer.

But for reasons scientists haven't figured out, more and more people are joining the estimated 500,000 Americans with the disease—a recent study shows a 49% jump in occurrences over the past decade.

Fortunately, another new study shows that changing your dietary mixture of fatty acids—the building blocks of fat—might keep ulcerative colitis out of your life.

Linoleic Acid Burns the Gut

Researchers in the UK analyzed four years of health data from more than 200,000 Europeans, aged 30 to 74. They found that those with the highest intake of *linoleic acid* were 2.6 times more likely to develop ulcerative colitis, compared with those with the lowest intake. Linoleic acid is a polyunsaturated

omega-6 fatty acid found in beef and pork, in vegetable oils such as corn and safflower and in many margarines.

Red flag: Many fried foods served in restaurants are cooked in oils loaded with linoleic acid.

The researchers also found that those with the highest intake of *docosahexaenoic acid* (DHA) were 77% less likely to develop the disease. DHA is an omega-3 polyunsaturated fatty acid found in fatty fish that live in cold water, such as salmon, mackerel and sardines.

The average age of those in the study diagnosed with ulcerative colitis was 60—and the researchers estimate that 30% of those and other new cases of ulcerative colitis might be caused by high dietary intakes of linoleic acid.

Why is linoleic acid a risk factor for ulcerative colitis?

Theory: In the body, linoleic acid turns into *arachidonic acid*...which is incorporated into the lining of bowel cells...where it breaks down into three inflammatory compounds...all of which are found in high levels in people with ulcerative colitis.

DHA, on the other hand, helps produce compounds that calm inflammation.

Bottom line: A diet lower in linoleic acid might not only help prevent the disease—it might help control the disease in people who already have it, say the researchers.

Protect Against Inflammation

"The omega-6 to omega-3 ratio of the typical diet is about 15-to-1," says Floyd Chilton, PhD, a professor at Wake Forest University in Winston-Salem, NC, and author of *Inflammation Nation* (Fireside). "If we change that ratio to be closer to 5-to-1—and, ideally, to 2-to-1—we can make changes that are very protective against inflammation."

"There are many ways you can increase your intake of omega-3 fatty acids and decrease your intake of omega-6s," says Jennifer Adler, CN, nutritionist, natural foods chef, and adjunct faculty member at Bastyr University in Seattle, Washington.

Their recommendations...

● **Limit vegetable oils.** Cut back on vegetable oils and margarine, says Dr. Chilton.

Smart idea: If a recipe calls for vegetable oil, use olive oil instead. Use "light" or 100% pure olive oil for high-heat cooking.

● **Eat fish with over 500 mg of omega-3 per serving.** These include mackerel, canned albacore tuna, canned sardines, canned wild Alaskan salmon and canned skinless pink salmon.

● **Eat grass-fed beef.** In our modern society, cows are typically fed on a diet of corn and soy, which increases the meat's content of linoleic acid.

Better: Purchase grass-fed beef, which is low in linoleic acid and high in omega-3s. "One study put the omega-6 to omega-3 ratio in conventional beef at 4-to-1, compared with 2-to-1 in grass-fed beef," says Dr. Chilton.

"Look for a label that says, '100% Grass-Fed,' which means the animal has been fed on grass their entire life," says Adler. "Otherwise, the animal may have been fed on corn for the last 90 days of its life—increasing linoleic acid and decreasing omega-3s."

● **Take cod liver oil.** "I frequently recommend that a client take a cod liver oil supplement to increase the intake of omega-3s," she says. "One reason I like cod liver oil more than omega-3 fish oil supplements is that it is also loaded with vitamins A and D."

Product: Carlson's (*www.carlson/labs. com*, 888-234-5656) or Nordic Naturals (*www. nordicnaturals.com*, 800-662-2544). "These brands have third-party testing to guarantee that they are free of contaminants," says Adler. "And they both have a range of flavored products, so the cod liver oil doesn't have an objectionable taste."

Recommended amount: Two tablespoons a day.

● **Make bone broth.** "Simmering bones for 12 hours produces a broth that is rich in collagen, elastin and gelatin, protein compounds that help heal a damaged intestinal tract," says Adler. "For someone with ulcerative colitis, I recommend one to three cups of the broth a day."

Use bone broth instead of water in soup, or in making rice and other grains, says Adler. Or you can drink it like a tea, salting to taste.

To make the broth: Fill a large soup pot with water, leftover bones from a roasted or baked chicken, four carrots, ½ bunch of celery and one or two whole onions. Bring to a gentle boil, then lower heat. Simmer slowly for 12 hours. Strain and refrigerate or freeze for future use.

Floyd Chilton, PhD, professor, physiology and pharmacology, Wake Forest University, Winston-Salem, North Carolina, and author of *Inflammation Nation* (Fireside).

Jennifer Adler, CN, nutritionist, natural foods chef and adjunct faculty member at Bastyr University in Seattle, Washington.

Slow Down Deadly Hepatitis C with a Cup of Coffee

The hepatitis C virus (HCV) infects the livers of an estimated four million Americans, killing 10,000 every year—in many cases when the damaged liver develops cancer.

Another 27,000 people die each year from advanced cirrhosis of the liver, in which the liver becomes fibrotic, so scarred (by excessive alcohol intake, or by a disease such as cystic fibrosis) that it can't function anymore.

People with HCV or cirrhosis might want to buy a new coffee machine.

In the last decade, research has linked coffee and liver health. *Studies show that...*

● Compared with people who don't drink coffee, people who drink one or two cups a day have a 30% lower risk of liver cancer, and people who drink three or more cups a day have a 70% lower risk;

● Coffee drinkers with HCV have a 69% lower risk of developing liver cancer, compared with people with HCV who don't drink coffee and

• People who drink two cups of coffee a day are 40% less likely to die from cirrhosis than people who don't drink coffee.

Those studies were retrospective—they analyzed what people did or didn't do, and linked those habits to health. Now, for the first time, researchers have conducted two prospective studies on coffee and the liver—they tracked coffee drinking while it was happening and matched the amount consumed to the advance of liver disease.

Refill your cup with java and read on…

More Coffee, Less Scarring

In one study, researchers at the Liver Diseases Branch of the National Institutes of Health (NIH) studied 121 people with HVC and 56 people without HVC but with cirrhosis.

First, they gave them a liver biopsy to assess the degree of scarring (*fibrosis*), a measurement of the severity of liver disease. Next, they tracked their coffee intake for six months. Then they gave them a second liver biopsy.

Among people with HVC, those who drank at least two cups of coffee a day had an 81% lower risk of developing additional scarring over the six months.

Among people with cirrhosis but not HVC, drinking two cups of coffee a day was linked with a 67% lower risk of scarring.

When researchers looked at black tea, green tea and decaffeinated coffee intake, they found no link.

In another study, researchers at NIH tracked the coffee intake of 766 people with hepatitis C who had failed to respond to treatment with antiviral drugs.

After nearly four years, those who drank at least three cups of coffee a day were 53% less likely to suffer the severe symptoms of advancing liver disease, such as accumulation of fluid in the abdomen (*ascites*), hemorrhages of veins in the esophagus and stomach, damage to the nervous system and brain (from an accumulation of ammonia in the blood), fibrosis, liver cancer and death.

Why it works: It's probably the caffeine—"the most widely consumed pharmacologically active substance in the world," say German researchers, who explain exactly how this everyday "drug" works in the liver.

Caffeine "degrades" genes named Smad2 and Smad3…which in turn "impairs" signals sent from transforming growth factor beta (TGF-beta), a master controller of cellular growth…and the interference with signaling then "inhibits" the production of connective tissue growth factor in liver cells—and with less growth factor, scars don't form and liver cancer doesn't get going.

The amount of caffeine necessary for the job: About 300 milligrams or two to three cups of coffee a day.

Coffee Is Beneficial

"There is now a lot of scientific literature suggesting that coffee is beneficial in people with liver disease," says Anurag Maheshwari, MD, a gastroenterologist at the Institute for Digestive Health and Liver Disease at Mercy Medical Center in Baltimore, Maryland.

• **Consider coffee.** "It's too soon to recommend that everyone with liver disease go out and drink two or three cups of coffee a day," he adds. "But if a patient asks me about the studies on coffee, I say, 'Yes, these findings are real, and increasing coffee intake is something you can do that may help slow the progression of your disease.'"

Red flag: Don't start drinking coffee or increase your intake if you have high blood pressure, heart arrhythmias or heart disease, says Dr. Maheshwari. Extra caffeine speeds the heart rate, which could worsen heart problems.

Also helpful: A low-salt diet, abstaining from alcohol, eating a balanced diet (without an excess of calories, fat or sugar) and exercising for thirty minutes at least three times a week are also good "lifestyle modifications" for people with liver disease, says Dr. Maheshwari.

Anurag Maheshwari, MD, gastroenterologist at the Institute for Digestive Health and Liver Disease at Mercy Medical Center, Baltimore, Maryland.

Digestive Disorders

How Sand Castles Cause Food Poisoning

You know the most common sources of food poisoning from E. coli bacteria, right? Beef and shellfish. Chicken and eggs. Lettuce and tomatoes. Beach sand.

Beach sand?!?

Surprising: In the last decade, researchers have found that sand from lake and ocean beaches around the US is loaded with E. coli bacteria, one of the most common bacterial causes of gastrointestinal (GI) illness. In fact, the levels in beach sand are typically much higher than the levels in the water right off the beach. (The suspected sources of E. coli in beach sand are bird feces and rotting algae.)

Now, studies are showing that the E. coli in beach sand can increase your risk of digestive problems…

Unsanitary Sand

Researchers from the US Geological Survey (USGS) asked study participants to handle sand from Lake Michigan beaches for one minute. Then they measured E. coli levels on their fingertips—and found levels high enough to close the beach! They estimated that about 1% of people ingesting that fingertip's worth of sand residue would end up with GI illness.

But they also found that submerging the E. coli–coated fingertips in water a couple of times removed more than 90% of the bacteria.

In another study, researchers at the University of North Carolina–Chapel Hill interviewed more than 27,000 people at four lake and three ocean beaches about their "sand contact" at the beach, and then called those same people 10 to 12 days later.

People who had been digging in the sand were 13% more likely to develop GI illness (nausea and stomachache) and 20% more likely to develop diarrhea, compared with people at the beach who didn't dig.

Those who were playfully buried in the sand were 23% more likely to develop GI illness and 24% more likely to develop diarrhea. (Those who were buried were also twice as likely to get sand in their mouths.)

And when the researchers focused their analysis on three ocean beaches, they found even higher rates of digestive difficulty—23% higher levels of GI illness and 43% higher levels of diarrhea for the diggers, and 32% higher levels of GI illness and 47% higher levels of diarrhea for the buried.

Fact: There was no difference in GI illness or diarrhea between those who had gone swimming at the beach and those who hadn't.

After the Beach, Wash Up

"Your mother was right—cleaning your hands before eating really works to reduce disease, especially after handling sand at the beach," says Richard Whitman, PhD, a research ecologist with the USGS, who led the Lake Michigan study.

● **Scrub your hands.** "Simply rinsing your hands before you eat may help reduce the risk," says Dr. Whitman. "But a good scrubbing before you eat is the best way to avoid illness."

You could also use an antibacterial hand sanitizer, such as Purell, he added.

"It's a good idea to wash your hands or use a hand sanitizer after digging or playing in the sand," agrees Christopher D. Heaney, PhD, the leader of the University of North Carolina study.

Red flag: Sand isn't the only problem. Algae in fresh water is loaded with E. coli and other types of pathogens. "You should never touch it," warns Dr. Whitman.

Richard Whitman, PhD, research ecologist with the US Geological Survey.

Christopher D. Heaney, PhD, Kellogg Health Scholar, Department of Epidemiology, University of North Carolina.

The Supplement That Stops Hemorrhoid Pain

If you're 50 or older, chances are fifty-fifty that you have one or more hemorrhoids, swollen and inflamed veins in your lower

148

rectum or anus—because one out of every two adults develops them. "Hemorrhoids are one of the most common medical problems," says Peter Rohdewald, PhD, of the University of Münster, in Germany.

Common causes include straining at stool (usually because of constipation); sitting in a chair for hours every day, day after day; and pregnancy.

A hemorrhoid can painlessly bleed a bit, leaving bright red spots on toilet paper or turn the toilet water red. It can itch. Worst-case scenario is that an internal hemorrhoid can turn into an external hemorrhoid, protruding outside the anus and becoming intensely painful for two or three days—a hemorrhoid "attack."

Treatments range from over-the-counter ointments that soothe everyday pain and itching, to surgery that removes a protruding, bleeding, severely painful hemorrhoid.

And now there's a new and uniquely effective treatment for this most common of anal ailments—a nutritional supplement that can both defuse a hemorrhoid attack and clear up a case of chronic hemorrhoids.

Pycnogenol for Pain Relief

The supplement is *Pycnogenol,* an extract from the bark of the Maritime Pine, a species found in southwest France.

Studies on Pycnogenol show that it can help a condition called *chronic venous insufficiency*—weak veins in the legs that cause varicose veins and leg ulcers. Other studies show it can treat eye disease and kidney problems in people with diabetes…high blood pressure…high cholesterol…arthritis…memory problems in older people…cramps and muscle pain…hot flashes in menopause…jet lag…side effects from radiation in cancer treatment…and many other conditions.

How can one supplement improve so many problems?

Pycnogenol improves *microcirculation*— the movement of blood through tiny vessels called *capillaries*—by strengthening the capillary wall. Pycnogenol is a powerful antioxidant, reducing oxidation, the rustlike

biochemical process that damages cells. And Pycnogenol is anti-inflammatory, dousing the chronic low-grade inflammation that causes and complicates many diseases.

Because of those proven benefits and abilities, a team of Italian researchers that had conducted more than a dozen studies on Pycnogenol theorized the supplement might help hemorrhoids too.

To find out, they studied 84 people in the midst of a hemorrhoid attack, dividing them into two groups.

One group took 300 milligrams (mg) of Pycnogenol for four days and then 150 mg for the following three days. The other group took a placebo.

Both groups also received lifestyle management to relieve constipation—they were advised to eliminate constipating foods such as cheese, take a fiber supplement or stool softener, increase fluids and exercise regularly.

During and after the treatment, the researchers evaluated all the hemorrhoid patients—and Pycnogenol turned out to be a lot more powerful than the placebo…

● **Pain.** After two weeks, those taking Pycnogenol had a 93% decrease in severe hemorrhoidal pain—on a four-point pain scale, their pain levels plummeted from 3.2 to 0.8. Those taking the placebo had a 45% decrease, from 3.4 to 1.9.

● **Bleeding.** This symptom stopped completely in the Pycnogenol group—but continued in those taking the placebo.

● **Everyday activity.** Needless to say, a hemorrhoid attack can interfere with everyday activity, such as working and spending time with family and friends. After two weeks, those on Pycnogenol had much less "impairment of work performance," much less "embarrassment and social withdrawal" and much less impairment in sitting, walking and standing, say the researchers.

● **Long-term control.** Only 5% of those taking Pycnogenol had another hemorrhoid attack within the month, compared with 19% of the placebo group.

"Pycnogenol represents an effective way of controlling the common, disabling problem of acute hemorrhoidal attacks and preventing future acute outbreaks," wrote Gianni Belcaro, MD, PhD, the study leader, in *Phytotherapy Research*.

"Pycnogenol may help relieve hemorrhoid attacks and offer pain relief," agrees Dr. Rohdewald.

Complete Healing

"If you've never been affected by hemorrhoids, you can't imagine what people with the problem go through," says Dr. Rohdewald. "Hemorrhoids can affect every aspect of your daily routine—sitting, walking, standing, your work, your social life—and this study suggests that Pycnogenol can help with all major symptoms."

Suggested intake: For an acute attack, take 300 mg a day for four days, and 150 mg for three days, says Frank Schönlau, PhD, an expert in the use of Pycnogenol. For prevention of acute attacks, and for healing a chronic hemorrhoid, take 150 mg a day.

"Take the Pycnogenol until the healing process is complete—until you no longer have bleeding, or any other symptoms from hemorrhoids," he adds.

About 3% of people who take Pycnogenol experience mild stomach upset. To avoid this side effect, take the supplement with or after a meal, says Dr. Schönlau.

Pycnogenol is available from many different supplement manufacturers.

Peter Rohdewald, PhD, professor, Institute of Pharmaceutical Chemistry, University of Münster.

Gianni Belcaro, lead researcher, Department of Biomedical Sciences, University of Chieti, Italy.

Frank Schönlau, PhD, biochemist and researcher specializing in Pycnogenol, Horphag Research. *www.pycnogenol.com.*

Why You Must Keep Your Kidneys Healthy

There's a big threat to your kidney that doesn't get much press. It's chronic kidney disease (CKD), an unheralded epidemic that is damaging and destroying the kidneys of more than 26 million Americans—one in every eight of us.

But you should know about CKD—so you can prevent it or stop it from getting worse.

Healthy kidneys filter and clean the blood, help maintain the body's acid-alkaline balance, manufacture hormones that regulate blood pressure and produce a form of vitamin D that strengthens the bones, explains Katherine Tuttle, MD, clinical professor of medicine in the Division of Nephrology at the University of Washington School of Medicine.

"They are absolutely essential to health," she says. "And it is essential that you maintain their function."

That's because *end-stage renal failure* (ESRF)—the last stage of CKD, which can appear suddenly after decades of steady, symptomless decline in kidney function—is a health disaster.

If you're one of the nearly 500,000 Americans with ESRF, you'll need dialysis, the regular cleaning of your blood by a machine. And you may join the queue for a kidney transplant—a line that now has approximately 50,000 people in it.

As for likely symptoms—as unfiltered toxins build up in your blood, you feel tired and generally sick…your skin itches…you're nauseated, with little appetite, and lose weight…your hands and feet swell with excess fluid…you bruise easily…you're thirsty all the time…and your bones hurt.

And 86,000 people with ESRF die every year.

Fact: If you're given a diagnosis of Stage 3 CKD (ESRF is Stage 5), your chances of survival are the same as if you were given a diagnosis of lung cancer.

Several standard tests can detect a decline in kidney function, the hallmark of CKD. If it's declining, your doctor can take appropriate measures. And medications can help control the two diseases that cause 60% of all cases of CKD—type 2 diabetes and high blood pressure.

Important: Anyone with diabetes or high blood pressure should have a test for *glomerular filtration rate* (GFR)—the standard measurement for determining kidney function—as part of their annual physical, says Dr. Tuttle. "But the rate of physicians performing this test is woefully low, with less than 50% of people with diabetes and high blood pressure receiving it."

But aside from appropriate medical care, several new studies show that self-care can help prevent or slow a decline in kidney function.

Newest Research

It's surprisingly easy to be nice to your kidneys...

• **Drink less diet soda.** Drinking two or more diet sodas a day may double your risk of declining kidney function, says Julie Lin, MD, an assistant professor of medicine at Brigham and Women's Hospital, Boston.

Dr. Lin analyzed 11 years of health and dietary data from more than 3,000 women and found that those who drank two or more diet sodas a day were twice as likely to have a 30% decline in GFR, compared with women drinking less than two sodas a day. (And this finding was independent of other factors that might cause kidney decline, such as diabetes and high blood pressure.)

She and her colleagues didn't find any link between decline in kidney function and sugar-sweetened beverages.

What to do: You may want to limit your intake of diet soda to no more than one a day, says Dr. Lin.

Consider drinking other, healthier beverages, such as water, tea and fruit juice within reasonable limits, says Dr. Tuttle.

• **Use less salt.** In her research, Dr. Lin also found that women with the most sodium (salt) in their diet had a 52% higher risk of a significant decline in GFR, compared with women getting the least sodium.

What to do: If you have a concern about a decline in kidney function—if you have diabetes, high blood pressure or GFR tests that show a decline—think seriously about following a low-sodium diet, says Dr. Lin.

"Taking the salt shaker off the table is the first step in restricting sodium," says Stephen Sinatra, MD, a cardiologist in private practice in Manchester, Connecticut, assistant clinical professor at the University of Connecticut Medical School and author of *Lower Your Blood Pressure in Eight Weeks* (Ballantine).

But he points out that an estimated 80% of sodium intake is from hidden sources—mostly packaged and prepared foods, such as frozen meals, soups, ice cream, bread, canned vegetables and pickles. "I encourage my patients to keep a food diary for several days, and then go back and look up the sodium content of each item on their list. They're usually shocked to find that they've been consuming between 5 and 10 grams of sodium every day—without sprinkling a single grain of salt on their food! I advise them to limit their sodium intake to 2 to 3 grams a day."

Red flags: Other packaged and processed foods that are typically high in sodium include salted nuts, potato chips, most crackers (unless labeled "unsalted" or "no added salt"), processed meats, olives, anchovies, soy sauce, bacon, most cheeses, most peanut butters, canned or bottled tomato juice, creamed cottage cheese, instant puddings and most instant hot cereals.

• **Exercise a little.** Researchers at the VA Healthcare System in Salt Lake City analyzed health data from more than 15,000 people and found that active people with CKD were 56% less likely to die than inactive people. But even a little bit of activity helped—people with CKD categorized as "insufficiently active" were 42% less likely to die than the fully inactive.

What to do: Walk one mile a day, or about 20 minutes at a brisk pace, says Dr. Sinatra. "Walking is the easiest, safest exercise."

Smart idea: Buy a pedometer—a small device that is clipped onto your waistband or belt and measures the amount of steps you take. A review of studies on pedometers, involving nearly 3,000 people, shows that using a pedometer can increase the amount of walking by almost exactly 1 mile per day (2,491 steps). The study was published in the *Journal of the American Medical Association.*

• **Lose a few pounds.** Researchers at the Cleveland Clinic analyzed studies on weight loss in overweight people with CKD. They found that losing just eight pounds significantly slowed decline in kidney function. The findings were in the *Clinical Journal of the American Society of Nephrology.*

What to do: "Small changes are the key to weight-loss success," says James Hill, PhD, cofounder of the National Weight Control Registry, and director of the Center for Human Nutrition at the University of Colorado. "You don't have to achieve your weight-loss goal right away. You just have to keep moving toward your goal, step by small step. The small changes are the way to get to—and sustain—the big change of permanent weight-loss."

Three small changes…

• **Eat a bowl of soup.** "The next time you feel hungry, try a large soothing bowl of broth-based soup," says Barbara Rolls, PhD, a professor of nutrition at Pennsylvania State University, and author of *The Volumetrics Eating Plan* (HarperCollins). "If you have it as a first course at lunch, it will be easier to eat fewer calories during lunch, and you probably won't eat more at dinner. If you have it as a first course at dinner, you're likely to eat less at that meal, too."

• **Eat slowly.** Research shows that people who eat slowly eat about 200 calories less a day than people who eat fast. "That's a big difference in calorie intake," says Kathleen Melanson, PhD, RD, an assistant professor in the Department of Nutrition and Food Sciences at the University of Rhode Island, who conducted the study. To eat slowly, put down your utensil between bites.

• **And remember to wear that pedometer.** A study by Italian researchers shows that people wearing and using pedometers were more likely to lose 10% of their weight than people who didn't wear them.

Katherine Tuttle, MD, clinical professor of medicine in the Division of Nephrology at the University of Washington School of Medicine.

Julie Lin, MD, assistant professor of medicine at Brigham and Women's Hospital, Boston.

Stephen Sinatra, MD, cardiologist, assistant professor, University of Connecticut Medical School.

James Hill, PhD, cofounder of the National Weight Control Registry and director of the Center for Human Nutrition at the University of Colorado.

Barbara Rolls, PhD, professor of nutrition at Pennsylvania State University, and author of *The Volumetrics Eating Plan* (HarperCollins).

Kathleen Melanson, PhD, RD, assistant professor, Department of Nutrition and Food Sciences, University of Rhode Island.

When to Worry About Constipation And Diarrhea

Bowel movements are hardly the stuff of polite dinner table conversation, so it's not surprising that many people don't know exactly what healthy, normal bowel habits are. The reality is that "normal" varies from person to person. And whatever normal is, it needs to stay that way in order for you to avoid other health challenges down the road. What changes might be worrisome?

Normal or Not?

Bowel movements vary in their degree of regularity, color, texture, odor and difficulty. It can be normal to have three a day or as few as three a week. The normal, healthy stool color is dark butterscotch, says Andrew L. Rubman, ND, but that can be affected by what you eat—especially if you had spinach or beets, for instance. The shape should be something like a sausage—soft but solid… relatively easy to pass…and emerging in one nearly continuous movement, as the different segments of the colon consecutively empty.

Constipation and Diarrhea: When to Worry

Constipation and diarrhea are the most common complaints, affecting most people from time to time, and not particularly worrisome on an occasional basis. You qualify as *constipated* if you have fewer than three bowel movements a week, with stools that are hard, dry and difficult to pass. There's often related abdominal discomfort and bloating as well. Dehydration, inadequate dietary fiber and a lack of exercise are the usual causes, according to Dr. Rubman.

As many people already know, you can help move matters along by eating more fiber-rich foods (e.g., whole grains, vegetables and fruits) and fewer processed foods. Various fiber supplements may also be helpful. Discuss with your doctor what type you should take. Exercising about 30 minutes most days of the week will also help ease constipation.

Diarrhea refers to loose, watery stools more than three times in a day. It's usually temporary—perhaps caused by food, antibiotics or the stomach flu—and typically clears on its own without treatment. In the meantime, good foods to eat include bananas, rice, applesauce and toast (called the BRAT diet) and Dr. Rubman also recommends egg drop soup, since diarrhea depletes not only water but salt and albumin (protein) as well. Consult your doctor if diarrhea persists longer than three days...if you become dehydrated...or you see blood, frothiness or large amounts of mucus.

What Changes Do You Need to Report?

Occasional digestive disturbances are part of life, but if you notice significant changes in regularity, color, texture or experience difficulty in passing stool for longer than a few weeks, it's time to take notice. Dr. Rubman suggests keeping a journal to help you identify what is different, including dietary factors, and advises seeing your doctor. Such changes may signal any of a number of digestive challenges—e.g., hemorrhoids, irritable bowel syndrome, ulcerative colitis or colorectal cancer (especially if you're 50 or older). In particular, always call your doctor if you see blood in the stool. Any abnormal color that lasts more than a few days and can't be traced to something you ate is a reason to call your doctor—most especially if it is accompanied by other symptoms, such as abdominal pain or unexplained weight loss. The earlier you diagnose and address any gastrointestinal disorder, the more successful the treatment.

Keep Your Digestive Tract on Track

To keep digestion on the right track, Dr. Rubman advises that you watch your diet and get regular exercise....avoid prolonged use of antacids or anti-inflammatory drugs such as ibuprofen, naproxen or aspirin...refrain from alcohol or tobacco use...chew food thoroughly...and limit water with meals. If you notice changes or are concerned about any symptoms, a naturopathic physician, specially trained and attuned to digestive issues, will be able to examine the state of your digestive function by ordering diagnostic tests, recommending diet and lifestyle changes and prescribing medicines, such as nutrients in which you are deficient. If necessary, he/she will refer you to a gastroenterologist for further treatment.

Andrew L. Rubman, ND, medical director, Southbury Clinic for Traditional Medicines, Southbury, Connecticut. *www.naturopath.org.*

Natural Ulcer Treatments

Gastric ulcers are a perfect illustration of the way medical thinking can change dramatically over a relatively brief period of time. It wasn't long ago that most people—including doctors—believed stomach ulcers were the result of intemperate living, primarily caused by spicy foods and stress. Scientists then discovered that in many cases, the real culprit was *Helicobacter pylori bacteria,* so that became the new target of treatment. Then they learned that killing off H. pylori can increase risk of cancer, so now the latest thinking represents another shift—instead of aiming for eradication of H. pylori altogether, the goal is control of the bacteria so that it remains in a healthy balance. This, it's believed, can fortify the digestive system…and ultimately support optimal overall health.

What Causes Ulcers?

One important role of the linings of the stomach and intestine is to protect against stomach acid and bacteria, but when intestinal balance is disturbed—for example, when H. pylori bacteria run rampant and begin replicating uncontrollably—the digestive tract becomes irritated and inflamed (*gastritis*), a condition that over time weakens and damages the protective mucus coating. If a sore or erosion then develops in the lining of the stomach or *duodenum* (the first part of the small intestine), you have an ulcer. In addition to H. pylori, other possible causes of ulcers include a high intake of aspirin, ibuprofen or other NSAIDs (non-steroidal anti-inflammatory drugs), alcohol use or smoking. Some people believe stress contributes to ulcers, but scientists continue to debate the issue.

Whatever their cause, ulcers are painful and can disrupt your life. To prevent that from happening, treatment for serious ulcers generally consists of seven to 10 days of prescription proton pump inhibitors (PPIs) to suppress stomach acid and give the tissue a chance to heal, plus a longer course of antibiotics to suppress H. pylori bacteria. Taking PPIs for much longer than 10 days—a common mistake—can backfire and alter the natural acid-producing abilities of the stomach. As for antibiotics, bacteria are becoming increasingly resistant to these drugs, which makes it all the more important to identify other means of treatment.

Give Your Stomach a Rest

Andrew L. Rubman, ND, stresses that the single most important rule in treatment and recovery is to give your stomach and digestive tract a rest. Just as you need additional rest to recover from illness or injury, Dr. Rub-

man advises taking measures to allow your digestive system to heal. He said that natural care is also beneficial, even as an adjunct to the pharmaceutical drugs necessary to treat severe ulcers. Specific advice includes eating smaller meals, three or four times a day, consisting of light proteins with easier to digest fats, like boiled eggs and steamed chicken…fresh low-fiber vegetables and their juices…and soft rice. Chew food slowly and thoroughly…limit fluid with meals…don't eat within two hours of bedtime…don't smoke or take NSAIDs…and avoid stomach irritants such as heavy animal protein (including beef, lamb and others), fatty and fried foods, stimulating spices like black pepper, spicy dishes, refined sugars, colas, caffeine and alcohol.

In his practice, Dr. Rubman also prescribes some combination of the following to ulcer patients…

● **L-Glutamine.** In a study at Beth Israel Deaconess Medical Center in Boston, mice that were infected with H. pylori and given supplemental L-glutamine experienced a significant improvement in gastric inflammation and early immune response, which helps to minimize further inflammation and damage. Dr. Rubman prescribes this simple amino acid to support mucosa and protect against gastric damage. Take it in the form of gelatin capsules, apart from meals in a little applesauce.

● **Botanical medicines.** To soothe the stomach and speed healing of delicate mucus membranes, Dr. Rubman prescribes Glyconda, a ready-made mixture of Turkey rhubarb root, cinnamon and goldenseal (you can buy it under the name Neutralizing Cordial O at *www.eclecticherb.com*). Dr. Rubman tells his patients to dissolve 10 to 20 drops in two ounces of warm tea or water and drink before meals. Ask your doctor about the right dosing for you.

Preventive Strategies

Digestive enzymes can help you better absorb nutrients by working alongside the natural enzymes produced by your body to break down chemical bonds in foods. This process helps re-establish a more balanced environment in the gastrointestinal tract so your gastritis and the scar left by the ulcer will heal completely. Though it may seem counterintuitive to take additional acids when your stomach lining is irritated, supplemental digestive enzymes properly prescribed can in fact be helpful to the digestive process for middle-aged and older individuals whose natural stomach acid levels are waning. Dr. Rubman often prescribes DuoZyme by Karuna (*www.karunahealth. com*) due to its combination of assorted enzymes. Take the dose prescribed by your doctor at the beginning of meals (check whether you should adjust for meal size and composition). Don't self-prescribe—taking the wrong amount can cause inappropriate acid release when the stomach is empty, of particular concern for those with a history of acute gastritis or ulcers.

• **Ulcers are dangerous.** Dr. Rubman emphasizes the importance of not undertaking treatment—natural or otherwise—on your own. It's far better and more effective, he said, to work with a physician who is expert in digestive issues and can help you learn to encourage your body's own natural healing processes to successfully cope with ulcers and other stomach and digestive challenges.

Andrew Rubman, ND, director, Southbury Clinic for Traditional Medicines, Southbury, Connecticut. *www.natur opath.org.*

The Power of Pickles

Foods that are pickled (fermented) dish up serious health benefits. Specifically, they are really good for soothing digestive discomfort of all kinds. Counterintuitive as it may be, eating fermented foods—not only pickled cucumbers, but also peppers, tomatoes and sauerkraut—is a simple and tasty way to resolve heartburn, bellyaches and other intestinal distress.

Pickling is an ancient preservation technique with healthful results. British seamen ate sauerkraut to ward off scurvy...Bulgarians were believed to live longer because they drank fermented milk...and Koreans today eat more than 40 pounds per year of *kimchi* (a blend of cabbage, garlic, chilis and other ingredients) both for taste and to ease digestion.

Pickling Promotes Digestion

The fermentation of foods takes place through the breakdown of carbohydrates by live microorganisms such as bacteria (for instance, *Lactobacillus acidophilus* or *Lactobacillus bulgaricus*), yeasts and molds. Kimchi, pickles, sauerkraut and the like act as probiotics, encouraging the growth of positive intestinal microbes. These fermented foods promote efficient digestion, support immune function and boost good nutrition overall. They support availability of B vitamins in certain foods and essential amino acids. They also serve to counteract the ill effects of antibiotics.

According to Dr. Rubman, fermented foods are far better than the over-the-counter antacids or the proton pump inhibitors (PPIs) people routinely swallow to relieve heartburn and stomach upset, which end up causing more harm than good. While they may provide temporary relief, use of antacids or PPIs can backfire because you need acid to efficiently digest foods...and insufficient stomach acid can upset the proper environmental balance of intestinal flora. In contrast, fermented foods encourage the growth of good gut flora while also helping to neutralize the small amounts of stomach acid left in the system between meals, which is a common problem for people with gastritis and GERD.

Pick a Peck...

Eating fermented foods a few times a week can make a real difference in how well your digestive system functions. It's easy enough to do—you can spice up stews with a ¼ cup of kimchi, enjoy a bowl of miso soup, slice pickled cucumbers or peppers onto sand-wiches or spoon yogurt over fresh fruit. *To find fermented foods, visit your local health or gourmet store or shop online…*

• **Order fermented foods from farms such as Wills Valley Farm Products** (*www. willsvalley.com*) in Lancaster County, Penn-sylvania, which offers fermented vegetables including kimchi, red cabbage, red beets and ginger carrots. Other American picklers in-clude Adamah Farm in Falls Village, Connect-icut (*www.isabellafreedman.org/adamah/ products*) and Alexander Valley Gourmet in Healdsburg, California (*www.alvalgourmet. com*). In New York City, classic Lower East Side vendors Russ & Daughters (*www.russ anddaughters.com*) and Pickle Guys (*www. nycpickleguys.com*) are great sources. You can find many more online.

• **Visit food festivals that celebrate pick-ling,** such as New York City's International Pickle Day (*www.nyfoodmuseum.org*).

• **Go international.** Explore fermented foods from around the world, such as the pickled Asian plums known as *umeboshi*. In Japan, these have been consumed for thou-sands of years for their purported ability to counter nausea, stimulate the digestive sys-tem and promote the elimination of toxins. Find them in Asian and gourmet markets and on Web sites such as *www.kushistore.com.*

• **Choose carefully.** Read labels and buy fermented products that are low in sugar and contain live or active cultures. Dr. Rubman warns that most brands of yogurt, in par-ticular, are loaded with sugar and artificial flavoring, but he notes that Stonyfield Farm and Nancy's are two organic brands that contain live bacterial cultures and no artifi-cial ingredients.

In cases of active intestinal disturbances such as irritable bowel syndrome or gastritis, Dr. Rubman sometimes prescribes ferment-ed foods and/or probiotics (supplements that you can take if you don't enjoy the taste of fer-mented foods), but he does not recommend that you try this on your own. See a quali-fied and experienced naturopathic physician who can assess your condition and prescribe an appropriate dosage. But if you're in good health, pile pickles on your plate…pucker up…and enjoy.

Andrew L. Rubman, ND, medical director, Southbury Clinic for Traditional Medicines, Southbury, Connecticut. www.naturopath.org.

Probiotics Combat Celiac Disease

Researchers from the National Spanish Research Council have found that pro-biotics, healthful bacteria, can reduce inflammation and improve the quality of life for patients with celiac disease (CD), a digestive disorder that damages the small intestine and interferes with absorption of nutrients from food. Even people with CD who control the dis-order by eating a gluten-free diet can benefit from a probiotic—to help them avoid symptoms when they digest even a small amount of gluten. CD patients can speak to their physicians about tak-ing a probiotic containing healthy bac-teria such as *Bifidobacteria*.

Mark A. Stengler, NMD, naturopathic medical doctor in private practice, La Jolla, California, and author of the Bottom Line/Natural Healing newslet-ter. www.drstengler.com.

Avoid Air Pollution to Prevent Appendicitis

Air pollution has long been linked with respiratory problems including asth-ma and emphysema, and studies have also associated it with cardiovascular disease. The latest finding by Canadian researchers suggests there may be a link between pollu-tion and appendicitis.

At the University of Calgary, Gilaad G. Ka-plan, MD, MPH, and his colleagues studied the records of more than 5,000 adults hospitalized for appendicitis between 1999 and 2005. Next, using figures from Canada's National Air Pollution Surveillance (NAPS) Network, they looked for possible links between the occurrence of appendicitis and daily air levels of ozone, nitrogen dioxide, sulfur dioxide, carbon monoxide and particulate matter pollutants. Investigators found that...

• **On days with the highest ozone concentration compared with days of lowest ozone concentration, people were approximately 15% more likely to be hospitalized for appendicitis.**

• **The impact of air pollution levels was most dramatic in the summer when people spend more time outside.** During the summer months, exposure to high concentrations of nitrogen dioxide and ozone were significantly associated with admission to a hospital for appendicitis, even after adjusting for temperature and humidity.

Earlier research demonstrates that exposure to these sorts of air pollutants may contribute to disease through an increase in inflammation and oxidative stress, causing the formation of free radical molecules. Dr. Kaplan believes that these same mechanisms may bring on appendicitis. Further research is necessary to corroborate this association and to determine the importance of this connection and what short- and long-term effects pollution may have on disease processes, including appendicitis.

What to Do

What can we do in the meantime? Andrew L. Rubman, ND, points out that the proper nutrients help the body to defend itself against even insults like smog. "The appendix functions with aid from well-digested, healthy foods that contain a broad range of nutrients and antioxidants. So your best bet is to rely on smart eating and professional oversight to help your natural defenses with multivitamin supplementation."

Beyond that, make sure you follow all the usual advice about avoiding air pollution as much as you reasonably can. You can check local air quality reports daily at airnow.gov.

Gilaad G. Kaplan, MD, MPH, assistant professor of medicine, departments of medicine and community health sciences, University of Calgary, Calgary, Alberta, Canada.

Andrew L. Rubman, ND, medical director, Southbury Clinic for Traditional Medicines, Southbury, Connecticut. *www.naturopath.org.*

Popcorn, Nuts and Corn Okay After Diverticular Disease

One of those long-standing "rules" in medicine has been that people who've had diverticular disease should not eat nuts, popcorn or corn. But as with so many medical conventions, this one is being called into question. New research finds no evidence to support the recommendation...and in fact, suggests that some of these nutrient-packed foods may actually help reduce the risk of diverticulitis.

Challenging Conventional Wisdom

Diverticular disease is a common digestive disorder, affecting about half of Americans over age 60. *Diverticulosis* is a condition where bulging pouches (diverticula), about the size of a pea or larger, form in the large intestine or colon wall...while diverticulitis refers to infection or inflammation that can cause symptoms such as abdominal pain, fever and nausea. Ten to 25% of people with diverticulosis develop diverticulitis.

Researchers at the Harvard School of Public Health and Harvard Medical School in Boston and the University of Washington School of Medicine in Seattle looked into the connection between consumption of nuts, popcorn and corn and diverticular disease in more than 47,000 men. At the outset, none of the participants (age 40 to 75) had diverticulosis or its complications, cancer or inflammatory bowel disease. From 1986 to 2004, the men filled out questionnaires on their medical status every two years and on their diet every four years.

In the 18 years of follow-up, 801 men developed diverticulitis and 383 experienced diverticular bleeding. Assistant professor, division of gastroenterology at University of Washington School of Medicine, Lisa L. Strate, MD, MPH, who led the research team, reveals the surprising findings.

• Nuts, popcorn and/or corn consumption is not associated with an increased risk of diverticulitis or diverticular complications.

• Men who ate nuts at least twice a week experienced a 20% lower risk of diverticulitis, compared with those who consumed nuts less than once a month.

• Men who ate popcorn at least twice weekly experienced a 28% lower risk of diverticulitis, compared with those who consumed popcorn less than once a month.

Results of this study were published in the *Journal of the American Medical Association*.

The theory behind the old recommendation was that foods like popcorn, nuts and corn are only partially broken down by digestion. The concern was that the remaining kernels and particles were abrasive and might get lodged within diverticula, where they could cause blockage or bleeding.

Based on the results of this study, Dr. Strate believes this advice should be reconsidered. Of course, if you know you are allergic or intolerant to nuts or other foods, you should continue to avoid them. But if these foods have not caused problems before and you enjoy them, you can probably continue to do so even after a bout with diverticular disease—check with your doctor to make sure.

Lisa L. Strate, MD, MPH, assistant professor, division of gastroenterology, University of Washington School of Medicine, Seattle, Washington.

Chapter 8

EYES, EARS & TEETH

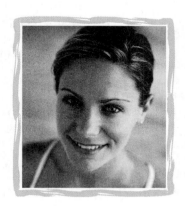

Supplements That Slow (Or Stop!) Age-Related Macular Degeneration

Aging isn't kind to your eyes.

Twenty percent of Americans aged 65 to 74...and 35% over age 75... have *age-related macular degeneration* (AMD)—the number-one cause of vision loss and blindness.

What happens: At the back of the eyeball is the retina, which converts light into electrical impulses that are sent to the brain. In the center of the retina is the *macula*, a tiny collection of cells that deliver your sharpest vision. In AMD, the cells of the macula begin to break down—along with your eyesight.

Doctors divide AMD into early and advanced stages. In early AMD, there may be bent or wavy lines in the center of your vision. The lines gradually widen to a blotch that is blurry, blank or dark. In advanced AMD, the blotch slowly spreads like a fog, enveloping everything in a hazy, sight-erasing monochrome—the pages of a book, the faces of family and friends, the TV screen, the stairs, a road sign, the road.

(There are two types of AMD that produce these symptoms—the slow-progressing *dry* type or the fast-progressing *wet* type. Ninety percent of people with AMD have the dry type. Wet AMD is a medical emergency. If you have AMD symptoms, an examination by an ophthalmologist can determine if you have wet or dry.)

Good news: Several recent studies show that specific nutritional supplements and foods can dramatically slow—or even stop—the progression of AMD from early to advanced.

Newest Research

Researchers at Queen's University Center of Vision and Vascular Science in Belfast, Ireland, studied 400 people with early AMD, dividing them into two groups.

One group took a supplement containing several macula-protecting nutrients that included…

- **Lutein and zeaxanthin,** pigments (known as carotenoids) found in dark green and yellow vegetables that work in the macula like internal sunglasses, shielding its cells from damage.

- **Vitamin C, vitamin E and zinc,** three powerful antioxidants that protect macular cells from oxidation, a kind of biochemical rust.

The other group took a placebo.

After five years, those taking the supplement had a much slower progression from early to advanced AMD—and far less loss of eyesight.

How it works: The supplement works by preserving *macular pigments,* coloring in the retina that absorbs cell-damaging ultraviolet light, explains Usha Chakravarthy, MD, the study leader.

In another recent study on AMD, researchers at the Laboratory for Nutrition and Vision Research at Tufts University in Boston analyzed eight years of diet and health data from nearly 3,000 people with early AMD, aged 55 to 80.

Those with diets richest in *docosahexaenoic acid* (DHA) and *eicosapentaenoic acid* (EPA)—omega-3 fatty acids found in fatty fish such as salmon and mackerel—were 26% less likely to progress to advanced AMD, compared with those with diets poorest in the fatty acids. The findings were in the *British Journal of Ophthalmology.*

How it works: Omega-3 fatty acids may protect the cells of the macula in several ways, say researchers from the government's National Eye Institute—by boosting circulation, reducing the cell-harming effects of sunlight, cutting inflammation and improving the efficient communication within cells (*cell signaling*) that helps keep them healthy.

Formulas That Work

- **Take an eye-protecting nutritional supplement.** "I think everybody over 50 should take a macula-protecting vision support nutritional formula similar to that used by the Irish researchers," says Marc Grossman, OD, LAc, an optometrist in private practice in Rye and New Paltz, New York. "Not only can it help slow the progression of macular degeneration—it can also help prevent the eye disease, and reduce the risk of cataracts.

Several products contain a formula similar to the one used in the Irish study (which is not yet available commercially), says Dr. Grossman.

They include…

- **PreserVision with Lutein Eye Formula,** from Bausch & Lomb.

- **VitEyes AREDS Formula Plus Lutein,** available at *www.viteyes.com,* or call 800-890-3937.

- **Macular Health** (which a recent two-year study shows improves the vision of people with AMD by an average of 17%), available at *www.macularhealth.com,* or call 800-980-6551.

- **Dr. Grossman's Advanced Eye & Vision Support Formula,** available at *www.natural eyecare.com,* or call 845-255-8222.

- **Increase your intake of omega-3.** "Eating two to three servings of fatty fish such as salmon, tuna, mackerel and herring every week would achieve the recommended daily intake of DHA and EPA linked in our study to a decreased risk of advanced AMD," says Chung-Jung Chiu, DDS, PhD, a study researcher from Tufts University.

But the majority of Americans don't eat this much fish, he adds. "If changing dietary habits isn't easy, supplementation with omega-3 fatty acids is an option."

Recommended intake: A daily supplement that supplies 2,000 mg of DHA and EPA, says Dr. Grossman. "In my practice, I use the brands Carlson and Nordic Naturals, because they're high-quality and not pricey."

Both companies manufacture several formulations containing omega-3s. The Carlson Web site is *www.carlsonlabs.com,* or call 888-234-5656. The Nordic Naturals Web site is *www.nordicnaturals.com*, or call 800-662-2544. Both brands are widely available in retail stores.

•**Eat more whole grains.** The *glycemic index* (GI) is a measurement of how quickly carbohydrates break down into blood sugar. Unrefined carbohydrates that break down slowly—like whole-wheat bread—are "low" GI. Refined carbohydrates that break down quickly—like white bread—are "high" GI. In their study, the Tufts researchers found that people eating a low-GI diet were 24% less likely to progress to advanced AMD.

How it works: The rapid rise in blood sugar triggered by refined carbohydrates results in cellular damage, injuring eye tissues, explains Dr. Chiu.

A daily substitution of whole-grain breads for white bread can reduce the risk of developing advanced AMD, he says.

"Many cases of AMD could be prevented by eating a low-GI diet," says Allen Taylor, PhD, the study leader.

Marc Grossman, OD, LAc, optometrist in private practice, Rye and New Paltz, New York. *www.drgrossman2020.com*.

Chung-Jung Chiu, DDS, PhD, assistant professor, Tufts University School of Medicine.

Usha Chakravarthy, MD, professor of ophthalmology, Queens University, Belfast, Northern Ireland.

Allen Taylor, PhD, director, Laboratory for Nutrition and Vision Research, Jean Mayer USDA Human Nutrition Research Center on Aging, Tufts University.

At Midlife—You *Can* Keep Wearing Contact Lenses

Many middle-aged individuals find contact lenses increasingly impractical or uncomfortable. Don't give up! Here's how to handle common complaints.

•**Blurred close-up vision.** *Presbyopia*, a reduced ability to focus on nearby objects, results from loss of elasticity in the eye's crystalline lens. *Options…*

•Multifocal contacts function much like trifocal or progressive eyeglasses. Tell your eye doctor whether close-up vision or distance vision is most important to you—this helps determine the appropriate lens design. Many people adapt quickly to multifocals, but others experience dizziness and/or distorted vision. Ask to try a sample pair for a week before committing to buy. Multifocals reduce but may not eliminate blurring, so reading glasses or distance glasses also may be needed at times.

•Monovision means that one eye is fit with a lens for distance vision and the other eye is fit with a lens for close-up vision.

Drawback: You lose some depth perception. Again, some users adjust easily and others don't.

•**Dry, irritated eyes.** Especially for women after menopause, hormonal changes may alter the lubricating film of tears. *To try…*

•Use lubricating eyedrops before inserting contacts. Through the day, apply rewetting drops as needed. Stay hydrated by drinking plenty of water and limiting caffeine. Women should remove eye makeup before bed. Place a warm, wet washcloth across your closed eyes for a few minutes… then gently massage the eye area with your fingertips to stimulate tear production.

•Swallow two grams of fish oil daily (don't put it in your eyes!). Its omega-3 fatty acids may reduce eye inflammation and promote a healthy tear film.

•Angle your chair away from any air conditioner, fan or heat vent. Blink often while working at a computer…and put the monitor at eye level.

•You may have developed a sensitivity to your cleaning solution or type of lens. Ask your eye doctor about switching solutions and/or lenses.

•Even with a cleaning solution labeled "no rub," it is best to gently rub lenses to remove irritating debris and deposits.

161

• For severe dryness, ask your eye doctor about Restasis, a prescription eyedrop used twice daily to increase tear production.

Kelly K. Nichols, OD, MPH, PhD, associate professor, Ohio State University College of Optometry, Columbus, and author of numerous journal articles on optometry.

Eye Drops That Help Reverse Cataracts

Cataracts, which are a clouding of the lens of the eye, are the leading cause of vision problems in the US. Risk factors include obesity, age, sun exposure, family history, smoking and radiation exposure (including from X-rays). A diet rich in fruits and vegetables, and supplements, such as vitamins C and E and lutein, can decrease the risk for cataracts and may slow their formation. Patients also may benefit from eyedrops containing the nutrient *N-acetyl carnosine*. Can-C eyedrops might help reverse cataracts in some patients. The dosage is two drops in each eye twice daily for a minimum of six months. Use these drops only under the supervision of a physician or eye specialist so that he/she can monitor how the eye responds to treatment. Can-C eyedrops are available from a number of distributors, including Natural Eye Care (845-255-8222, *www.naturaleyecare.com*).

Mark A. Stengler, NMD, naturopathic medical doctor in private practice, La Jolla, California, and author of the *Bottom Line/Natural Healing* newsletter. *www.drstengler.com*.

Common Eye Myths— And Fixes for Everyday Eye Strains

Almost one-quarter of all American adults are nearsighted, and everyone over age 40 will have increasing difficulty reading fine print or seeing clearly in dim light.

Most people understand that age is the main reason for declines in eye health and vision, but there's still a lot of confusion about other factors that help or hurt the eyes. *Common myths...*

Myth: Sitting too close to the TV hurts the eyes.

Reality: Generations of mothers have scolded their children for sitting too close to the television. This might have made sense in the 1940s, when TVs emitted fairly high levels of radiation, but it isn't a factor anymore.

Today you could sit with your nose pressed against the screen, and it wouldn't hurt your eyes. If you do watch TV up close, you might experience eyestrain because the eyes aren't designed for prolonged, short-distance viewing. This may result in a headache, but apart from this, there aren't any risks associated with up-close TV watching.

Myth: You'll damage your eyes if you read in dim light.

Reality: Using your eyes, even under difficult viewing conditions, doesn't hurt them. You won't damage your vision by reading in dim light any more than you could hurt your ears by listening to quiet music, but you may develop eyestrain.

Myth: Computer monitors cause eye damage.

Reality: Computer monitors are no more likely than TVs to damage the eyes. However, people who spend a lot of time in front of the computer might experience an increase in eye dryness.

People don't blink normally when they're engaged in prolonged, up-close focusing. When you're working on the computer, you might blink less than once every 10 seconds. That's not enough to lubricate the eyes.

Infrequent blinking causes additional problems in older adults because their tear film is effective for only about seven or eight seconds between blinks—about half as long as in younger adults.

Recommended: During computer sessions, take an "eye break" at least once an hour. Shift your vision to something farther away, and consciously blink every few seconds. Use an over-the-counter natural teardrop to remoisturize your eyes. Good brands include Systane, Optive, Soothe XP and Refresh.

Myth: Using stronger reading glasses than you need weakens vision.

Reality: No, it is not true that using a stronger power than you need makes your eyes come to need that power. You can wear any power reading glasses that you want. You need to choose reading glasses based on the distance at which you work. You may want a stronger power for reading the newspaper than for working on the computer.

Myth: Redness means infection.

Reality: Eye infections are relatively infrequent compared with the cases of red eyes from noninfectious causes. Viral infections (which do not respond to antibiotics) occur somewhat more often but also are relatively uncommon.

Eye redness usually is due to simple irritation of the surface of the eye—from allergies or from dryness, for example, or from *blepharitis,* an inflammation of the eyelid, which also can cause dry eyes.

Self-test: The eye will be very red if you have an infection (bacterial or viral). With a bacterial infection, you might notice a thick yellow-white discharge. A viral infection is likely to have a clear, continuous watery discharge. Viral conjunctivitis (commonly called *pink eye*) results in a very irritated, very red eye, which often spreads to the other eye in one to three days. Typically, people with pink eye have had a cold recently or have been exposed to someone with pink eye.

Pink eye is very contagious and can quickly spread to family members and coworkers. To reduce the spread of infection, limit your contact with other people and wash hands frequently. Unlike bacterial conjunctivitis, which is treated with antibiotic eyedrops, there is no treatment for viral pink eye except lubricating eyedrops to reduce discomfort.

Myth: Extended-wear contacts are safe to keep in when you sleep.

Reality: The Food and Drug Administration (FDA) has approved extended-wear contact lenses that you can keep in when you sleep, but I see a lot of patients with eye inflammation caused by these lenses.

The cornea, the transparent front of the eye, takes in oxygen all the time. Wearing a contact lens for extended periods reduces oxygen at the eye surface. Silicone hydrogen lenses allow much more oxygen to get to the cornea, but even they can cause irritation and infection when worn too long.

Always follow your doctor's instructions. If your contact lenses are designed to be worn for two or four weeks, then change them at the recommended frequency. If you are wearing your contacts overnight and your eyes become irritated or red, stop wearing them and see your eye doctor. Generally, if you take your contacts out each night, there's less risk for infection and irritation.

Irritation sometimes can be caused by multipurpose or cleaning solutions. Multipurpose solutions (Opti-Free, ReNu) include chemicals designed to kill bacteria, and some people become sensitive to these products. I recommend a product called Clear Care. The active ingredient, hydrogen peroxide, kills bacteria and other germs. Then, after six hours of soaking, the solution turns into saline.

For people who have trouble wearing contacts, one-day disposable lenses are another possibility. They are more expensive than the extended-wear lenses but don't require disinfectant solutions.

Brett Levinson, MD, ophthalmologist, director of the Cornea and Anterior Segment at Select Eye Care in Baltimore and clinical instructor in ophthalmology at University of Maryland School of Medicine.

Good Mood = Good Vision

Y̶ou know how to improve your vision… Don a pair of glasses. Put in your contact lenses. Or just turn up the light.

Well, researchers at the University of Toronto have discovered a new way to improve vision—improve your mood!

A Wider Window on the World

"Our study shows that when you are in a positive mood, your visual cortex—the part of the brain that processes visual images—take in more information, while a negative mood results in tunnel vision," says Adam Anderson, PhD, an associate professor in the Department of Psychology at the University of Toronto, and a study researcher. "Good and bad moods literally change how we see."

The researchers studied 16 people with normal vision.

Can Supplements Protect Your Eyes?

There's evidence that nutritional supplements can help eye patients who have already been diagnosed with age-related macular degeneration. A National Institutes of Health study found that patients with the disease who took a daily combination of beta-carotene (15 mg), vitamin C (500 mg), vitamin E (400 IU), zinc (80 mg) and copper (2 mg) were 25% less likely to progress to an advanced form of the disease.

This was an impressive finding, but there is no solid evidence that nutritional supplements prevent macular degeneration or other eye problems in healthy people.

Exception: Fish oil. Studies show that patients with mild-to-moderate eye dryness usually improve after taking oral supplements of fish oil. Brett Levinson, MD and opthalmologist, advises patients to buy a product that contains both *docosahexaenoic acid* (DHA) and *eicosapentaenoic acid* (EPA) and follow the dosage instructions on the label.

First, they showed them pictures intended to create either a positive or negative mood—such as a picture of adorable puppies for the positive mood, and a picture of burning one hundred dollar bills for the negative.

Next, they showed them a series of images with a face in the middle and a house interior or exterior in the background. As each image flashed by, the participants were asked to focus on the face, identifying its gender—but also say whether the background was an interior or an exterior.

Results: Those in a positive mood successfully identified the faces and the backgrounds. Those in a negative mood could only identify the faces.

While all this was going on, the researchers were observing the real-time functioning of the brain of each participant, through *functional magnetic resonance imaging* (fMRI). They found that those in a negative mood had less activity in the *parahippocampal place area*—the part of the brain that responds to new information.

"Good moods enhance the literal size of the window through which we see the world," says Taylor Schmitz, PhD, the study leader. "We can see things from a more global, or integrative perspective.

"Bad moods, on the other hand, may keep us more narrowly focused, preventing us from integrating information outside of our direct attention."

Be Kind to Your Eyes

After 40 years of clinical research, Roberto Kaplan, OD—a behavioral optometrist and author of *Conscious Seeing: Transforming Your Life Through Your Eyes* (Beyond Words)—wasn't surprised by the results of this unusual experiment.

"Emotional states and seeing are correlated," he says.

Vision is information coming in through the eye that is processed by the retina, the light-sensitive tissue lining the inner surface of the eye, he explains. The center of the retina (the *macula*) is responsible for clarity and logic. But the periphery of the retina is responsible for feeling.

"A negative emotional state leads to suppression of feeling, an absence of retinal participation and awareness, and a narrowed visual field," he says.

Dr. Kaplan describes an experiment he conducted with near-sighted patients who watched a positive video (a smiling, happy mime) and a negative video (a mime simulating violence). "I measured the eyesight of the patients before and after they watched these two videos—and after watching the violent video, their eyesight worsened."

●**Nurture yourself.** There are many ways to improve your vision through improving your mood—listening to music you like, participating in an engaging hobby, watching a humorous DVD, spending time with a loved ones and friends. *But maybe you feel like taking care of yourself is selfish...*

"There's no need to feel guilty about pursuing pleasure and play," says Alice Domar, PhD, director of the Domar Center for Mind-Body Health in Waltham, Massachusetts, and author of *Self-Nurture* (Penguin). "Take an hour to read a book, or call up friends on a whim and convince them to go out and do something. Nurture yourself—care for yourself, and put yourself on your own list of priorities." *Two of her recommendations to do just that...*

●First thing in the morning. "Every morning, when your alarm goes off, spend 30 seconds thinking about what you can do that's nice for yourself that day. Whether it's buying yourself a fabulous piece of fruit you love, or calling a great friend—anything!"

●During the day. "Every day, at least once a day, when you start feeling stressed out, stop yourself and say, 'What do I need right now?' It may be something simple as taking a two-minute relaxation break looking up a joke on the Internet, or calling a friend, or going for a walk or deciding to order a pizza for dinner."

●**Nurture your eyes.** Dr. Kaplan encourages people to boost their feelings by nurturing their eyes. *Some of his suggestions...*

●Cupping. Rub your hands rapidly together to create warmth in your palms. Put your left hand over your left eye and your right hand over your right eye, in a cuplike or hatlike shape. Feel the warmth, like a blanket over your eyes.

●Affirmations. *While cupping, say these affirmations to yourself:* "I am nurturing my eyes. I have a relationship with my eyes that is one of health. My eyes do a wonderful job and I love them."

●Relaxation. "The eyes have six huge, strong muscles—and overfocusing leads to a buildup of tension in those muscles," he says.

To counteract that tension, he suggests this simple exercise:

1. Sit comfortably and breathe easily in and out.

2. Performing cupping, or visualize your eyes covered by a warm, comforting blanket.

3. As your breath out, visualize the tension around your eyes traveling down your body and flowing out through the toes.

Resources: You can find out more about behavioral optometry at Dr. Kaplan's Web site, *www.beyond2020vision.com*, where he offers coaching to improve eyesight, and "insights" to help you understand how eye problems reflect your life as a whole.

You can also find a behavioral optometrist near you by visiting the Web site of the College of Optometrists in Vision Development, at *www.covd.org* and entering your zip code into the "Locate A Doctor" feature on the homepage.

Adam Anderson, PhD, associate professor in the Department of Psychology at the University of Toronto. *www. aclab.ca.*

Taylor Schmitz, PhD, researcher, Department of Psychology, University of Toronto.

Roberto Kaplan, OD, behavioral optometrist and author of *Conscious Seeing: Transforming Your Life Through Your Eyes* (Beyond Words). *www.beyond2020vision.com.*

Alice Domar, PhD, director of the Domar Center for Mind-Body Health in Waltham, Massachusetts, and author of *Self-Nurture* (Penguin). *www.domarcenter.com.*

Secrets to Keeping Your Teeth Forever

By the time we reach middle age, most of us have had a few root canals—or worse. Years of use make our teeth weaker and more vulnerable to decay and breakage.

Surprising statistic: At least two out of every 10 older Americans (about 20 million people) are toothless.

But strong, healthy teeth are important: If you have dental pain or denture problems, it can be difficult to eat fruits and vegetables, which are crucial for adequate nutrition. In addition, numerous studies have linked gum (periodontal) disease—a primary cause of tooth problems—to a variety of serious ailments, including heart disease, diabetes, dementia and some forms of cancer. *How to optimize the health of your teeth...*

- **Use sugarless candy or gum to stimulate saliva.** Salivary flow decreases as we age, creating an ideal environment for mouth bacteria to flourish. Many heart drugs, antidepressants and other medications may further decrease saliva production.

To help lubricate your dry mouth, your doctor may have suggested that you suck on mints or other small candies. But the sugar in such candies—including so-called breath mints—feeds bacteria in the mouth, accelerating tooth decay you may not even see.

Advice: Switch to sugarless candies—or chew sugarless gum. Also avoid "sticky" foods, such as dried fruit (including raisins and prunes), that tend to promote tooth decay.

- **Bite carefully.** Our teeth become more fragile as we age, and any tooth that has had a root canal, crown or filling is more brittle than an intact tooth. A crown (a custom-made, thimble-like structure that fits over a trimmed-down tooth that has decayed) typically lasts for seven to 10 years, but the longevity of natural teeth, crowns and fillings may be shortened if you don't take the right precautions.

Advice: If you have crowns, fillings and/or veneers (facings applied to the front of teeth to improve their shape and/or color) in the front of your mouth, biting into an apple, carrot or even a crusty piece of bread could shatter them.

Instead, bite with your side teeth to shift the force on to them. Better yet, cut up apples, carrots or hard bread into bite-sized pieces so you can chew with the teeth in the back of your mouth (molars), which are usually the strongest.

Caution: Never chew ice—even molars can be shattered with one good crunch. Also, don't use your teeth as tools to do such things as open plastic packages, cut thread or crack nut shells.

- **Pamper your gums.** Most people have some degree of gum recession (in which the gums have pulled back, exposing the roots of the teeth). It results from brushing too aggressively or from gum disease. Receding gums make teeth more susceptible to cavities at the roots and increase their sensitivity.

Smart Idea: If you have receding gums and use "sensitive" toothpaste (such as Sensodyne or Colgate Sensitive), apply it with your finger to the sensitive area, count to 60 (to ensure good absorption), then brush.

Advice: To minimize gum recession, most people know to use a "soft" or "ultrasoft" toothbrush, but it's also important for these brushes to be replaced at least every three to four months. After that point, the bristles usually flare out and become less effective. When brushing, use light pressure. Dennis P. Tarnow, DDS, recommends electric toothbrushes only if you have arthritis in your hands or some other condition that affects manual dexterity.

- **Be vigilant about self-care.** Up to 30% of the population is genetically predisposed to gum disease, which is a major cause of tooth loss. Even people who are not genetically primed for gum disease may wind up with bacterial infections in the tissues surrounding the teeth as a result of changing hormone levels, poor self-care or other health problems.

Advice: For adults with healthy teeth, twice-daily thorough brushing is fine. If you have gum disease or its precursor (gingivitis), which causes such symptoms as swollen gums, bad breath and gums that bleed easily when brushing or flossing, brush your teeth after every meal—or, if that's inconvenient, at least swish your mouth with water after you eat.

Important: Brush for a full two minutes with any fluoride toothpaste. When you floss (any type is fine), be sure to remove the plaque from the sides of every tooth.

Important: Since many people now drink bottled water instead of tap water, which is fluoridated in most municipalities, some experts fear that the incidence of tooth decay may increase. If you live in a community that does not have fluoridated water, look for bottled water brands that are fluoridated. Many companies, including Culligan and Natural Springs, produce fluoridated bottled water.

For a list of companies: Consult the International Bottled Water Association, 800-928-3711, *www.bottledwater.org/public/flu orida.htm.*

• **Opt for an implant.** In the old days, when you lost a tooth, your dentist would crown the teeth adjacent to an empty space and create a "bridge" to hold a replacement tooth. An implant (a metal post and abutment that are surgically anchored into the jawbone to provide support for a crown) generally is a better option because its placement does not require cutting down adjacent teeth. However, the price of a bridge may be lower than implants initially, and some insurance companies balk at covering the cost of an implant.

Advice: If your dentist recommends a bridge, ask whether an implant can be used instead. If cost is an issue, work out a payment plan with your dentist.

Helpful: If your dental insurance does not cover implants, insist that your case be reviewed by a dentist. About half the time, such appeals result in at least partial reimbursement. Or ask the insurance company

to pay you its standard reimbursement for a bridge and apply it to your implant.

If the cost is still too high: Go to a nearby dental school, where students are supervised by professors and the cost is about half of that charged at a private practice.

Dennis P. Tarnow, DDS, periodontist and prosthodontist (a dentist who specializes in the fitting and placing of implants, bridges and dentures) and chairman of the Department of Periodontology and Implant Dentistry at New York University College of Dentistry.

Eliminate Canker Sores Once and for All

A t first glance, canker sores seem like a trivial complaint. These small sores inside the mouth aren't life-threatening or contagious. They don't leave a scar and usually go away within a week. What's the big deal?

The problem is that many people have recurrent canker sores that occur several times a month. Because the nerves in the mouth are so sensitive, canker sores, which occur on the tongue, inside the cheek and/or behind the lips, cause a lot of pain. If you have recurrent canker sores, it can be extremely painful to eat—or even speak.

Unlike cold sores, which are triggered by the herpes simplex virus and can be treated with antiviral medications, most canker sores result from a localized immune reaction brought on by stress, a food allergy, nutritional problems or trauma, such as biting your tongue or lip. *If you have recurrent canker sores...*

• **Consider allergy testing.** You may develop a canker sore because your mouth becomes irritated within a matter of hours of eating a highly acidic meal that includes tomatoes, citrus or chocolate—or after drinking coffee, black tea or carbonated beverages. With a food allergy, the reaction may not occur for several hours—or it may be immediate. If you get recurrent canker sores, it's wise to get an immunoglobulin G (IgG) food allergy blood test to identify the specific foods that weaken your immune system and trigger an allergic reaction. If it's not convenient for you to get allergy testing, try avoiding the most common offending foods—one at a time for one week each—to identify those that trigger an allergic reaction in you. In my practice, wheat, garlic, nuts, soy and citrus are the most frequent allergens among canker sore sufferers.

• **Check for a nutritional deficiency.** If you have a deficiency of vitamin B-12, the B vitamin folic acid or iron, you are likely to develop recurrent canker sores. Even if you already take a daily multivitamin, you can safely add 600 micrograms (mcg) in supplemental folic acid and an 800-mcg supplement of vitamin B-12 daily. Try these supplements for one month to see if they effectively keep cancer sores at bay.

Caution: Be sure to get your iron levels tested if you suspect an iron deficiency. Taking an iron supplement unnecessarily can lead to liver damage.

• **Take precautions if you're under stress.** Stress leads to canker sores because it reduces digestive function, decreases immune health and increases inflammation. If you are prone to canker sores, add more bland foods, such as brown rice, baked potatoes, lightly steamed vegetables, poultry and fish, to your diet when you're under stress. Bland foods are easier to digest and less likely to irritate the mouth and digestive tract.

• **Use herbal remedies.** If you develop a canker sore, you can speed healing by taking two slippery elm capsules every four hours on an empty stomach. In addition, drink three cups of licorice root tea daily. Both these herbs moisten and soothe the mucous membranes of the mouth and digestive tract.

Caution: if you have high blood pressure, avoid licorice—which can adversely affect blood pressure in some people.

Jamison Starbuck, ND, is a naturopathic physician in family practice in Missoula, Montana.

Natural Cures for Cold Sores

They swell up…blister…scab. Cold sores that sprout on or near the lips are a year-round annoyance. Sun exposure increases their frequency. Other triggers include stress…a cold or fever…menstruation…and irritation, such as severely chapped lips.

The cause of most cold sores is a virus—herpes simplex type 1. (Type 2 typically causes genital herpes but also can cause cold sores.) The herpes simplex type 1 virus is spread by person-to-person contact, including kissing or touching someone else's cold sore or saliva. Once in your body, the virus never goes away, which means that you will be forever vulnerable to cold sores.

Note: Those who have strong immune systems are less susceptible to cold sores.

Several natural substances may help heal or prevent cold sores…

• **L-lysine.** This amino acid can prevent a cold sore outbreak or reduce its severity. Take 1,000 milligrams (mg) three times daily without food as soon as you feel a cold sore developing. Take it until the problem has resolved. If prone to outbreaks, you can use L-lysine preventively (500 mg to 1,000 mg twice daily without food) for two to three months and then again as needed. There are no side effects. Avoid foods such as nuts and egg yolks that are high in the amino acid L-arginine, which can cause cold sores.

• **Balms.** Natural balms can soothe the pain of cold sores and speed up healing. Look for balms with these ingredients—aloe vera…zinc sulfate…lemon balm. Apply to the cold sore four times daily. Although these ingredients are safe, they can cause a reaction (usually redness in the area). If you are sensitive to one ingredient, try a product with another ingredient. Protect your lips from the sun with a sunblock balm.

Mark A. Stengler, NMD, naturopathic medical doctor in private practice, La Jolla, California, and author of the *Bottom Line/Natural Healing* newsletter. *www.drstengler.com.*

Refreshing Solutions for Dry Mouth

Xerostomia (dry mouth) is a common condition with many possible causes, including regular consumption of caffeinated beverages (such as coffee and tea) and/or alcohol—all of which can have a dehydrating effect. Dry mouth also can be a side effect of over-the-counter pain/sleep medications (such as Tylenol PM and Advil PM) and antihistamines as well as certain prescription diuretics, antidepressants and medications for overactive bladder and Parkinson's disease. In addition, medical conditions such as diabetes and the autoimmune disorder Sjögrens syndrome can be to blame.

To alleviate dry mouth, drink more water (aim for at least 32 ounces daily) and limit or avoid alcohol, caffeinated soda, coffee and tea, salt and salty foods. During the winter, set your thermostat at the lowest comfortable temperature and use a humidifier. If you suspect that medication may be causing your dry mouth, ask your doctor if there are alternatives that you could take. Products such as Biotène mouthwash and toothpaste for dry mouth also can provide relief. If your dry mouth persists or worsens despite taking these steps, see your physician. If left untreated, dry mouth can reduce your sense of taste and raise your risk for gum disease, heartburn and other problems.

Thomas Lackner, PharmD, professor of pharmacy, College of Pharmacy, University of Minnesota, Minneapolis.

The Gargle That Douses Burning Mouth

Burning mouth syndrome (BMS) causes persistent pain in the mouth that usually is not relieved by conventional pain medications.

New finding: In a small study, half the patients who gargled twice daily with a solution of two teaspoons of the laxative milk of magnesia (sold under many brand names) mixed with one-half cup of water reported significant reduction in mouth pain. Larger studies are under way.

Theory: Milk of magnesia stimulates touch and taste receptors that can inhibit pain.

If you suffer from BMS: Ask your doctor about gargling twice daily with this mixture.

Alan R. Hirsch, MD, director, Smell & Taste Treatment and Research Foundation, Chicago.

Banish Bad Breath— For Good

If a whiff of your breath makes others wince, it may be more than a social problem—often it suggests a medical problem, too. Here's what you need to know about *halitosis*, or bad breath.

● **Blame occasional bad breath on diet.** *What to do...*

●Minimize food odors with herbs. Onions, garlic, cabbage and spices contain strong-smelling compounds that break down during digestion, are absorbed into the bloodstream and travel to the lungs. To reduce production of smelly intestinal gases, along with the offending foods, swallow one of the following—one-eighth teaspoon of dried caraway seeds (chew them first)...six ounces of hot water mixed with one-quarter teaspoon of powdered caraway...one caraway capsule...or one parsley oil capsule.

●Mask the smell. For a quick temporary fix, chew a clean mint leaf or sprig of fresh parsley, or suck on a sugar-free breath mint.

●**Chronic halitosis usually is caused by bacteria in the mouth.** *Fixes...*

● Prevent dry mouth. Saliva helps flush out bacteria. Cut back on alcohol and caffeine, which are dehydrating...drink more fluids... chew sugarless gum or suck on sugarless hard candy to stimulate saliva production. Antihistamines, antidepressants, blood pressure drugs and diuretics contribute to dry mouth, so ask your doctor about alternatives. Use a humidifier in your bedroom, especially if you are a nighttime mouth-breather.

• Clean your tongue. The tongue's surface has tiny protuberances called *papillae* that create havens for bacteria. Use a tongue scraper ($10 or less at drugstores) once a day...or try the Colgate 360 toothbrush, which has soft tongue-cleaning knobs on the back of the head.

• Use antibacterial mouthwash. Good nonprescription antibacterials include zinc, found in TheraBreath Plus and Tom's of Maine Natural Tartar Control Mouthwash... or chlorine dioxide, found in ProFresh.

Avoid: Mouthwashes with alcohol, such as Listerine, which are drying.

• Try antimicrobial toothpaste. The only toothpaste with the effective antimicrobial *triclosan* is Colgate Total.

Also important: Floss teeth daily!

• **Disease-related bad breath may stem from a dental problem** or from a systemic (body-wide) medical condition. *Solutions...*

• See your dentist. When plaque-filled pockets form between teeth and gums, trapped bacteria create foul odors. Your dentist may recommend a cleaning, antibiotics and/or surgery. *If that does not fix the problem...*

• See your primary care doctor. Do not wear cologne or scented lotion to your appointment—these mask odors that could help your doctor make a diagnosis.

Warning signs: Diabetes makes breath smell overly fruity...gastric cancer produces a fecal odor...kidney disorders create an ammonia-like smell...liver problems lead to fishy breath...lung disease causes a putrid smell...postnasal drip leads to sulfurous breath.

Good news: When the underlying disorder is addressed, breath freshens up, too.

Violet I. Haraszthy, DDS, PhD, associate professor of oral biology and restorative dentistry, University of Buffalo School of Dental Medicine, Buffalo, New York, and leader of a study on bad breath.

How Beverages Can Harm Your Teeth

We know that candy and sugar-filled foods are bad for the teeth. But it's easy to overlook how much harm can be done by what we drink.

Hazards of Popular Beverages

American Dental Association (ADA) spokesperson Richard Price, DMD, says that even beverages passing briefly through your mouth bathe the teeth in sugar, chemicals, acid and coloring agents. *He describes how various drinks affect the teeth...*

• **Soft drinks.** One 12-ounce can of soda contains the equivalent of 10 to 12 teaspoons of sugar and 20-ounce bottles are loaded with 17 teaspoons. While you would never dream of shoveling this amount of sugar into your mouth, it goes down pretty easily in a soft drink. More sugar brings more risk of decay...and the acid content may cause even more harm. Both regular and diet sodas commonly contain phosphoric or citric acid that erodes tooth enamel and can lead to softening, demineralization, erosion (the wearing away of enamel), cavities and tooth sensitivity. Acid erosion and heavy consumption of dark-hued soft drinks such as cola also stains teeth.

• **Juices and juice drinks.** In terms of overall health, pure juices are a better choice than sugar-filled juice drinks, but both pose problems for teeth. Fruit juices are naturally high in sugar (higher than fruit, in fact, since the pulp and fiber are removed) and may have even more sugar than some juice drinks sweetened with high fructose corn syrup. Not only that, but citrus-based lemonade, orange juice, grapefruit juice, etc., are high in acid. Dark juices (especially grape) cause staining.

• **Sports and energy beverages.** Sports beverages, energy drinks and vitamin waters may promise a surge of power on the playing field or at the office, but they, too, are frequently laced with sugar, acid and food coloring.

- **Coffee and tea.** There are plenty of health benefits to both coffee and tea, but be aware that just as they stain teacups, they can also stain teeth. Sweetening them with sugar can also contribute to decay.

- **Milk.** Even though it contains lactose (milk sugar), milk is also high in calcium, which makes it a better beverage choice for teeth. Calcium strengthens tooth enamel and can neutralize the effects of acid.

- **Alcohol.** Alcoholic beverages are made from fermented sugars and often contain significant residual sugar, and the mixers used with them also contain sugar and acid, so Dr. Price notes that in excess these can be harmful to the teeth. If you drink enough to lead to a hangover, the resulting dehydration and dry mouth can be detrimental to oral health since it produces conditions favorable to decay. Red wine is notorious for staining teeth. To offset this effect, alternate sips of wine with sips of water. Although white wine by itself is not a "stainer," it may make teeth more susceptible to staining by other beverages, i.e., grape juice, tea, coffee, etc. If you choose these drinks, it's actually better for your teeth to have them with meals rather than in-between.

Keep Your Teeth Pretty and Healthy

After consuming beverages, swish water around in your mouth—and don't brush your teeth. It may seem counterintuitive, but brushing at this point does more harm than good. By softening enamel, acids in beverages such as cola, sports and energy drinks or citrus drinks make teeth more susceptible to abrasion from toothpaste. Wait at least 30 minutes before brushing.

More strategies to protect your pearly whites include...

- **Use a straw.** To minimize staining and exposure to sugar and acid, use straws to keep the liquids from swishing around in your mouth.

- **Near bedtime, avoid soda, sports drinks and juices.** Saliva production decreases while you sleep, and since saliva is what neutralizes acid and tames bacteria that cause decay, nighttime sweet drinks may be especially damaging.

- **Do not brush your teeth vigorously.** Use a soft-bristled, ADA-approved toothbrush that is gentler on enamel.

- **Consider dental sealants.** Especially if you are cavity-prone, dental sealants—protective plastic coatings on the chewing surfaces of the back teeth—can help stave off decay.

- **Review the medications you take with your dentist.** Many drugs (including antihistamines, antidepressants, high blood pressure and asthma medications) cause dry mouth as a side effect, which in turn can lead to decay and erosion.

Richard Price, DMD, American Dental Association spokesperson, retired from private practice in Boston.

Whiten Teeth Naturally

There are several natural options when it comes to whitening teeth. David Banks, DDS, a holistic dentist in San Marcos, California, explains that most darkening of teeth is due to the accumulation of stains over time.

First: Brush with a quality low-abrasion toothpaste.

His favorites: PerioPaste by Bio-Pro, which contains antibacterial herbs and essential oils, such as peppermint, calendula flower and olive leaf (866-924-6776, *www.docharrison.com*) and PowerSmile Enzyme Brightening Oral Pre-Rinse by Jason Naturals, with papaya and pineapple enzymes (877-527-6601, *www.jason-natural.com*). Both contain calcium carbonate, sodium bicarbonate and colloidal silica—low-abrasion tooth-cleaning compounds that help with stains. Beyond that, if you want still whiter teeth, a bleaching process may be necessary.

Best: Have your dentist perform an in-office procedure, which limits the duration of exposure to the bleaching chemicals.

Mark A. Stengler, NMD, naturopathic medical doctor in private practice, La Jolla, California, and author of the *Bottom Line/Natural Healing* newsletter. *www.drstengler.com.*

The Toothpaste Made by Mother Nature

You probably know aloe vera as the cactuslike plant on your kitchen's windowsill. A squeeze of one of its succulent leaves yields a dab of gel, good for soothing minor burns and other boo-boos—so good, in fact, that two common names for aloe vera are "burn plant" and "first aid plant."

Well, maybe aloe should also be dubbed "periodontal plant"—because new research shows aloe vera gel can kill the microbes that cause gum disease.

Aloe Vera Kills Germs

A team of Indian researchers tested an aloe vera gel toothpaste to see if it had the same microbe-fighting power as two commercial toothpastes, Colgate and Pepsodent.

And no matter which mouth-inhabiting, disease-causing germ they tested it against—a range of seven bacteria and fungi—aloe vera held its own, killing as many germs as the commercial toothpastes.

The findings were in *General Dentistry.*

A Great Alternative

"Aloe vera contains *anthraquinones*, antimicrobial and anti-inflammatory compounds that kill bacteria and fungi, stop pain and heal tissue," says Dilip George, MDS (Master of Dental Surgery), the study leader. "And because aloe vera doesn't contain the abrasive elements typically found in commercial toothpaste, it's a great alternative for people with sensitive teeth and gums."

However: Not all aloe vera tooth gel contains the effective form of aloe vera.

"To be effective, the product must contain the stabilized gel located in the center of the plant," says Dr. George. "And during manufacturing the gel can't be filtered or treated with excessive heat, which reduces or destroys the active compounds in the gel."

Recommended: Forever Bright Aloe Vera Toothgel, from Forever Living (888-440-2563, *www.foreverliving.com*), the product tested in the study.

Forever Bright Aloe Vera Toothgel is also available at *www.bestaloeveraproduct.com, www.bonanzle.com* and other Web sites.

Also helpful: "An aloe vera gel placed directly on gum tissues after periodontal surgery will promote faster healing and prevent infection," says Laura Torrado, DDS, a cosmetic dentist in New York City.

She also recommends applying aloe vera gel any time gum tissue has been "scratched or traumatized."

Dilip George, MDS, senior lecturer, Department of Pedodontics and Preventive Dentistry, Pushpagiri College of Dental Sciences, India.

Laura Torrado, DDS, cosmetic dentist in New York City. *www.drlauratorrado.com.*

Convertibles, Golf Clubs And Other Weird Causes Of Hearing Loss

Hearing loss muffles the daily lives of nearly 40 million Americans, one-third of them over 65.

Most hearing loss is *sensorineural*—damage to the hair cells within the *cochlea*, the nerve-rich part of the inner ear that translates sound vibrations into electrical impulses that are sent to the brain.

There are two main causes of sensorineural hearing loss, explains Michael Seidman, MD, director of otologic/neurotologic surgery and otology research at the Henry Ford Health System in Detroit, Michigan, and author of *Save Your Hearing Now: The Revolutionary Program That Can Prevent and*

May Even Reverse Hearing Loss (Wellness Central).

●**Aging.** A cause so common it has its own name—*presbycusis.*

●**Noise.** The nerves of the inner ear are battered from a lifetime of loudness—from hair dryers and garbage disposals, lawn mowers and chainsaws, rock concerts and (literally) deafening work environments.

"Hearing loss can be insidious and irreparable," warns Dr. Seidman. "It develops slowly—even imperceptibly. And once you lose it, it may be gone forever."

To reduce your risk of sensorineural hearing loss, you need to reduce your exposure to loud noise and noisy environments, he says. But several new studies show that some of those environments aren't what you might expect—from a golf course to the front seat of a Porsche.

Newest Research

Fresh research—most of it reported at a recent annual meeting of the American Academy of Otolaryngology–Head and Neck Surgery—reveals unexpected risks to your hearing…

●**Convertible cars.** Driving a car with the top down may increase your risk for hearing damage, says Philip Michael, MD, a UK researcher.

He and his colleagues measured noise levels in convertibles at 50, 60 and 70 miles per hour.

The cars tested were:

- Toyota MR2
- Maxda Miata MX5
- Audi A4 Cabriolet
- Morgan plus 4 Roadster
- Porsche 997 Carrera
- Aston Martin V-8 Vantage
- Bentley convertible

They found that drivers in convertibles are continuously exposed to between 88 and 90 decibels (dB), with a high of 99—and the faster the speed, the louder the noise.

(To put those decibels into context: a whisper is 20dB, a normal conversation is 50 to 60, a typical vacuum cleaner is 75, a hair dryer or a quiet lawn mower is 85 to 90, a power saw is 100, a snowmobile engine or jackhammer is 120, a jet takeoff is 135, a gunshot or emergency siren is 140.)

"Repeated or long exposure to sounds over 85 dB causes permanent hearing loss," says Dr. Michael.

Self-defense: "Simply keeping the car windows raised on a convertible significantly reduces noise exposure levels to 82 dB, even with the top down," says Dr. Michael.

And don't drive your convertible all the time. "It's unlikely you'll damage your hearing during short trips," he says. "But if you spend the entire summer driving around with the top down—particularly on highways, which we found generated more noise than driving on city streets or rural roads—you increase your chances of hearing loss."

If you're intent on driving a convertible, find out if wearing earplugs while driving is legal in your state, advises Paul Dybala, PhD, an audiologist in Texas and editor-in-chief of the Web sites *www.healthyhearing.com* and *www.audiologyonline.com.* "Go with the hear-through variety," he says. "These earplugs enable you to hear the sounds of potential danger while blocking out the sound of the wind rushing by."

Product: EAR Arc Flash Earplugs, which are widely available.

●**Titanium golf clubs.** In England, a team of ear, nose and throat specialists and audiologists treated a 55-year-old man with sensorineural hearing loss in his right ear—but not in his left. They found out that the right-hander had been playing golf three times a week for 18 months with a titanium golf club. The man commented that the noise of the club hitting the ball was "like a gun going off." In fact, the sound had become so unpleasant he stopped using the club.

After conducting hearing tests and reviewing the patient's medical history, the researchers firmly concluded that the man's hearing loss "was attributable to the noise of the golf club."

In their report on the case in the *British Medical Journal*, they explain that "thinner-faced titanium clubs (such as the King Cobra LD the man was using) deform on impact more easily...resulting in a louder sound."

And when they went a step further and conducted tests on the sound levels produced by 12 drivers—comparing six thin faced titanium drivers to six standard stainless steel clubs—they found the titanium clubs produced much louder sounds, typically above 120 dB, and as high as 128 dB.

"Our results show that thin faced titanium drivers may produce sufficient sound to induce temporary, or even permanent, hearing damage," say the researchers. "Caution should be exercised by golfers who play regularly with thin faced titanium drivers, to avoid damage to their hearing."

Self-defense: "Ear protection should be used whenever you are exposed to loud noise of any kind—including from golf clubs," says Dr. Seidman. "There is very little difference between the sound of that club striking a ball and the sound of a jackhammer.

"Invest in earplugs—they are tiny enough to be carried everywhere, and they are easy to use."

Trap: "Don't try to use cotton balls to protect your ears," says Dr. Seidman. "Cotton is completely ineffective at protecting against noise. It reduces sound by a mere 5 to 7 dB."

● **Subways and buses.** 33 million people safely ride mass transit systems to and from work every day. But are their ears safe?

Researchers from Columbia University Mailman School of Public Health measured dB levels on all types of mass transit in New York City—and found levels as high as 101 and 102 at bus stops and subway platforms. On average, levels in commuter trains (such as the PATH train between New Jersey and New York) were around 75, and subways around 80.

"The noise levels on subway platforms could cause hearing loss in some people with as little as two minutes of exposure per day," says Robyn Gershon, DrPH, the study leader.

And the hazard isn't only to your hearing, she says. Excessive noise is a stress—and can cause or complicate high blood pressure, heart disease and sleep disorders.

Self-defense: "If you're riding on mass transit 30 to 60 minutes a day or more, for four or five days a week, you should wear hearing protection, such as earplugs," says Dr. Gershon.

Smart idea: Buy a small and inexpensive noise meter called a noise dosimeter, available at outlets such as RadioShack (often sold as a sound-level meter), says Dr. Gershon. "In a situation that seems noisy, check the meter. If it's above 75 dB, put in your earplugs."

● **XY chromosomes beware.** That's right guys—hearing loss seems to be sexist. When US researchers analyzed hearing data from more than 5,000 people, they found men were 2.5 times more likely than women to develop noise-induced hearing loss.

Self-defense: What to do? Maybe eat more spinach.

A team of researchers from the Channing Laboratory at Harvard Medical School recently discovered that men over 60 with the highest dietary intake of the B-vitamin folate were 20% less likely to develop hearing loss, compared with men with the lowest intake. (They don't know why folate may protect hearing.)

Foods high in folate include: leafy green vegetables such as spinach, romaine lettuce, collard greens and turnips greens; broccoli and asparagus; beans of all kinds, such as pinto, garbanzo, navy and black, and lentils and folate-fortified cereals and breads.

Michael Seidman, MD, director of otologic/neurotologic surgery and otology research at the Henry Ford Health System in Detroit, Michigan.

Paul Dybala, PhD, audiologist in Texas and editor-in-chief of the Web sites *www.healthyhearing.com* and *www. audiologyonline.com.*

Philip Michael, MD, ear-nose-throat surgeon at Worcestershire Royal Hospital, UK.

Robyn Gershon, DrPh, associate dean for research resources, Mailman School of Public Health, Columbia University.

Biofeedback for Tinnitus Relief

An estimated 35 million Americans have tinnitus—a lifetime of exposure to loud noises (the most common cause) produces noises inside your head, such as buzzing, hissing, clicking or whooshing.

There are a lot of treatments for tinnitus, including drugs, surgery and tinnitus-masking devices—but few are consistent at solving the problem.

Now, a new study from Germany shows that biofeedback may help control the problem...

Less Noise and Annoyance

German researchers treated 130 people with tinnitus, dividing them into two groups.

One group was treated with biofeedback—they were hooked up to a machine that emitted signals when muscles in the head and neck were tense, allowing them to identify and relax those muscles.

The other group was told they were on a waiting list for biofeedback.

After 12 sessions, biofeedback was "highly effective" in reducing the perception of the inner sound and feelings of annoyance about it. And when the researchers evaluated the patients six months later, they found these "improvements were maintained."

The findings were in the *British Journal of Clinical Psychology*.

The Most Effective Therapy

"Biofeedback is the most effective therapy for tinnitus," says Murray Grossan, MD, an ear-nose-and-throat specialist in Mission Hills, California.

Why it works: "Being bothered by tinnitus is based on what I call 'the tiger response,'" says Dr. Grossan. "Our primitive ancestors were genetically programmed to react to sounds—such as the snap of a twig in the jungle from an approaching tiger—with a reflex that flooded the body with adrenaline and instantly created tense muscles for fighting or fleeing the tiger. That same stressed, anxious response automatically kicks in with tinnitus—but there isn't any tiger!

"The result of that sustained anxiety is constant and fretful concern about the inner sound and a heightened perception of its loudness."

But overcoming the tiger response is easy, says Dr. Grossan. "Simply identify and relax the tense muscles, through biofeedback. When muscles relax, anxiety disappears.

"When you use biofeedback to get rid of your 'tiger response' to tinnitus, the noise becomes a slight, background annoyance that you hardly notice, like a tight belt," says Dr. Grossan.

Good news: You don't need a biofeedback machine to do biofeedback.

• **Mirror biofeedback.** "Instead of using a machine for biofeedback, use a mirror, observing the tense muscles in your face and shoulders and allowing them to relax," says Dr. Grossan. *Here's how to do it...*

1. Breathe deeply, counting to four on each inhale and six on each exhale.

2. Notice the tight muscles in your jaw.

3. Breathe deeply.

4. Watch your jaw relax.

5. Notice your tense shoulders.

6. Breathe deeply.

7. Watch your shoulders fall and relax.

8. Repeat those seven steps until you feel very relaxed.

"Practice this biofeedback technique about five minutes a day, says Dr. Grossan. "Soon, you'll get the message that there isn't any tiger!"

(See appendix page 358 for more information on biofeedback.)

Murray Grossan, MD, ear-nose-and-throat specialist in Mission Hills, California. *www.grossan.com.*

Chapter 9

HEART DISEASE

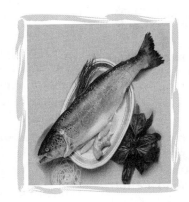

You Can Cure Heart Disease—with Plant-Based Nutrition

In the mid-1980s, 17 people with severe heart disease had just about given up hope. They had undergone every available treatment, including drugs and surgery—all had failed. The group had experienced 49 cardiovascular events, including four heart attacks, three strokes, 15 cases of increased angina and seven bypass surgeries. Five of the patients were expected to die within a year.

Twelve years later, every one of the 17 was alive. They had had no cardiovascular events. The progression of their heart disease had been stopped—and, in many cases, reversed. Their angina went away—for some, within three weeks. In fact, they became virtually heart-attack proof. And there are hundreds of other patients with heart disease who have achieved the same remarkable results. *What you need to know...*

How the Damage Is Done

Every year, more than half a million Americans die of coronary artery disease (CAD). Three times that number suffer heart attacks. In total, half of American men and one-third of women will have some form of heart disease during their lifetimes.

Heart disease develops in the *endothelium*, the lining of the arteries. There, endothelial cells manufacture a compound called *nitric oxide* that accomplishes four tasks crucial for healthy circulation...

- Keeps blood smoothly flowing, rather than becoming sticky and clotted.

- Allows arteries to widen when the heart needs more blood, such as when you run up a flight of stairs.

- Stops muscle cells in arteries from growing into plaque—the fatty gunk that blocks blood vessels.

- Decreases inflammation in the plaque—the process that can trigger a rupture in the cap or surface of a plaque, starting the clot-forming, artery-clogging cascade that causes a heart attack.

The type and amount of fat in the typical Western diet—from animal products, dairy foods and concentrated oils—assaults endothelial cells, cutting their production of nitric oxide.

Study: A researcher at University of Maryland School of Medicine fed a 900-calorie fast-food breakfast containing 50 grams of fat (mostly from sausages and hash browns) to a group of students and then measured their endothelial function. For six hours, the students had severely compromised endothelial function and decreased nitric oxide production. Another group of students ate a 900-calorie, no-fat breakfast—and had no significant change in endothelial function.

If a single meal can do that kind of damage, imagine the damage done by three fatty meals a day, seven days a week, 52 weeks a year.

Plant-Based Nutrition

You can prevent, stop or reverse heart disease with a plant-based diet. *Here's what you can't eat—and what you can…*

●**What you cannot eat…**

●No meat, poultry, fish or eggs. You will get plenty of protein from plant-based sources.

●No dairy products. That means no butter, cheese, cream, ice cream, yogurt or milk—even skim milk, which, though lower in fat, still contains animal protein.

●No oil of any kind—not a drop. That includes all oils, even virgin olive oil and canola.

What you may not know: At least 14% of olive oil is saturated fat—every bit as aggressive in promoting heart disease as the saturated fat in roast beef. A diet that includes oils—including monounsaturated oils from olive oil and canola oil—may slow the progression of heart disease, but it will not stop or reverse the disease.

●Generally, no nuts or avocados. If you are eating a plant-based diet to prevent heart disease, you can have moderate amounts of nuts and avocados as long as your total cholesterol remains below 150 milligrams per deciliter (mg/dL). If you have heart disease and want to stop or reverse it, you should not eat these foods.

●**What you can eat…**

●All vegetables.

●Legumes—beans, peas, lentils.

●Whole grains and products that are made from them, such as bread and pasta—as long as they do not contain added fats. Do not eat refined grains, which have been stripped of much of their fiber and nutrients. Avoid white rice and "enriched" flour products, which are found in many pastas, breads, bagels and baked goods.

●Fruits—but heart patients should limit consumption to three pieces a day and avoid drinking pure fruit juices. Too much fruit rapidly raises blood sugar, triggering a surge of insulin from the pancreas—which stimulates the liver to manufacture more cholesterol.

●Certain beverages, including water, seltzer water, oat milk, hazelnut milk, almond milk, no-fat soy milk, coffee and tea. Alcohol is fine in moderation (no more than two servings a day for men and one for women).

●**Supplements**

For maximum health, take five supplements daily…

●Multivitamin/mineral supplement.

●Vitamin B-12—1,000 micrograms (mcg).

●Calcium—1,000 milligrams (mg) (1,200 mg if you're over 60).

●Vitamin D-3—1,000 international units (IU).

●Flaxseed meal (ground flaxseed)—one tablespoon for the omega-3 fatty acids it provides. Sprinkle it on cereal.

The Cholesterol Connection

If you eat the typical, high-fat Western diet, even if you also take a cholesterol-lowering statin drug, you will not protect yourself from heart disease—because the fat in the diet will damage the endothelium cells that produce nitric oxide.

In a study in *The New England Journal of Medicine*, patients took huge doses of statin drugs to lower total cholesterol below 150 but didn't change their diets—and 25% experienced a new cardiovascular event or died within the next 30 months.

Recommended: Eat a plant-based diet, and ask your doctor if you should also take a cholesterol-lowering medication. Strive to maintain a total cholesterol of less than 150 and LDL ("bad" cholesterol) below 85.

Moderation Doesn't Work

The most common objection physicians have to this diet is that their patients will not follow it. But many patients with heart disease who find out that they have a choice—between invasive surgery and nutritional changes that will stop and reverse the disease—willingly adopt the diet.

Why not eat a less demanding diet, such as the low-fat diet recommended by the American Heart Association or the Mediterranean diet?

Surprising: Research shows that people who maintain a so-called low-fat diet of 29% of calories from fat have the same rate of heart attacks and strokes as people who don't.

Plant-based nutrition is the only diet that can effectively prevent, stop and reverse heart disease. It also offers protection against stroke...high blood pressure...osteoporosis...diabetes...senile mental impairment...erectile dysfunction...and cancers of the breast, prostate, colon, rectum, uterus and ovaries.

Caldwell B. Esselstyn, Jr., MD, surgeon, clinician and researcher at The Cleveland Clinic for more than 35 years. He is author of *Prevent and Reverse Heart Disease: The Revolutionary, Scientifically Proven, Nutrition-Based Cure* (Avery). *www.heartattackproof.com.*

Is Sugar Poisoning Your Heart?

The American Heart Association (AHA) has become specific (finally!)—their most recent statement (as of 2009) about sugar and CVD (cardiovascular disease, the umbrella term for heart disease and stroke) explains why excess sugar is bad for your heart, and then recommends a safe upper limit for "added sugar" in your diet. (The AHA defines "added sugar" as the sugars, and sugary syrups such as high-fructose corn syrup, that are added to food during processing or preparation.)

22 Teaspoons a Day

In the 2000s, Americans increased their intake of sugar by an average of 22.2 teaspoons (355 calories) a day, mostly from soft drinks, according to the recent "Scientific Statement" in the AHA journal *Circulation*.

The "statement" says that this increased sugar could be causing high blood pressure...high triglycerides (a blood fat that can damage arteries)...and low levels of "good" artery-cleaning HDL cholesterol. And, they note, a sugar overload can also cause overweight, a risk factor for type 2 diabetes—and three out of four people with type 2 diabetes die of CVD.

Newest research: Researchers at the University of Colorado Denver Health Sciences Center analyzed diet and health data from more than 4,500 people with no history of high blood pressure—and found that those who ate and/or drank more than 74 grams a day of fructose (the amount in 2½ 12-ounce sodas) were 36% more likely to develop high blood pressure.

Based on its analysis, the AHA issued these new guidelines...

• **Women should eat no more than 100 calories of added sugar per day, or six teaspoons.**

• **Men should eat no more than 150 calories, or nine teaspoons.**

Example: A 12-ounce can of cola contains 8 teaspoons of sugar, or 130 calories.

Problem: "Eating too much sugar is an addiction," says Jacob Teitelbaum, MD, author of *Beat Sugar Addiction Now!* (Fair Winds). "Sugar gives you an initial high, you crash several hours later, and this leaves you wanting more sugar. If you crave sugar, telling you to cut your intake is like telling an addict to stop taking a drug."

Beating Sugar Addiction

"The goal of beating sugar addiction isn't to get you off sugar," says Dr. Teitelbaum. "The goal is to get you healthy—not only lowering your risk for CVD and diabetes, but also reducing anxiety, depression, fatigue, chronic sinus problems, irritable bowel syndrome and other health conditions that are often caused or complicated by excessive sugar intake."

His recommendations can work for everybody...

• **Use sugar substitutes.** "They give you the pleasure of sugar without the side effects," says Dr. Teitelbaum. He favors stevia, and also *sugar alcohols* (erythritol, isomalt, lactitol, maltitol, mannitol, sorbitol and xylitol).

Smart idea: Stevia and erythritol are combined in the products PureVia and Truvia.

• **Cut out excess caffeine.** It aggravates the symptoms of sugar addiction.

• **Choose whole foods that don't fuel sugar cravings.** That includes vegetables, unprocessed fruit, whole grains, beans and meat.

• **Take a multivitamin/mineral supplement.** Inadequate levels of nutrients trigger food cravings.

• **Drink water.** "You'll have a tougher time kicking sugar if you don't stay hydrated," says Dr. Teitelbaum.

Smart idea: Check your mouth and lips every so often. If they're dry, you need to drink more water.

• **Get enough sleep.** "Adequate sleep optimizes energy, decreases appetite and slashes sugar cravings," he says.

Best: Seven to nine hours.

Smart ideas: Go to bed and wake up at the same time. Cut out caffeine intake after 2:00 p.m. Don't drink alcohol right before bed. Keep the bedroom cool. Don't exercise within an hour of bedtime.

Jacob Teitelbaum, MD, author of *Beat Sugar Addiction Now!* (Fair Winds). *www.endfatigue.com.*

The Best Way to Use Heart-Healthy Margarine

Some plants have very high cholesterol. Or rather, they have very high *sterols*, a chemical cousin to cholesterol that does the same thing for a plant that cholesterol does for you—maintains and strengthens cellular membranes, the envelope around every cell.

When you eat plant sterols (or *stanols*, their twin) they act in your body as if they were dietary cholesterol, blocking the real thing at every turn—beating it to the punch before it's absorbed through the intestines... and shoving it aside before it's packaged into the lipoproteins that carry it through the bloodstream (LDL stands for low-density lipoprotein).

Dozens of studies show that a daily intake of 2.5 grams (2,500 milligrams [mg]) of plant sterols can help lower LDL cholesterol levels up to 15%—dramatically lowering your risk of heart disease. In fact, if you're taking a cholesterol-lowering statin, adding a goodly amount of plant sterols to your diet is more effective than doubling the dose of the drug.

To get more plant sterols, you just eat more plants, right?

Well, our hunter-and-gatherer ancestors managed to consume only about 1.2 grams (1,200 mg) of plant sterols a day, as they spent endless hours munching and crunching their way through a diet of seeds, berries, leaves and the like. Today even the most determined vegetarians consume no more than 500 mg a day. The average American eats about 250 mg.

To make up for the shortfall, food scientists began enriching everyday foods with plant sterols—starting with heart-healthy margarines such as Benecol and Take Control, and expanding to sterol-enriched salad dressings, yogurts, chocolate bars, juices and a supermarket aisle's worth of other sterol-filled products.

But are each of those foods equally effective at lowering LDL cholesterol?

Latest development: New research shows that some sterol-enriched foods do a much better job than others at lowering LDL—and that *when* you eat sterols can make all the difference in whether or not sterols work to protect your heart.

Sterols with Fat Work Best

A team of researchers at McGill University in Montreal, Canada, analyzed 59 studies on the cholesterol-lowering ability of sterol-enriched foods.

They found the highest reduction in LDL when plant sterols were combined with fat—in margarine, mayonnaise, salad dressing, milk or yogurt.

They found the lowest reduction from other sterol-enriched foods, such as croissants, muffins, orange juice, nonfat beverages, cereal bars, chocolate and meat.

They also found that eating all your sterols at one meal—such as spreading sterol-enriched margarine on your toast at breakfast, and then calling it a day—failed to lower LDL.

Best: Eating sterol-enriched foods two or three times a day.

A confirming study conducted a few months later showed that eating sterol-enriched margarine three times a day lowered cholesterol 6% more than eating the same amount of margarine once a day.

Two Servings Are Better Than One

• **Eat in divided dosages.** "If you want the biggest cholesterol-lowering bang for your buck, eat sterols in smaller doses, two or three times a day, rather than in one, large dose," says Peter Jones, PhD, the lead researcher on those studies, and professor of nutrition and food science at the University of Manitoba, Canada.

• **Focus on fat.** "Our research shows that the most effective way to ingest plant sterols is in the company of fat," says Dr. Jones. "That might seem odd, because fat is supposedly bad for your heart. But we have to eat some fat to live, and research shows the right kinds of fats, eaten in moderation, are actually good for your heart.

Recommended: A sterol-rich margarine that also includes heart-protecting monounsaturated and omega-3 fatty acids, such as Smart Balance.

"Smear the margarine liberally on a piece of toast at breakfast, and on your sandwich bread at lunch," says Dr. Jones. "You get the sterols, you get the benefits of the good fats in the margarine and your timing maximizes the cholesterol-lowering power of the sterols."

The greatest reduction in LDL cholesterol is from 2.5 grams of sterols a day.

Trap: Eating more than 2.5 grams a day doesn't cut cholesterol any further.

• **Or take a sterol supplement.** If you don't like margarine, Dr. Jones recommends a sterol supplement, taking 2.5 grams a day, in two doses.

Best: For maximum cholesterol-lowering power, look for a supplement in a soft gel (rather than a pill), with the sterols suspended in a healthy oil (such as omega-3 or mono-unsaturated fat).

Peter Jones, PhD, professor of nutrition and food science at the University of Manitoba, Canada.

Can Sex Really Cause A Heart Attack?

Many people wonder whether sex can cause a heart attack. The answer may surprise you.

The sex-heart attack connection: For a healthy, middle-aged man, sexual intercourse, performed at a typical level of exertion, translates into a risk for heart attack of about one to two in one million. (There are no comparable statistics for healthy, middle-aged women—virtually all studies on heart attack and sex have focused on men.)

Why is the risk so low? It's because sex typically isn't strenuous enough to trigger a heart attack. Vigorous exertion, however, raises heart attack risk because the heart has to work harder to supply blood to the body, increasing heart rate and blood pressure. If blockages in the heart's arteries prevent the heart from receiving enough blood to do its work, a person may suffer chest pain (angina) or a heart attack.

Red flag: If a healthy, middle-aged man has sexual intercourse with an unfamiliar and/or younger partner in unfamiliar surroundings, typical exertion levels may double—partly due to the man being motivated to try more vigorous sexual activity than usual. Feelings of heightened excitement, anxiety and/or guilt also can potentially raise the risk for a heart attack.

Sex After a Heart Attack

If you have recently suffered a heart attack, sex is probably the last thing on your mind. But once your condition has stabilized—for example, your blood pressure is normalized and any chest pain you may have experienced is controlled—you should discuss sexual activity with your cardiologist.

Good news: For most heart attack patients, sexual intercourse is rarely the cause of a subsequent attack.

What you need to know to safely engage in sex if you've had a heart attack—or you are at risk for one…

The Heart at Risk

While the risk factors described below are aimed primarily at heart attack patients, the recommendations also can serve as general guidelines for people who have had a stroke. *Levels of risk…*

● **Low risk**

You may be in this category if…

● You've been diagnosed with heart disease but have no more than two identifiable risk factors, such as high cholesterol, high blood pressure, diabetes, a sedentary lifestyle or smoking, or…

● You have coronary artery disease (blockage in one or more arteries of the heart severe enough to prevent the heart from getting sufficient blood) but no history of heart attack, or you had a heart attack more than six weeks ago.

Bottom line: If you don't have shortness of breath or pains that could be due to the heart not getting enough blood (including pain in the chest, left shoulder and arm or neck) with normal activity (such as climbing one or two flights of stairs), you are most likely in the low risk category and can probably resume sexual intercourse.

● **Intermediate risk**

You may be in this category if…

● You had a heart attack two to six weeks ago, or…

● You've been diagnosed with heart disease and have three or more risk factors (such as those described earlier), or…

● You have moderate angina or heart failure that causes shortness of breath with moderate or greater exertion, such as playing tennis or shoveling snow or…

● You had a stroke two or more weeks ago.

Bottom line: You should not have sexual intercourse until your cardiovascular disease is under control and you are considered at low risk. Other physical expressions of affection, such as kissing, hugging and foreplay, are reasonably safe.

● **High risk**

You may be in this category if…

● You had a heart attack or stroke less than two weeks ago, or…

● Your angina is unstable (described above), or…

● You have uncontrolled high blood pressure, or…

● You have been diagnosed with congestive heart failure (severe enough to limit normal activities)…a life-threatening arrhythmia (an irregularity of heart rhythm)…hypertrophic obstructive cardiomyopathy (increased thickness of the heart muscle that limits the amount of blood pumped out to the rest of the body)…or moderate-to-severe heart valve disease (a dysfunction in one or more of the four valves that help regulate blood flow into and out of the heart).

Bottom line: As with intermediate risk, do not have sexual intercourse until your cardiovascular problem is under control.

Help Your Heart

Even men who are at low risk can decrease their chance of a heart attack during sex by minimizing strain on the heart. *That means…*

● **Digest first, make love later.** The heart works harder after you eat, pumping blood to the stomach, intestines, pancreas and other digestive organs. Wait one to three hours after a meal before having sexual intercourse.

● **Delay sex if you've been under stress.** Stress makes the heart work harder. Don't have sex right after you've had an argument, done your taxes or even watched the news. Instead, relax for several hours before engaging in sexual intercourse.

Henry G. Stratmann, MD, clinical professor of medicine at Saint Louis University and a cardiologist in private practice in Springfield, Missouri. He is coauthor with his wife, Maryellen Stratmann, MD, of *Sex and Your Heart Health* (Starship).

Heart Drug Dangers

Widely used heart medications can cause erectile dysfunction (ED) in 1 to 2% of men who take them, according to Henry G. Stratmann, MD. *These include…*

Beta-blockers, which slow the heart rate…*thiazide diuretics*, which reverse fluid retention…and *clonidine*, which relaxes blood vessels.

If you develop ED after taking one or more heart medications, talk to your doctor about using a lower dose that would still be effective but might not cause ED…or ask about changing to a different kind of heart medication.

If you must use a heart medication that causes ED, ask your doctor about taking an ED medication, such as *sildenafil* (Viagra), *vardenafil* (Levitra) or *tadalafil* (Cialis).

Do not use any of these ED drugs if you also take a nitrate medication for angina, such as *isosorbide mononitrate* (Imdur) or nitroglycerin. Check with your doctor for further advice.

Go Ahead and Exercise!

Before beginning any exercise program, check with your doctor. You've read those words before. In fact, you've probably read them dozens of times—they're the standard advice given whenever exercise is recommended, meant to keep folks with heart disease from jogging out the door… and dropping dead.

But do most people really have to see a physician before making the heart-healthy switch from a sedentary lifestyle to regular exercise?

Probably not, according to a recent study.

Who Needs a Stress Test

To make sure you're good-to-go for exercise, doctors often order a stress test (also called an *exercise stress test* or *exercise tolerance test*)—you exercise on a treadmill or stationary bike, while medical technicians monitor your blood pressure, heart rhythms and possible symptoms of heart disease (such as chest pain or shortness of breath).

If your stress test indicates heart problems, the doctor conducts more tests to figure out if you have heart disease and, if you do, how serious it is.

If you're planning to start vigorous exercise, the American College of Cardiology says you should have a stress test if you're a man over 45, a woman over 55, or have diabetes.

However, in a scientific statement, the American Heart Association points out that the recommendation doesn't cover nonvigorous exercise (like walking)...isn't strongly supported by scientific evidence...and is therefore "controversial."

To clarify the situation, a team of Israeli researchers conducted an in-depth "decision analysis," looking at data from hundreds of thousands of people to find out whether stress tests really reduce the risk of heart attacks and sudden death in people starting an exercise program. *Their findings...*

In people at low risk for heart disease (nonsmoker, total cholesterol below 200, HDL cholesterol above 40, blood pressure 120/80 or lower, no diabetes, normal weight, no family history of heart disease), a stress test produced no statistical reduction in heart attacks or sudden cardiac death from exercise.

In fact, stress tests *harmed* people! Dozens of low-risk folks had false positives, underwent medically risky procedures—and died. The researchers point out that more low-risk people died because of the process initiated by the stress test than died exercising without the stress test!

In people at high risk (known heart disease, or diabetes, or over age 65 with two or more risk factors such as high LDL cholesterol and high blood pressure) or intermediate risk (over age 65, with one risk factor), a stress test did reduce exercise-related heart attacks and deaths. But, as with the low-risk group, it increased the total number of deaths—because after their stress test, a number of people died during angiography, an invasive procedure test that corrects arterial blockage.

Bottom line: "Routine screening before initiating regular exercise is not recommended for the purpose of reducing the risk of sudden death during exercise training," say the researchers, in the *Journal of General and Internal Medicine.*

On balance, they add, exercise-induced death is a "dramatic but rare event" that is "far less common than the mortality resulting from a sedentary lifestyle, a leading cause of death."

In other words, it's usually a lot safer to start exercising than it is to have a stress test!

Go Ahead and Walk

● **Walk without worry.** "Anyone can start a walking program—you don't need clearance from a physician to do that," says Carl J. Lavie, MD, medical director of Cardiac Rehabilitation and Prevention, and director of the Stress Testing Laboratory at the Ochsner Heart and Vascular Institute in New Orleans, Louisiana.

"Start slowly, and gradually increase the intensity of your walking routine," advises Mayer Brezis, MD, the study leader, and professor of medicine at Hadassah Hebrew University Medical Center, in Jerusalem.

Example: A 60-year-old, sedentary woman might start with a 10-minute walk at a pace with "no extra effort," he says. (You know you're exercising with extra effort if you're having any difficulty speaking while walking. For that reason, it's best to start walking with a friend or spouse, says Dr. Brezis.)

● **Increase your walk by five minutes every three days, until you reach 30 minutes daily.** At that point, increase the intensity for the last five or 10 minutes—walk at a rate where you have slight difficulty talking during exercise.

Gradually increase that level of intensity to half the time you walk, and then to most or all of the time.

Red flag: If you start walking and experience any possible symptoms of heart disease, such as shortness of breath or chest pain—walk home very slowly, and call your doctor for an appointment. The physician will probably order a stress test—which, in this case, you definitely need.

If you match these criteria, see your doctor before exercising. If you've been sedentary and you have intermediate-to-high risk for heart disease and you're thinking of starting an exercise program more vigorous than walking (such as jogging, swimming laps, outdoor cycling at faster than 10 miles an hour, tennis or aerobic dancing), see your physician before you start, says Dr. Lavie. "It's moderate to high intensity exercise that really poses a risk for heart attacks and sudden cardiac death, not low to moderate intensity."

Trap: "When an unfit person suddenly does high-intensity exercise—such as shoveling after a heavy snowfall—they increase their risk of heart attack or sudden cardiac death 10- to 20-fold," says Dr. Lavie.

"Any person who has angina or suffered a heart attack should exercise under close supervision at a cardiac rehabilitation center," adds Dr. Brezis.

Carl J. Lavie, MD, medical director of Cardiac Rehabilitation and Prevention and director of the Stress Testing Laboratory at the Ochsner Heart and Vascular Institute in New Orleans.

Mayer Brezis, MD, professor of medicine at Hadassah Hebrew University Medical Center, in Jerusalem.

Can't Tolerate Statins? Try Red Yeast Rice

Statins work—really well. By reducing high blood levels of artery-clogging "bad" LDL cholesterol, they can reduce the risk of a heart attack by up to 40%, compared with people not taking statins.

That's why more than 15 million Americans take the drug. Or at least start taking it.

Because two out of five people who start a statin—a drug intended to be a lifelong therapy—stop it within a year.

The likely reason—a side effect.

The most common statin side effect (bothering three out of five people who reported a side effect to the Statin Effects Study, at the University of California–San Diego) is muscle pain and weakness, or *myalgia*. In fact, some people who take a statin find their muscles become so achy and fatigued they can no longer exercise!

Other side effects commonly reported in the Statin Effects Study include digestive upset...cloudy memory and thinking...*neuropathy* (burning, tingling and numbness in the hands and feet)...irritability...insomnia...and sexual problems such as erectile dysfunction or low libido.

And switching from one statin to another isn't necessarily a solution—nearly 60% of people who develop myalgia from their first statin still have it after switching to a second or third.

Are there any LDL-lowering alternatives for people who can't handle statins? Yes, says a team of physicians from the University of Pennsylvania School of Medicine.

The ancient Chinese heart remedy, red yeast rice.

Red yeast rice is the granddaddy of all statins. When the yeast *monascus purpureus* grows on rice, it produces compounds called *monacolins* that block the action of HMG-CoA reductase, an enzyme with a key role in manufacturing cholesterol.

A few decades ago, Western scientists took a closer look at this intriguing Chinese heart medicine, identified its active ingredients, synthesized one (monacolin K), and produced *lovastatin* (Mevacor)...which was followed by *simvastatin* (Zocor), *atorvastatin* (Lipitor), *rosuvastatin* (Crestor) and all the other statins...now the most-prescribed medicines in the US.

Same Effect, but No Side Effects

The researchers tested the effectiveness of red yeast rice in 62 people (average age 61) who had stopped taking a statin because of myalgia, and whose muscle pain cleared up after they discontinued the drug.

They divided them into two groups, giving one red yeast rice and the other a placebo. (Those taking red yeast rice also attended classes in "therapeutic lifestyle changes," learning about a low-fat Mediterranean diet, regular exercise and relaxation techniques.)

Results: After six months, LDL cholesterol in the red yeast rice group fell from 163 mg/dL (milligrams per deciliter) to 128, a 21% drop. In the placebo group, LDL fell from 165 to 150, a 9% decline.

Total cholesterol fell in the red yeast rice group from 245 to 208, or 15%. In the placebo group, it dropped from 246 to 230, or 5%.

And what about myalgia?

Red yeast rice is a statinlike supplement—it caused myalgia in 2 people, who stopped taking it. But the other 27 people taking red yeast rice were myalgia-free!

"Red yeast rice significantly decreased LDL and total cholesterol levels compared with the placebo, and did not increase the incidence of myalgias," summed up the researchers, in the *Annals of Internal Medicine.* "The regimen of red yeast rice," they continued, "may offer a lipid-lowering option for patients with a history of intolerance to statin therapy."

In an earlier study, the researchers conducted a head-to-head test of Zocor and red yeast rice (along with the therapeutic lifestyle changes and fish oil supplements) in 74 people with high LDL.

After three months, those taking the red yeast rice had a 42% drop in LDL; those taking the Zocor, 40%.

But can red yeast rice prevent heart attacks like statins?

Latest development: Researchers at the Peking Union Medical College in Beijing treated more than 1,500 older individuals who had suffered a heart attack with either red yeast rice or a placebo. *After four years, red yeast rice had...*

• Reduced the risk of heart attack by 38% and

• Reduced the risk of death from heart disease by 29%.

The findings were published in the *Journal of Clinical Pharmacology.*

Supplement with Supervision

The University of Pennsylvania researchers note that the amount of lovastatin delivered by red yeast rice is equivalent to 6 mg of Zocor, which is usually given in 20 to 40 mg doses. So why does red yeast rice work as well as Zocor? And why is it less likely to cause myalgia? Nobody knows for sure, but there are theories.

"Red yeast rice has several monacolins in small amounts," says Joshua Levitt, ND, a naturopathic physician in private practice in Hamden, Connecticut. "They might work additively or synergistically, accomplishing the same effect as a pharmaceutical product with only one agent. Also, red yeast rice has compounds other than monacolins, which might enhance their effectiveness."

Suggested dosage: 1,800 mg, twice a day.

Products: The study doctors used a red yeast rice manufactured by Sylvan Bioproducts, which is available at GNC stores (*www.gnc.com*) as Red Yeast Rice, from Traditional Supplements. The Sylvan formulation is also used in Naturals Organic Red Yeast Rice, at *www.naturals-supplements.com*, or call 866-352-7520.

In his practice, Dr. Levitt uses the product Choleast, from Thorne Research, which includes both red yeast rice and the antioxidant CoQ10 (a nutrient often recommended to counter statin side effects). It is available at many Web sites, including *www.thorne.com* (or call 800-228-1966), *www.amazon.com* and *www.pureprescriptions.com* (or call 800-860-9583).

Red flags: "Just because red yeast rice is a natural, over-the-counter product doesn't mean it's safe," says Dr. Levitt. "It has statin-like activity, and carries the risk of all the same side effects, including rare but serious conditions that can cause extensive muscle damage.

"I feel very strongly that this supplement should be taken only under the supervision of a licensed health professional, who can monitor your health, which includes periodic laboratory tests to ensure that there is no liver damage—a possible risk of statins—and that the therapy is effectively lowering LDL."

There have also been questions about the purity and potency of over-the-counter red yeast rice supplements, says Dr. Levitt—some have been contaminated with toxins, and some contained only minuscule amounts of monacolins.

The Sylvan Bioproducts formulation used in the study and the product recommended by Dr. Levitt both have strict quality controls.

Joshua Levitt, ND, naturopathic physician in private practice in Hamden, Connecticut. *www.wholehealthct.com.*

The Hidden Path to Cardiac Wellness— Your Lymphatic System

We're all familiar with the circulatory system that transports oxygen-rich blood to the tissues of the body, including the heart. But there's another major system that is largely overlooked by patients—and doctors—when it comes to heart health.

The lymphatic system, which is widely known for its ability to help our bodies fight infection, may have a much greater impact on the heart than previously recognized.

New thinking: Most scientists agree that low-level, chronic inflammation can be a significant underlying cause of heart disease.

Some now believe that impaired lymph circulation may be what allows inflammatory substances to irritate blood vessel walls and promote *atherosclerosis* (fatty buildup in the arteries). Impaired lymph flow also can cause cholesterol to remain longer inside blood vessel walls, which contributes to the formation of plaque and increases risk for heart attack and stroke.

The lymphatic hypothesis of cardiovascular disease isn't widely embraced by mainstream physicians, but it's supported by several laboratory studies.

A leading proponent of this hypothesis is Gerald M. Lemole, MD, a heart surgeon who worked closely with the cardiac-surgery pioneers Michael DeBakey, MD, and Denton Cooley, MD, and was a member of the surgical team that performed the first successful heart transplant in the US, in 1968. Since then, Dr. Lemole has performed or overseen close to 20,000 cardiac-surgery procedures.

Here Dr. Lemole explains the ways in which the lymphatic system may affect heart health.

Sluggish Lymph Flow

Our bodies contain more lymph than blood, and we have more miles of lymph vessels than blood vessels. Normally, all of the lymph in the body circulates through the lymphatic system about once every two days. This turnover means that inflammatory cytokines and other irritating substances are swept out of circulation and to the liver for disposal—ideally, before these substances are able to damage adjoining arterial linings.

• **Stress, poor diet and a sedentary lifestyle impair lymph drainage.** Because these lifestyle factors are so prevalent in the US, many Americans are thought to have *lymph stasis,* in which lymph flow is slower than normal.

• **In people who have lymph stasis, pools of lymph essentially stagnate.** Irritating substances suspended in lymph have more time to damage nearby blood vessels, which is thought to contribute to the buildup of LDL "bad" cholesterol and other substances that promote atherosclerosis.

Even though lymph flow in humans has been measured only in research settings, cardiac surgeons have long noted that atherosclerosis develops mostly in blood vessels on the surface of the heart. In this area, lymph flow is relatively weak. Atherosclerosis usually doesn't occur in deeper coronary tissues, where the beating of the heart presses against lymph ducts and promotes rapid lymph drainage.

While the blood circulatory system is largely powered by the heart, the lymphatic system depends mainly on muscle and respiratory movements to supply the pressure changes that are needed for lymph circulation. In addition, the flow of lymph is thought to be enhanced by antioxidants (such as those in green tea) that dilate lymph vessels.

To Keep Lymph Moving

Even though the link between lymph and cardiovascular disease still is theoretical, it may be possible to reduce the risk for heart disease by up to 30% by enhancing lymph circulation—in part because the same things that promote lymph circulation (regular exercise, stress management and a healthful diet) also can help lower blood pressure, inflammation and other proven cardiovascular risk factors. *Actions you can take...*

• **Go for brisk walks.** Muscle movements from walking or other forms of exercise press against the lymph ducts and increase circulation. For example, a daily walk (about 20 to 30 minutes) can double or triple lymph flow.

This may be one reason why people who exercise tend to have lower cholesterol and better immunity than those who are sedentary.

Advice: When performing exercise (such as walking), open your arms as wide as you can and then bring them back together in front of your body (roughly in sync with your breathing). This arm movement opens the chest cavity and allows the lungs to expand more fully, which enhances lymph circulation.

• **Practice deep breathing.** It's the best way to promote lymph circulation in the heart. Taking deep breaths produces pressure in the chest cavity, which makes it easier for lymph to flow through tissues in the heart. Deep breaths also massage the thoracic duct (which carries lymph through the chest and into the bloodstream) and promote better lymph circulation.

Advice: Set aside about 10 minutes a day for deep breathing. Take slow, deep breaths, exhaling completely at the conclusion of each one. You can combine deep breathing with walking and/or other forms of exercise.

Helpful: To ensure proper movement of the diaphragm, make sure that your posture is erect when performing deep breathing, whether you are sitting or standing.

• **Try Daflon-500.** This supplement is marketed under brand names such as Detralex and Arvenum 500. It is available online and in some health-food stores. Originally designed to improve damaged blood vessels in patients with hemorrhoids as well as other venous disorders, such as leg cramps, the supplement contains *bioflavonoids*, plant chemicals that promote lymph flow.

Advice: If you are at high risk for cardiovascular disease, ask your doctor about trying Daflon-500. Follow the label directions—the usual dose is 500 mg, two to three times daily.

• **Drink green tea.** The flavonoids in green tea promote *peristalsis* (contractions) of the lymph ducts. The same chemicals inhibit the activation of the inflammatory cytokines that are closely linked to heart disease.

Advice: Drink three or more cups of green tea daily—the amount shown to confer the most benefit. Water (six to eight glasses daily, between meals) also helps promote lymph flow.

• **Get regular massages.*** The lymph ducts that are located in deeper tissues get a natural massage every time you breathe or move your muscles. However, those closer to the surface may not receive enough muscle pressure for optimal lymph circulation.

Advice: Get a massage from a massage therapist or a friend or your spouse at least once a month to keep lymph moving.

*Caution: If you have scar tissue due to an injury or surgery or if you have recently received radiation treatments, ask your doctor if massage is safe for you.

What Is the Lymphatic System?

This drainage network of vessels, nodes and fluid (*lymph*) helps the body fight infection. Lymph collects excess fluid that seeps from the bloodstream. As lymph passes through several hundred nodes located throughout the body (primarily in the neck, armpits and groin), toxins are filtered out before the cleansed fluid is returned to the bloodstream.

Best: A lymphatic massage, a specialized form of massage that promotes lymph circulation.

(For more information on massage as a healing therapy, see appendix page 353.)

Also helpful: Take a few minutes every day to rub your neck, shoulders, chest, etc. Exert enough pressure to compress the muscles, which will stimulate lymph flow.

Gerald M. Lemole, MD, professor of surgery at Jefferson Medical College, Thomas Jefferson University in Philadelphia and medical director of the Preventive Medicine and Rehabilitation Institute in Wilmington, Delaware. Dr. Lemole is author of *The Healing Diet: A Total Health Program to Purify Your Lymph System and Reduce the Risk of Heart Disease* (William Morrow & Company).

Tune Up Your Heart— With the Right Music

"**M**usic hath charms to soothe a savage breast, to soften rocks, or bend a knotted oak," wrote William Congreve, seventeenth-century English poet and playwright.

"Music induces a continuous, dynamic change in the cardiovascular system," concluded Luciano Bernardi, MD, twenty-first-century Italian scientist.

It's taken a couple of centuries, but the scientists have finally caught up to the poets—they've proved that music can soothe a breast, chest and the heart inside it, providing a buffer against high blood pressure, heart disease and stroke.

Louder Music, Faster Heartbeat

In 2006, researchers in Italy conducted a study in which they found that music with a fast tempo sped up heart rate, boosted blood pressure and triggered more rapid breathing—and that music with a slow tempo had the opposite effect.

In their most recent study, the same researchers played several tracks of classical music (from Puccini, Bach, Verdi and Beethoven) to 24 people, while monitoring the electrical activity of their hearts. This time, they wanted to see how the heart responds to crescendos and decrescendos—gradual increases and decreases in the volume of music.

Result: Like fast music, the crescendos increased heart rate...narrowed blood vessels...increased blood pressure...and increased the respiration rate. And the louder the crescendo, the greater the changes. In the decrescendo, all of those parameters returned to normal.

But Dr. Bernardi isn't the only scientist studying music's effect on the heart.

Standout scientific evidence: Researchers at the Art and Quality of Life Research Center at Temple University, Philadelphia, recently analyzed 23 studies that looked at how music affects stress and anxiety level in people with heart disease. "Music listening can have a beneficial effect on blood pressure, heart rate, respiratory rate, anxiety and pain in persons with coronary heart disease," the researchers concluded.

Entraining Your Heart to Health

"Music can calm the heart because of the principle of entrainment—just as nearby metronomes equalize to the same beat, so the rhythms of the body, such as heartbeat and breathing, quickly synchronize or 'entrain' with the tempo and mood of a piece of music," says Alice H. Cash, PhD, LCSW, a clinical musicologist and social worker in Louisville, Kentucky.

"Music alone isn't going to prevent or reverse heart disease," she adds. "But it can be one of many tools for protecting and improving the health of the heart." *Her recommendations…*

• **Change your "musical diet" from stressful to restful.** "If you're trying to prevent or control heart disease, you're probably focusing on changing your diet," says Dr. Cash. "Well, you can also focus on changing your 'musical diet,' as a way of calming down, and reducing the stress that can cause or complicate heart problems.

"Become aware of the music that calms you, relaxes you and makes you smile—whether it's classical, country or another style—and listen to more of that."

• **Use music to help you exercise.** Regular exercise is crucial to the health of your heart—and music can make regular exercise a lot more enjoyable, says Dr. Cash. "I always listen to music when I exercise. I particularly like athletics-inspired music, such as 'Chariots of Fire' from Vangelis, or the theme from *Rocky*."

Newest research: German researchers divided 20 people into two groups—one group exercised on a treadmill while listening to music through headphones, and one did the same exercise without music. Those listening to the music had less of a sense of unpleasantness during exercise and exercised harder.

• **Listen to calming music before, during, and after angioplasty or heart surgery.** People who are undergoing a stressful heart procedure such as angiography or heart surgery should listen through headphones to relaxing music with a slow, steady, heart-calming tempo of sixty beats per minute, such as music by the baroque composers Bach, Handel and Pachelbel, says Dr. Cash.

"Studies show that you will probably need less anxiety medication before the surgery, less anesthesia during surgery, less pain medication after the surgery and that you'll recover faster."

Important: Research shows that at some level of awareness you do hear sound during surgery, even though you're supposedly "unconscious," says Dr. Cash. That's why it's necessary to listen to music before, during and after surgery.

Resource: The "Surgical Serenity System"—a pair of self-contained, wireless headphones that are preloaded with calming "surgical music." You can also program the headphones with music of your own choosing. It's available at *www.surgicalhead phones.com*, or 502-419-1698.

Newest research: Swedish researchers studied forty people the day after open-heart surgery—half listened to soft, relaxing music through an MP3 player, and half didn't. The music group had higher levels of *oxytocin* (a hormone linked to feelings of relaxation and peace), and said they felt more relaxed. "Music intervention should be offered…to patients who have undergone cardiovascular surgery," they conclude.

In another Swedish study, patients who listened to music before surgery had a greater decrease in anxiety than those who took anti-anxiety medication.

Luciano Bernardi, MD, professor of internal medicine, University of Pavia, Italy.

Alice H. Cash, PhD, LCSW, clinical musicologist and social worker in Louisville, Kentucky. *www.healingmusicen terprises.com*.

Eat More Dark Chocolate —Survive a Heart Attack

Nobody wants to have heart disease or a heart attack, but a lot of us do.

Fact: More than 100 million Americans have high, artery-clogging levels of cholesterol, and every year nearly one million people have their first heart attack, with 141,000 dying.

Maybe you've been diagnosed with heart disease, but haven't had a heart attack. If so, you might want to start eating more chocolate—now.

Eight Years of Protection

A team of researchers from the Karolinska Institute in Sweden and Harvard Medical School surveyed more than 1,100 nondiabetic people who lived through their first heart attack, finding out how much chocolate they ate in the year before the attack. Then they tracked their health for the next eight years.

Surprising: The more chocolate they had eaten in the year before a heart attack, the less likely they were to die of heart disease in the eight years after the attack.

Compared with people who hadn't eaten any chocolate, eating chocolate reduced the risk of dying from heart disease by...

- 66%, eating chocolate twice or more a week
- 44%, eating chocolate once a week
- 27%, eating chocolate less than once a month

Why it works: Dark chocolate is packed with what the study authors call *beneficial bioactive compounds*—flavonols (like those found in red wine and green tea) that are antioxidant and anti-inflammatory. Oxidation (a kind of internal rust that damages cells) and chronic low-grade inflammation (similar to acute inflammation after an injury) are two factors that drive heart disease.

Kenneth Mukamal, MD, a study author and associate professor of medicine at Harvard Medical School, says that other studies show chocolate can lower blood pressure, an effect that might account for the reduced the risk of heart-related deaths in this study.

Standout Scientific Evidence

Many recent studies add to the scientific evidence that chocolate is good for your heart:

- **Lower blood pressure.** Researchers in Germany analyzed data from 10 studies on flavanol-rich chocolate (dark chocolate) and blood pressure. On average, dark chocolate lowered blood pressure by up to 6 points systolic (the upper reading) and 4 point diastolic (the lower reading). This analysis "confirms the blood pressure-lowering capacity of flava-nol-rich cocoa products," say the researchers, in the *American Journal of Hypertension*.

- **Decreased risk of stroke.** Canadian researchers analyzed diet and health data from more than 44,000 people and found that those who ate chocolate once a week were 22% less likely to have a stroke, compared with those not eating chocolate. In another study, people who ate chocolate once a week were 46% less likely to die after a stroke.

- **Reduced inflammation.** Researchers in Spain studied 42 people with heart disease (average age 70), dividing them into two groups. One group drank chocolate milk (skim milk and flavanol-rich cocoa powder) and one didn't. After one month, the chocolate group had less activity in genes that contribute to inflammation, and lower levels of inflammation-sparked biochemicals that play a role in forming blood clots. "These anti-inflammatory effects may contribute to the overall benefits of cocoa consumption against heart disease," say the researchers, in the *American Journal of Clinical Nutrition*.

- **Better circulation.** Researchers in Japan studied 39 healthy people, feeding them either "flavonoid-rich dark chocolate" or white chocolate (which doesn't contain any flavonols). After two weeks, those eating the dark chocolate had an improvement in blood flow of 22%. There was no improvement in those eating white chocolate.

Choose Your Chocolate Wisely

"Chocolate is high in fat and sugar, but it can be nutritious and delicious—as long as you choose your chocolate wisely," says Jessica Levinson, RD, a registered dietitian in New York City.

Here are a few options from nutritional experts...

- **Eat dark chocolate.** "Look for dark chocolate containing 70 to 85% cocoa solids, which contains about 150 calories, and a minimum amount of fat and sugar," says Roger Corder, PhD, professor of experimental therapeutics at the William Harvey Research

Institute in London, and author of *The Red Wine Diet* (Avery). Eat about 1 ounce a day.

●**Use unsweetened cocoa powder.** "The best way to get your chocolate is with unsweetened cocoa," says Deborah Klein, RD, a registered dietitian in California and author of *The 200 SuperFoods That Will Save Your Life* (McGraw-Hill).

"For maximum antioxidants, mix one tablespoon of unsweetened organic cocoa powder with a teaspoon of agave nectar, in a mug of hot water, with a dash of cinnamon—a delicious daily comfort drink!

"Not only is this great for heart health, but cocoa powder also stabilizes blood sugar levels, helping prevent diabetes."

●**Eat semi-sweet chocolate chips.** Replace chocolate bars with a handful of semi-sweet chocolate chips, says Klein. "A teaspoon of chips is only 4 grams of fat, instead of 13 grams from a 1.5 ounce chocolate bar."

Kenneth Makamal, MD, associate professor of medicine, Harvard Medical School.

Jessica Levinson, RD, registered dietitian in New York City (*www.nutritioulicious.com*).

Roger Corder, PhD, professor of experimental therapeutics, William Harvey Research Institute, London, and author of *The Red Wine Diet* (Avery).

Deborah Klein, RD, registered dietitian in California (*www.livitician.com*) and author of *The 200 SuperFoods That Will Save Your Life* (McGraw-Hill).

The Best Type of Garlic For Your Heart

The *Charaka-Samhita*—a medical text from ancient India—recommended garlic for treating heart disease.

A couple of thousand years later, medical experts are still pretty enthusiastic about garlic for your heart.

Hundreds of scientific studies show that a diet rich in this pungent herb can...

●Decrease the stickiness of blood components called *platelets*, reducing the risk of artery-clogging blood clots;

●Lower high blood pressure;

●Increase the flexibility of stiff, "hardened" arteries;

●Slow (and even reverse) the buildup of arterial plaque;

●Cool the chronic low-grade inflammation that fuels heart disease and

●Slow the advance of cardiovascular disease (CVD) in people with type 2 diabetes, most of whom die from CVD.

"Garlic consumption has a significant protective effect against atherosclerosis," concludes an international team of scientists in a recent review of the "vast scientific literature" about garlic and heart disease.

But what's the best type of garlic for your heart?

Raw or cooked? Whole, crushed or sliced? Garlic powder, flakes, oil or the aged extract found in many garlic supplements?

Now: A team of scientists at the Cardiovascular Research Center at the University of Connecticut School of Medicine may have found the answer.

Fresh vs. Powdered

The researchers conducted a study on laboratory animals, dividing them into three groups.

For one month, one group was fed raw, freshly crushed garlic; one group was fed processed, dried garlic and one group wasn't fed any garlic. (The amount of garlic was equivalent to two cloves a day for a person.)

The researchers anesthetized the animals, induced heart attacks and then restored blood flow—while carefully measuring the initial damage to the heart, the speed and strength of recovery from the heart attack and a wide range of cellular changes.

Results: Compared with the animals fed dried garlic, the animals fed raw, crushed garlic had less initial damage to their hearts, with fewer dead heart cells...the blood flow to their hearts was restored more quickly... the heart's ability to pump blood after the heart attack was stronger...there was less cell-damaging oxidation...and there was more activation of heart-protective genes.

The study showed "for the first time that freshly crushed garlic possess superior and diverse cardioprotective abilities compared with processed garlic," says Dipak Das, PhD, the study leader.

But *why* was fresh, crushed garlic more heart-protective than processed?

The *allicin* in garlic—often pointed to as the herb's active ingredient—breaks down into "volatile sulfur compounds," including *hydrogen sulfide*, explains Dr. Das. And the newest research from laboratories around the world shows that it's hydrogen sulfide that probably gives garlic most of its heart-protecting power.

"Although best known as the stuff that gives rotten eggs their distinctive odor, hydrogen sulfide also acts as a chemical messenger in the body, relaxing blood vessels and improving circulation," he says. It also protects heart cells and strengthens the heartbeat.

However: Processed and cooked garlic lose their ability to generate hydrogen sulfide.

Bottom line: "There is growing interest among heart patients in using natural and complementary medicine," says Dr. Das.

"The results of this study strongly suggest that using fresh garlic would provide maximal and added benefits to cardiovascular patients."

The Chefs Recommend

Here are recommendations from two top cookbook writers for putting more fresh, crushed garlic into your diet...

● **How to peel garlic.** "Many people find garlic difficult to peel, but that's because they don't know an important trick—you must crush the garlic before you peel it, says Sarah Pinneo, author of *The Ski House Cookbook* (Clarkson-Potter). *Her recommendation...*

● First, break several cloves off of the garlic bulb. Place the cloves one at a time on a cutting board. Then take a large chef's knife or cleaver and lay the flat side of the blade over the garlic clove, covering it. Hold the knife handle in your nondominant hand. Make a fist with your dominant hand. Pound your fist one time down on the flattened knife blade, taking care not to hit the blade edge with your skin. (If you are worried about this, you can substitute some other flat metal or plastic object for the knife.) When you remove the knife blade, you will have a crushed garlic clove from which the peel separates with just a gentle flick.

● **How to crush fresh garlic.** There are several ways to crush fresh garlic to use in recipes, says Elizabeth Hoiles-Menzel, a professional chef in Las Vegas, NV, and food editor for the book *Reservations Required: Culinary Secrets of Las Vegas Celebrity Chefs* (Huntington). *Her recommendations...*

Knife and Cutting Board: Roughly chop several cloves of garlic. Using the side of the blade and a pinch of coarse salt, grind the garlic into a paste. The garlic may then be placed in a bowl and mixed with the remaining ingredients in a recipe. "This is a great way to add garlic to tabbouleh or cucumber-yogurt salad," says Hoiles-Menzel.

Garlic Press: Garlic presses are also effective for adding crushed garlic directly to a recipe, she says. "After you're done, rinse the press immediately to keep the garlic from drying in the little holes of the press and making it difficult to clean."

Mortar and Pestle: Place several cloves of garlic into the mortar (a heavy bowl with a rough interior) and crush the garlic using the pestle, she says. Additional ingredients can be added to the mortar and the pestle to make a sauce, dip or topping. "This is a traditional way to make pesto sauces, fresh salsas and salad dressings."

Food Processor or Blender: Place the garlic cloves in the food processor and pulse the garlic until it reaches the desired size or puree, she instructs. You can add additional ingredients to the processor to make a finished sauce, dip, topping or even a green smoothie. "I find the processor a very effective way to make pesto sauces, garlic and herb blends to top salads and entrees, garlic-rich dips like baba ganoush or hummus or salad dressings."

Dipak Das, PhD, professor and director of the Cardiovascular Research Center, University of Connecticut.

Sarah Pinneo, author of *The Ski House Cookbook* (Clarkson-Potter).

Elizabeth Hoiles-Menzel, professional chef in Las Vegas and food editor for *Reservations Required: Culinary Secrets of Las Vegas Celebrity Chefs* (Huntington).

The Heart-Saving Secret In Chinese Herbs

The body's natural cardiovascular wonder drug. That's the description of nitric oxide in the book *No More Heart Disease* (St. Martin's) by Louis Ignarro, PhD, who won the Nobel Prize in 1998 for his discovery of how nitric oxide (not to be confused with nitrous oxide, or laughing gas) affects the heart.

Nitric oxide (NO, for short) is manufactured by the body in the endothelium, the single layer of cells that lines the arteries and veins. *And it's a "cardiovascular wonder drug" because it can...*

● Relax and expand blood vessels, lowering high blood pressure;

● Prevent the formation of artery-plugging blood clots, the trigger for many heart attacks and strokes;

● Slow the buildup of artery-clogging plaque and

● Protect the heart or brain from injury after a heart attack or stroke.

"Without a doubt, NO is the most important molecule in the cardiovascular system," says Nathan Bryan, PhD, of the Brown Institute of Molecular Medicine at the University of Texas Health Science Center in Houston.

Dr. Bryan's research is focused on developing strategies for enhancing the body's production of NO—and because several of his colleagues at the Institute have been trained in Traditional Chinese Medicine (TCM), they decided to see if herbs used by TCM to treat heart disease might work by generating nitric oxide.

1,000 Times Stronger

First, the researchers went to a local oriental herb and acupuncture shop in Texas and bought herbs commonly used in TCM to treat heart disease—DanShen, GuaLou, XieBai and six others.

Next, they tested each herb three ways...

1. Quantity of nitrite and nitrate, chemical precursors of NO

2. Ability to generate nitric oxide from nitrite and nitrate

3. Ability to relax the blood vessels of laboratory animals by stimulating the production of NO in the endothelium

Result: The herbs excelled in all three areas.

They contained lots of nitrate and nitrite. They were able to turn those compounds into nitric oxide—in fact, one herb did it at a level 1,000 times greater than the body does it. And they were very effective at relaxing and widening blood vessels through NO production.

"Traditional Chinese medicines that have been used for thousands of years have profound NO bioactivity," say Dr. Bryan and his fellow researchers, in the journal *Free Radical Biology & Medicine*.

Find the Best TCM Formulas

"This study is so affirming for the effectiveness of the herbs used in TCM to protect the heart," says Angelo Druda, a certified practitioner of Traditional Chinese Medicine in northern California and author of *The Tao of Rejuvenation: Fundamental Principles of Health, Longevity and Essential Well-Being* (North Atlantic).

Druda emphasizes that DanShen, GuaLou, XieBai and other herbs are usually used in combination, in a formula customized for the patient's unique pattern of imbalances, as understood by TCM. "No two people are exactly alike, and the best treatment is always a unique formula."

However: "Several experienced TCM practitioners have created companies that sell high-level, effective formulas to other practitioners of TCM, including heart formulas—and they can produce excellent results," he says.

●**Sources of healing herb combinations.** As an expert in Chinese herbology, Druda created the formula Cultivation, which increases blood production and circulation. It is available at *www.traditionalbotanical medicine.com* or call (707) 928-4126.

Other sources of excellent TCM formulas used by many certified practitioners include:

●The Institute for Traditional Medicine, *www.itmonline.org* or call 503-233-4907.

●Blue Poppy, at *www.bluepoppy.com*, or call 800-487-9296 or 303-447-8372.

●Health Concerns, at *www.healthcon cerns.com*, or call 800-233-9355 or 510-639-0280.

Find a certified practitioner of TCM. To find a competent practitioner of TCM who can either create or recommend a formula for you, Druda suggests looking for an individual who has been certified by a reputable organization.

You can find a practitioner certified by the National Certification Commission for Acupuncture and Oriental Medicine (NCCAOM) by visiting its Web site (*www.nccaom.org*) and clicking on "Find a Practitioner" on the home page. At their "Certification Registry" you can enter your state and zip code to find all the practitioners certified by the NCCAOM in "Chinese Herbology" and "Oriental Medicine."

Nathan Bryan, PhD, assistant professor, Brown Institute of Molecular Medicine at the University of Texas Health Science Center in Houston.

Angelo Druda, certified practitioner of Traditional Chinese Medicine and author of *The Tao of Rejuvenation* (Worth Atlantic).

The Verdict Is In—Fish Oil Can Save Your Life

What if there were just one food or one pill that could dramatically reduce your risk of the heart problems that bedevil and kill more Americans than any other disease...

●**Coronary artery disease,** the slow, toxic accumulation of arterial plaque, choking off the flow of blood and oxygen to the heart.

●**Heart attack,** the disastrous, and sometimes deadly, blockage of blood flow to the heart.

●**Sudden cardiac death,** electrical mayhem in the rhythms of the heart (*arrhythmia*), causing cardiac arrest.

●**Atrial fibrillation,** a quiver rather than a beat in the upper chambers of the heart, increasing the risk of blood clots and strokes.

●**Heart failure,** a weakened heart (perhaps damaged by one or more heart attacks) that can't pump blood normally, choking the body of oxygen.

Fortunately, there is one food and one pill that can help prevent or treat all these conditions.

The food is oily fish. The pill is a fish oil supplement.

Three Decades of Evidence

A recent "state-of-the-art" paper in the *Journal of the American College Cardiology*—by cardiologist and fish oil expert Carl Lavie, MD, medical director of Cardiac Rehabilitation and Prevention at the Ochsner Heart and Vascular Institute in New Orleans, Louisiana, and his colleagues—details three decades of studies on fish oil and heart health, involving more than 40,000 people.

And the scientific evidence that fish oil—specifically, the omega-3 fatty acids EPA (*eicosapentaenoic acid*) and DHA (*docosahexaenoic acid*)—is good for your heart isn't just "suggestive," as cautious scientists like to say. It's incontrovertible.

"We now have tremendous and compelling evidence from very large studies, some dating back 20 and 30 years, that demonstrate the protective benefits of omega-3 fish oil in multiple aspects of preventive cardiology," says Dr. Lavie.

Why it works: The body incorporates fish oil into the membranes (outer envelopes) of red blood cells and the cells of your blood vessels. *From there, it works to…*

● Reduce triglycerides, blood fats that can damage the heart;

● Stabilize plaque—crucial, because a chunk of plaque can break off an artery wall and become an artery-closing blood clot;

● Stop the deposition of collagen, a protein fiber that stiffens flexible arteries;

● Boost the functioning of the endothelium, the lining of the artery, which generates artery-relaxing, clot-dissolving nitric oxide;

● Reduce inflammation—and chronic, low-grade inflammation fuels heart disease;

● Lower blood pressure, a major risk factor for heart attacks and strokes;

● Thin the blood by decreasing platelet aggregation, the clumping of tiny structures in the blood that form blood clots;

● Prevent arrhythmias, the chaotic electrical episodes that can cause sudden cardiac death and

● Tone the autonomic nervous system, which controls the heartbeat—another way to decrease the risk of arrhythmia.

Two Fish Meals a Week

"You can get fish oil into your diet by eating oily fish, such as herring, mackerel, salmon, albacore tuna, sardines and oysters, or by taking fish oil supplements or cod liver oil," says Dr. Lavie.

Recommended intake: If you have heart disease, the American Heart Association recommends a daily dose of 1,000 milligrams (mg) (1 gram) of EPA and DHA.

If you don't have heart disease, the AHA recommends you eat two oily fish meals a week, which is the equivalent of about 500 mg a day of EPA and DHA—the amount linked to the lowest risk of developing heart disease.

As a cardiologist, Dr. Lavie adds these recommendations…

● **To prevent heart failure,** a supplement containing 800 to 1,000 mg a day of combined EPA and DHA.

● **To lower triglycerides,** supplements supplying 4 grams a day of EPA and DHA (a therapeutic dose taken with the approval and supervision of a doctor).

Dr. Lavie notes that your doctor can safely combine a high-dose fish oil supplement with statins, fibrates, niacin and other "lipid therapies."

Bottom line: "It's really good to get your fish oil through diet—because you replace bad food with good food, and you don't have to take a supplement," says Dr. Lavie.

However: "Very few people probably have two fish meals per week—the amount you need to get 500 mg a day," he says. And the dosage that showed benefits in heart disease would require five fish meals a week. So it may be far more practical to take a fish oil supplement.

"If you have heart disease, you should talk to your doctor about whether a fish oil supplement is needed, and what the right amount is for maximum heart protection in your case."

Smart idea: "I eat a lot of fish, including sushi," he says.

"And I take a supplement on the days I don't eat fish. If I ate sushi the evening before, I skip the supplement the next day."

Product: Dr. Lavie recommends Lovaza, a prescription omega-3 supplement, which is guaranteed to deliver the specified amount of DHA and EPA.

For over-the-counter brands, he prefers Nordic Naturals and GNC.

● **Don't worry about mercury.** You may be scared of eating a lot of fish—particularly if you're pregnant or nursing—because you've heard it's contaminated with mercury or other pollutants.

Not to worry, says Dr. Lavie.

"A study of nearly 12,000 British women during their pregnancy and beyond found that women who exceeded the US FDA recommendation for fish intake actually had offspring with better cognitive and behavioral development than the offspring of women who consumed less fish," he says. (DHA nourishes the brain and nervous system.)

Dr. Lavie also points to a risk-benefit analysis from researchers at Harvard Medical School that looked at hundreds of studies on fish and fish oil. It showed that oily fish and/or supplements reduced deaths from heart disease by 36% and premature deaths from any cause by 17%—and did not increase the risk of "subclinical neurodevelopmental deficits" in children caused by mercury, or the risk of cancer in adults caused by the fish-borne pollutants PCBs and dioxin.

"The most commonly consumed dietary sources of omega-3—salmon, sardines, trout, oysters and herring—are quite low in mercury," says Dr. Lavie. "And because mercury is water soluble and protein bound, it's present in the muscle of the fish but not in the oil, so fish oil supplements should contain negligible amounts of mercury."

Red flag: The Harvard researchers warn consumers away from three mercury-laden species—swordfish, shark and golden bass (tilefish) from the Gulf of Mexico.

Carl Lavie, MD, medical director of cardiac rehabilitation and prevention at the Ochsner Heart and Vascular Institute in New Orleans.

Juice Up Your Heart

"Juice has gotten a bad rap," says Gale Maleskey, RD, a clinical dietitian and author of *Nature's Medicines* (Rodale). "That's because when people heard soda was bad for you, many stopped drinking 32 ounces or more of soda a day and started drinking the same amount of juice. But drinking large quantities of any sugar-rich

beverage is not a healthy choice, because of the extra calories and the risk of diabetes."

However: Several recent studies show that drinking a glass or two a day of a juice packed with cell-nourishing, cell-protecting plant antioxidants called *polyphenols* can be a healthy choice—particularly for your heart.

Striking Research Findings

• **Tart cherry juice, a powerful antioxidant.** Researchers at the Kronos Longevity Institute in Phoenix, Arizona, asked 12 people, average age 69, to drink either 8 ounces of tart cherry juice twice a day, or a look-alike juice.

Two weeks later, those drinking the true cherry juice had triple the ability to resist *oxidative damage*, the injury to cells and genes from molecules called free radicals that is a main cause of heart disease.

"Tart cherries are very rich in protective antioxidants, such as flavonols and anthocyanins," says Tinna Traustadóttir, PhD, the study leader.

"It's often hard to eat four to five servings of antioxidant-rich fruit every day," Dr. Traustadóttir says. "This is a very convenient way of maximizing antioxidant intake."

Product: The product used in the study was CherryPharm, a 100% juice with 50 tart cherries per bottle. You can order the juice online at *www.cherrypharm.com* or use the Web site to find a retailer near you.

• **Pomegranate juice, for cleaner arteries.** Researchers at the University of Chicago studied 289 people, aged 45 to 74, all of whom had one or more risk factors for heart disease, such as high cholesterol. They divided them into two groups—one drank 8 ounces a day of pomegranate juice, and one didn't.

After one year, the pomegranate-drinkers with the most risk factors for heart disease had a much slower accumulation of artery-clogging plaque, compared with the high-risk folks not drinking the juice.

The findings were in *American Journal of Cardiology*.

"I was surprised by the results," says Michael Davidson, MD, the study leader and director of preventive cardiology at the University of Chicago Medical Center. "Pomegranate juice slowed the progression of atherosclerosis in the group most at risk for heart disease and stroke."

Theory: The powerful antioxidants in pomegranate juice slow or stop the oxidation of LDL cholesterol, the process that creates arterial plaque.

Dr. Davidson says that larger studies are needed to prove that pomegranate juice is truly protective against cardiovascular disease. But he calls the results "encouraging"—and recommends talking to your doctor about whether pomegranate juice is right for you.

Product: POM Wonderful was the juice used in the study.

Smart idea: If you're overweight or have diabetes, drinking 8 ounces of juice a day may not be advisable because of the amount of calories and sugar. If that's the case, says Dr. Davidson, you can get the same amount of pomegranate antioxidants found in an 8-ounce glass of juice by taking a one teaspoon liquid extract of the juice or a pomegranate extract pill, both called POM-X.

● **Orange juice, for lower blood pressure.** Research links a diet rich in flavonols, a class of polyphenols, to less risk for heart disease. French researchers decided to see if the most abundant flavonol in orange juice—*hesperidin*—might help control high blood pressure, a risk factor for heart disease and stroke.

To find out, they studied 24 men, aged 50 to 64, dividing them into three groups. One group drank 16 ounces of orange juice a day. One group drank a placebo beverage, and also took a pill containing 292 milligrams (mg) of hesperidin, the amount in 16 ounces of orange juice. And one group drank the placebo beverage and took a placebo pill.

After one month, those drinking the orange juice and taking the hesperidin had a significant drop in blood pressure. There was no change in the placebo group.

The researchers also noted that orange juice quickly increased levels of nitric oxide, a biochemical that relaxes and strengthens arteries.

And the men drinking OJ or taking hesperidin had more activity in hundreds of genes linked to control of CVD.

Important: "Whole fruit contains up to two times as much hesperidin as the equivalent amount of juice," says Christine Morand, PhD, the study leader. "Eating 1 to 1¼ oranges provides as much hesperidin as drinking 16 ounces of juice."

Juicing Judiciously

"These and other studies make clear that some juices have very unique polyphenols and drinking more of them is worthwhile," says Maleskey. *Her suggestions for drinking juice healthfully…*

● **Don't overdo it.** "Pure fruit juice can have more calories per ounce than soda—for example, 20 calories for grape juice, compared with 12 calories for cola," she says. "That's 160 calories for an 8-ounce glass of juice—a lot of calories, if you're trying to control or lose weight. Plus, it's easy to overconsume juice, because your body doesn't register 'fullness' the way it does with solid food."

What to do: Stick to 4 to 6 ounces a day, or ½ to ¾ of a cup.

Red flag: If you have diabetes, avoid juices. "They can upset your blood sugar levels," says Maleskey.

● **Drink unfiltered juice.** "It has a lot more heart-healthy polyphenols in it than filtered juice," says Maleskey. Unfiltered juice is usually cloudy in the bottle.

● **Drink juice with a high-fiber, high-protein snack.** A handful of nuts are a good choice, says Maleskey. Or drink juice with a meal. "With this strategy, the sugar from the juice enters the bloodstream more slowly, preventing an unhealthy spike of blood sugar."

● **Mix juice with a soluble fiber supplement.** "It helps slow the absorption of sugars—and reduces cholesterol, too. And a soluble fiber supplement made from methylcellulose doesn't thicken the juice, so you won't even know it's there."

Product: Benefiber, from Novartis.

Gale Maleskey, RD, clinical dietitian and author of *Nature's Medicines* (Rodale). *www.galemaleskey.com.*

Tinna Traustadóttir, PhD, associate director of exercise sciences, Kronos Longevity Research Institute (KLRI).

Michael Davidson, MD, director of preventive cardiology, University of Chicago Medical Center.

Christine Morand, PhD, senior research scientist, biochemist and nutritionist, Centre Hospitalier Universitaire, Clermont-Ferrand, France.

Keep LDL in Check With L-Carnitine

L DL cholesterol is known far and wide as the "bad" cholesterol, but that's a bad rap. The truth is we need cholesterol, including the LDL kind. But when free radicals in the body oxidize LDL cholesterol it does indeed turn from friend to foe, building up in artery walls—it is one of the substances that lays the foundation for dangerous plaque.

Recently an Italian study demonstrated that one way to reduce oxidized LDL levels is by supplementation with the amino acid derivative *L-carnitine.* Researchers randomly assigned 81 patients with diabetes (who are prone to cholesterol problems) to one of two treatment groups. One group received a placebo and the other received 2 grams of L-carnitine once daily. At the end of three months, the L-carnitine-treated patients showed a decrease of oxidized LDL levels compared with the placebo group.

The Many Uses of L-Carnitine

According to Mark Stengler, NMD, L-carnitine helps with various health problems and its benefits are not limited to people with diabetes. He notes that L-carnitine—or *carnitine* as it is also called—helps get energy to the heart muscles and is therefore beneficial to a number of cardiac conditions (angina, ischemia-induced arrhythmias, cardiomyopathy and congestive heart failure). It has also been used as therapy for myocardial infarction to help minimize muscle damage as a result of the oxygen reduction…it is helpful for chronic fatigue syndrome and kidney and liver disease…and there's more.

Studies have shown that carnitine (in the form known as acetyl-l-carnitine) may help ease the discomfort of *peripheral neuropathy*, a condition often triggered by diabetes or chemotherapy drugs that causes nerves in the feet and sometimes the hands to develop painful burning and stinging sensations. It appears that carnitine may even help peripheral nerves regenerate, though this is a preliminary finding.

A variety of small studies have looked at the possibility that carnitine also boosts athletic performance given its role in energy production, but so far none has shown any positive effect. However, Dr. Stengler states that his patients who engage in endurance sports such as long-distance running seem to benefit from it. Dr. Stengler says people with elevated LDL (but who do not have diabetes) can also benefit from taking carnitine to help prevent LDL oxidation.

How to Get Carnitine Into Your Body

Carnitine is naturally produced in the body by the liver and kidneys and is stored in the skeletal muscles, brain and heart, but, as is so often the case, production diminishes with advancing age. You can obtain carnitine through food, in particular red meat. Steak or hamburger has three times the amount of carnitine as pork, another high source. Lesser dietary sources include dairy products, chicken, fish and avocado. It may be a good idea for vegetarians and vegans to consider carnitine supplementation.

Additionally, Dr. Stengler says people who suffer from muscle fatigue and cramps may have a carnitine deficiency. For such complaints, he orders a blood test to measure carnitine levels in the tissue and red blood cells, weighs this data against patient symptoms, and treats accordingly.

Carnitine Supplementation

For adult patients who have chronic fatigue, congestive heart failure or angina, Dr. Stengler often prescribes dosages of 1,000 milligrams (mg), taken two or three times daily. Higher dosages of up to 2,000 mg a day may even be a good idea for people with high LDL levels, he says, but the body can't absorb any more than this at a time. A reported side effect is occasional digestive upset. Carnitine is considered quite safe. Dr. Stengler decreases the dosage or directs the carnitine to be taken with meals for those who find this to be a problem. As always, if you are interested in taking carnitine and most especially if you take any drugs or supplements, be sure to discuss this with your doctor before you start.

Mark Stengler, NMD, naturopathic medical doctor in private practice, La Jolla, California, and author of *Bottom Line/Natural Healing* newsletter. *www.drstengler.com.*

The New Blood Pressure Control Diet for Women

For the first time, high blood pressure that is uncontrolled is more common in women than in men—yet women are less likely to be prescribed treatment, such as blood pressure–lowering medication. High blood pressure, or hypertension, doesn't hurt or cause other obvious warning signs, but it damages arteries in ways that can lead to stroke, heart attack, kidney problems and cognitive impairment. *More concerns for women…*

• Hypertension now affects nearly one in four American women. Rates in women are rising even as rates in men are falling.

• About 35% of women with hypertension go untreated.

Blood pressure is the force that blood exerts against the arterial walls. It is reported as two numbers. The top number, or *systolic pressure*, is the pressure as the heart pumps. The bottom number, or *diastolic pressure*, is the pressure as the heart rests between beats. Normal, healthy blood pressure is below 120/80 millimeters of mercury (mmHg)… hypertension is diagnosed at 140/90 mmHg or higher.

Problem: Up to 70% of people who are told that they are fine because their blood pressure is in the "high normal" range actually are at serious risk. Systolic pressure of 120 to 139 and/or diastolic pressure of 80 to 89 indicates prehypertension—which often progresses to hypertension.

Good news: You can significantly reduce blood pressure by changing what you eat. You must do more than just cut back on salt—although following this common advice helps—but the simple strategies below are worth the effort.

If you already have hypertension or have "high normal" blood pressure…are at risk due to being overweight or having a family history of blood pressure problems…or simply want to be as healthy as possible, this diet is for you.

Bonus: These habits often lead to weight loss—which also lowers blood pressure.

Have more…

• **Berries.** Berries are high in polyphenols, micronutrients that relax blood vessels.

Study: Hypertension patients who ate berries daily for two months lowered their systolic blood pressure by up to seven points—which could reduce risk for heart-related death by up to 15%.

Action: Eat one cup of fresh or frozen berries daily.

• **Fat-free milk.** A study found that people who ingested the greatest amounts of low-fat dairy were 56% less likely to develop hypertension than those who ate the least.

Theory: The active components may be the milk proteins whey and/or casein, which help blood vessels dilate.

Action: Have eight to 16 ounces of fat-free milk per day. Evidence suggests that fat-free milk is best—higher fat milk and other dairy products may not work as well.

● **Potassium-rich produce.** Potassium counteracts the blood pressure–raising effects of sodium.

New study: Prehypertension patients with the highest sodium-to-potassium intake were up to 50% more likely to develop cardiovascular disease within 10 to 15 years, compared with those who had the lowest ratio.

Action: Among the generally recommended five or so daily servings of fruits and vegetables, include some potassium-rich choices, such as bananas, citrus fruits, lima beans, potatoes and sweet potatoes (with skin), tomatoes and yams. Talk to your doctor before increasing potassium if you take blood pressure or heart medication (diuretic, ACE inhibitor or ARB blocker) or if you have kidney problems.

● **Fiber.** Studies suggest that fiber lowers blood pressure, though the mechanism is unknown. The fiber must come from food —fiber supplements do not offer the same benefit.

Action: Check food labels, and aim for at least 25 grams of fiber daily.

Good sources: Whole fruits (juice has less fiber)…raw or lightly cooked vegetables (overcooking reduces fiber)…beans and lentils …high-fiber breakfast cereals…and whole grains, such as barley, brown rice, oats, quinoa and whole wheat.

Eat less…

● **Meat.** Often high in cholesterol and saturated fat, meat contributes to the buildup of plaque inside arteries—a condition called *atherosclerosis.* Hypertension significantly increases the risk that atherosclerosis will lead to a heart attack or stroke.

Action: If you have been diagnosed with both atherosclerosis and hypertension, a good way to reduce your cardiovascular risk is to adopt a vegetarian or near-vegetarian diet.

Also: Avoid other sources of saturated fats, such as high-fat dairy, and palm oil.

If you are concerned about getting enough protein, increase your intake of plant proteins.

Good sources: Soy foods (edamame, soy milk, tofu)…beans, lentils, peas…nuts and seeds.

If you have hypertension or prehypertension but no atherosclerosis, limit yourself to no more than three weekly four-ounce servings of animal protein, and stick with low-fat meat, fish or poultry.

● **Salt.** Sodium raises blood pressure by increasing blood volume and constricting blood vessels. Some people are more sensitive to salt than others—but limiting dietary salt is a good idea for everyone.

Recommended: Healthy people up to age 50 should limit sodium to 2,300 mg per day (about one teaspoon of salt)…older people and anyone with prehypertension or hypertension should stay under 1,500 mg daily (about two-thirds of a teaspoon of salt).

Action: Instead of salt, add flavor with pepper, garlic and other seasonings. Do not use seasoning blends that contain salt. Avoid processed and canned foods unless labeled "low sodium."

Pros and cons of…

● **Red wine.** Like berries, red wine contains heart-healthy polyphenols.

But: Polyphenols relax blood vessels only when exposure time is short, as with light-to-moderate alcohol consumption. Heavy drinking actually reduces the blood vessels' ability to relax, negating polyphenols' benefits.

Advised: If you choose to drink alcohol, opt for red wine and have no more than one glass per day.

Alcohol-free option: Polyphenol-rich unsweetened dark grape juice.

● **Coffee, tea and soda.** Some evidence links caffeine to increased blood pressure.

Advised: Opt for caffeine-free beverages.

Good choice: Herbal tea. A recent study suggests that drinking three cups daily of a blend that includes hibiscus can lower systolic blood pressure by about seven mmHg.

● **Chocolate.** Small studies suggest that dark chocolate helps lower blood pressure.

Theory: Cocoa contains antioxidant procyanidins, which boost the body's production of nitric oxide, a chemical that relaxes blood vessels.

But: Chocolate is high in sugar and fat, both of which contribute to weight gain.

Advised: If you want an occasional dessert, one-half ounce of dark chocolate is a good choice.

C. Tissa Kappagoda, MD, PhD, professor of medicine, director, cardiac rehabilitation program, University of California, Davis.

Home Blood Pressure Monitoring May Save Your Life

The twenty-first-century version of the standard doctor's advice may be "take your blood pressure twice a day and call or e-mail me in the morning."

As our collective blood pressure keeps rising and more and more research affirms the benefit of at-home monitoring to better manage hypertension, patients are being instructed to keep close track of their own highs and lows. According to new guidelines from the American Heart Association, the American Society of Hypertension and the Preventive Cardiovascular Nurses' Association, most Americans with known or suspected hypertension (74 million adults, at least) should take regular blood pressure readings at home—especially those with high blood pressure of 140/90 mm Hg or higher.

Not only will this help keep hypertension in check, but it also may be the only accurate way to get measurements for people who suffer from what's come to be known as "white coat hypertension," where the mere fact that a health care professional is checking makes blood pressure soar.

Hypertension and vascular specialist Mark C. Houston, MD, author of *What Your Doctor May Not Tell You About Hypertension: The Revolutionary Nutrition and Lifestyle Program to Help Fight High Blood Pressure* (Grand Central) explains the benefits of home pressure monitoring.

By providing a more accurate representation of day-to-day rises and falls, home monitoring can confirm suspected or newly diagnosed hypertension or it can be used to evaluate and fine-tune your response to antihypertensive treatment, says Dr. Houston. Continuous monitoring may also be valuable for people with borderline or pre-hypertension (between 120/80 and 139/89), as it can help determine whether to initiate treatment and at what level.

Best Buy: Digital Monitors

The two most common types of home monitors are aneroid and digital. Aneroid monitors are the old-fashioned ones that have a stethoscope, a bulb you pump to inflate, a cuff and a gauge. Digital monitors are more convenient and easier to use on yourself, with built-in sensors and easy-to-read number displays, plus most automatically inflate and deflate. According to Dr. Houston, the arm monitors are the most accurate. Although wrist and finger versions are also available, Dr. Houston does not recommend using them.

Those who are instructed to begin home monitoring should do it twice daily, as close to the same time as you can—once in the morning, before you take medication and again in the evening. If you plan to exercise or drink anything with caffeine—or have a cigarette, which you shouldn't be doing anyway—take your blood pressure first. Also, make sure to sit quietly for five minutes before taking a reading.

Monitors are widely available at pharmacies, medical supply stores and online. Prices vary from about $30 to over $100, depending on options (e.g., memory recall that allows you to view blood pressure history, built-in printers and a USB cable or AC adapter to hook up to a computer to transmit data directly to your doctor's office). Dr. Houston likes those by Omron (*www.omronhealth care.com*).

Whatever monitor you choose, make sure your doctor sees and approves it and also tests it against what's used in the office. Ask for some training in proper use as well. Establish in advance what type of reading merits a phone call or visit.

It may require a little extra work, but home blood pressure monitoring can pay off with a lower risk of serious complications and greater peace of mind.

Mark C. Houston, MD, associate clinical professor of medicine, Vanderbilt University School of Medicine, director, Hypertension Institute, and author of What Your Doctor May Not Tell You About Hypertension *(Grand Central).*

Peas Help Reduce Blood Pressure

Peas, once viewed as a starchy vegetable, are now being recognized as nutritional blockbusters, packed with protein, assorted nutrients and fiber and free of fat and cholesterol. Even better, Canadian food chemists have discovered a protein in yellow garden peas that shows promise in treating high blood pressure and chronic kidney disease (CKD).

While researching treatment options for patients with kidney disease, Rotimi Aluko, PhD, a professor in the department of human nutritional sciences at the University of Manitoba, in Winnipeg, Canada, and colleagues purified a mixture of proteins—pea protein *hydrolysate*—from yellow peas. They fed this to rats with severe kidney disease every day for eight weeks. At the end of this period, Dr. Aluko and his team found that...

Blood pressure decreased by 20% in rats who consumed the pea mixture, compared with a control group of rats who did not.

Urine production, which typically decreases with kidney disease, improved by 30% in treated rats, bringing it to a normal level.

Pea Pills for the Heart and Kidneys

Given these promising results, trials are now under way in humans with mild hypertension, and—subject to regulatory approval—Dr. Aluko estimates that an edible product derived from peas could be available in as little as two to three years. By 2012, you may be able to stroll into your local pharmacy or health food store and purchase pea extract in pill form or as a powder to add to food or beverages. As for eating peas themselves, Dr. Aluko explains that for this purpose pea proteins must be treated with special enzymes in order to become active. But he believes that they're healthy anyway—so tell the kids and adults at the table to eat their peas, please.

Rotimi Aluko, PhD, professor, department of human nutritional sciences, University of Manitoba, Winnipeg, Canada.

"Massage" Therapy For Angina

If climbing stairs, walking fast or running brings on a crushing pain in your chest, you may be experiencing angina. You should not treat this lightly. Angina is a symptom of *ischemia*, which occurs when blood flow to your heart slows, starving the muscle of the oxygen it needs. Though the pain typically subsides when you rest, it's not safe to ignore it. Angina is almost always a symptom of coronary artery disease, and it should be evaluated by your physician.

A Safe and Noninvasive Treatment

First-line therapy for angina typically involves addressing the underlying problem, according to C. Richard Conti, MD, a professor of medicine at the University of Florida in Gainesville, which is usually high blood pressure, high cholesterol or diabetes. Some patients have blocked arteries, which conventional Western medicine generally treats with angioplasty or stenting. Both of these can be effective, short-term solutions to open the arteries, but Dr. Conti said that some patients find they still experience angina. Also, there are some patients for whom such invasive treatments aren't advisable, due to underlying medical problems.

Fortunately, there's another solution that is quite effective—external counterpulsation (ECP) therapy, which significantly reduces or eliminates angina about 70% of the time.

In contrast to the other treatments available, ECP isn't all that complicated or high tech. The technology itself resembles a large, comfortable reclining chair. The patient sits and a technician wraps three pressure cuffs—similar to but slightly larger than standard blood pressure cuffs—around the calves, lower thighs and upper thighs or buttocks. The cuffs inflate and deflate, compressing and releasing blood vessels in the limbs to move blood toward the heart. This "unloads" the heart by relaxing pressure in the arteries while the heart is pumping, Dr. Conti explains. As the cuffs inflate and deflate in harmony with your cardiac cycle, they encourage optimal coronary blood and oxygen flow. This action relieves chest pain and improves exercise tolerance, which means that you can begin to work out again without discomfort—another plus for heart health.

A standard course of ECP treatment consists of 35 one-hour outpatient sessions over a period of seven weeks. This is a big time commitment, Dr. Conti acknowledges, but he finds that angina sufferers are willing to put in the time if it gets rid of their pain. If the treatment is successful but angina eventually recurs, it can be repeated. Outcome varies—some patients obtain relief that lasts for years.

Note: While ECP is generally safe, doctors do not recommend it for people who have conditions such as phlebitis, peripheral artery disease or a leaky aortic valve, because it can lead to complications.

More Extensive Use of ECP in the Future?

Health insurers generally cover ECP for angina but only after standard medical and surgical care fails to control it. Dr. Conti notes that treatment may be beneficial earlier, for example as a complement to medical management before surgery proves necessary. Since this has not been demonstrated in trials, it's not typically covered by insurance. Data also suggests that ECP may benefit people with heart failure, but again further study is needed. If new research continues to demonstrate expanded benefits, however, treatment—and coverage for treatment—is likely to be extended as well.

C. Richard Conti, MD, professor of medicine, Division of Cardiovascular Medicine, University of Florida, Gainesville, Florida.

Chapter 10

MEMORY

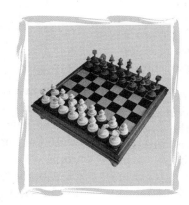

Reverse Brain Aging by Three Years—in Three Seconds a Day

Yes, three seconds—about the time you'd need to take a supplement of DHA (*docosahexaenoic acid*), an omega-3 fatty acid that recent research shows can erase years of aging from your brain.

Better Memory

Researchers studied 485 people, with an average age of 70. They were healthy, but they had a problem called *age-related memory loss*—even though their memory was normal for someone their age, it wasn't as reliable and ready as it once was. (About 40% of people over 60 have this problem.)

At the beginning of the study, the participants took a test that measured memory and learning ability. Then the researchers divided them into two groups, giving one group a daily supplement of DHA and the other a placebo.

Six months later, the study participants took the memory/learning test again—and those who had taken DHA scored 47% higher on the test than those who hadn't. (And the higher the DHA blood levels among the DHA-takers, the better they did on the test.)

"The benefit from taking DHA was roughly equivalent to having the memory and learning skills of someone three years younger," says Karin Yurko-Mauro, PhD, the study leader.

"Our study suggests that taking DHA would help slow or reverse the kind of memory loss that often bothers people as they age—not recalling a name, or not being able to locate your keys, or forgetting where you parked your car."

Latest development: In other new research, scientists from the University of Pittsburgh studied 280 people who were 36 to 55 years old. They measured their blood levels of DHA, and also had them take several tests that measured memory and other mental functions, such as reasoning and mental flexibility.

The higher the blood level of DHA, the better the performance on the tests.

"It is plausible that insufficient dietary intake of DHA is related to relatively poor cognitive abilities or performance," say the researchers, in the *Journal of Nutrition.* "DHA may favorably affect cognitive performance, and may do so throughout the lifespan," they conclude.

Why it works: DHA accounts for 97% of the omega-3 fatty acids in the brain, says Dr. Yurko-Mauro. It's found in high levels in the membrane or outer covering of brain cells (*neurons*)…in the mitochondria, or energy-generating structures within neurons…and in dendrites, the branchlike extensions of neurons.

DHA improves signaling between neurons…helps neurons repair and regrow…and protects neurons from the inflammatory and oxidative damage that ages the brain. "Optimal DHA levels are a must for optimal brain functioning," says Dr. Yurko-Mauro.

In fact, she says, more than a dozen studies that analyze DHA intake and health in large populations linked lower intakes of DHA with a higher risk for cognitive decline and Alzheimer's disease.

And animal studies show that DHA can block the production and accumulation of the protein plaques and tangles in the brain that are the main features of Alzheimer's.

A Guaranteed Intake

DHA is found in fatty fish, such as salmon, sardines, anchovies, mackerel, herring and tuna. But to get the amount of DHA used in the study—900 milligrams (mg) a day—you'd have to eat five fatty fish meals a week, something most people don't or won't do, says Dr. Yurko-Mauro.

For a guaranteed intake, she recommends taking a daily supplement containing 900 mg of DHA.

However: The DHA used in the study was not from fish oil. It was from algae, under the brand name Life's DHA. (Fatty fish supply DHA because they eat DHA-rich algae in the ocean.) This vegetarian source of DHA is produced in stainless steel vats in controlled facilities, so there's no risk of mercury or PCB contamination (which is a concern with fatty fish or fish oil).

Product: You can find algae-based fish oil under the brand name Algal 900 at major retailers, such as Walmart, CVS and Walgreens.

Red flag: You can also get DHA in fish oil, but check the supplement to make sure it supplies 900 mg. Most fish oil supplements contain more EPA (*eicosapentaenoic acid*), which is proven to help the heart but not the brain.

Karin Yurko-Mauro, PhD, associate director, clinical research, Martek Biosciences Corporation.

Superfoods, Superbrain

The aging American population is facing a sharp increase in diagnosed cases of dementia. Alzheimer's disease and other forms of dementia affect about 10% of people 65 and older. Among those in their mid-80s and older, up to half have a significant degree of cognitive impairment.

Millions of younger Americans suffer from less obvious mental impairments, including mild memory loss and diminished alertness, as well as brain-related disorders, such as depression and chronic anxiety.

According to Mark Hyman, MD, founder of, The Ultra Wellness Center, Lenox, Massachusetts, research clearly shows that some foods can improve mental performance and help prevent long-term damage. *Best choices…*

• **Sardines.** They have two to three times more omega-3 fatty acids than most other fatty fish. Our bodies use omega-3s for the efficient transmission of brain signals. People who don't get enough omega-3s in their diets are more likely to experience learning disabilities, dementia and depression.

Bonus: Omega-3s reduce inflammation and inhibit blood clots, the underlying cause of most strokes.

Fatty fish also are high in *choline,* a substance used to manufacture one of the main neurotransmitters (*acetylcholine*) involved in memory.

Recommended: Three cans of sardines a week. Sardines are less likely to accumulate mercury or other toxins than larger fish.

Caution: Many people believe that flaxseed is an adequate substitute for fish. Although it contains *alpha-linolenic acid* (ALA), a type of omega-3, only about 10% of ALA is converted to *docosahexaenoic acid* (DHA) or *eicosapentaenoic acid* (EPA), the most beneficial forms of omega-3s and the ones that are plentiful in fish oil.

If you don't like sardines, you can take fish oil supplements (1,000 milligrams twice a day).

• **Omega-3 eggs.** They're among the best foods for the brain because they contain folate along with omega-3s and choline. *Folate* is a B vitamin that's strongly linked to mood and mental performance. A Finnish study of 2,682 men found that those with the lowest dietary intakes of folate were 67% more likely to experience depression than those with adequate amounts.

Recommended: Up to eight eggs a week. Only buy eggs that say "Omega-3" on the label. It means that the chickens were given a fish meal diet. Eggs without this label contain little or no omega-3s.

• **Low-glycemic carbohydrates.** The glycemic index ranks foods according to how quickly they elevate glucose in the blood. Foods with low glycemic ratings include legumes (beans, lentils) and whole-grain breads. They slow the release of sugars into the bloodstream and prevent sharp rises in insulin.

Why it matters: Elevated insulin is associated with dementia. For example, diabetics with elevated insulin in the blood have four times the rate of dementia as people without diabetes. Elevated insulin damages blood vessels as well as neurons. The damage is so pronounced that some researchers call Alzheimer's disease "type 3 diabetes."

Recommended: Always eat natural, minimally processed foods. They're almost always low on the glycemic index. For example, eat apples instead of applesauce…whole-grain bread instead of white bread…or any of the legumes, such as chickpeas, lentils or soybeans.

• **Nuts.** They're among the few plant foods that contain appreciable amounts of omega-3 fatty acids. They also contain antioxidants, which reduce brain and arterial inflammation that can lead to cognitive decline.

Most of the fat in nuts is monounsaturated—it lowers harmful LDL cholesterol without depressing beneficial HDL cholesterol—important for preventing stroke.

Recommended: One to two handfuls daily. Walnuts and macadamia nuts are among the highest in omega-3s, but all nuts are beneficial. Avoid highly salted and roasted nuts (the roasting changes the composition of the oils). Lightly toasted is okay.

• **Cruciferous vegetables, such as broccoli, brussels sprouts, cauliflower and kale.** They contain detoxifying compounds that help the liver eliminate toxins that can damage the hippocampus and other areas of the brain involved in cognition.

Recommended: One cup daily is optimal, but at least four cups a week. Cooked usually is easier to digest than raw.

• **B-12 foods.** Meat, dairy products and seafood are our only source (apart from supplements) of vitamin B-12 in the diet. This nutrient is critical for brain health. A study published in *American Journal of Clinical Nutrition* found that older adults with low levels of vitamin B-12 were more likely to experience rapid cognitive declines. Older adults have the highest risk for B-12 deficiency because the age-related decline in stomach acid impairs its absorption.

Recommended: Two to three daily servings of organic lean meat, low-fat dairy (including yogurt) or seafood.

Also important: Dr. Hyman advises everyone to take a multinutrient supplement that includes all of the B vitamins.

● **Green tea.** It's a powerful antioxidant and anti-inflammatory that also stimulates the liver's ability to break down toxins. New research indicates that green tea improves insulin sensitivity—important for preventing diabetes and neuro-damaging increases in insulin.

Recommended: One to two cups daily.

● **Berries, including blueberries, raspberries and strawberries.** The darker the berry, the higher the concentration of antioxidant compounds. In studies at Tufts University, animals fed blueberries showed virtually no oxidative brain damage. They also performed better on cognitive tests than animals given a standard diet.

Recommended: One-half cup daily. Frozen berries contain roughly the same level of protective compounds as fresh berries.

Mark Hyman, MD, founder of The UltraWellness Center (*www.ultrawellness.com*) in Lenox, Massachusetts, and author of *The UltraMind Solution* (Scribner).

Blueberries Are Sweet To Your Brain

If you're 65 or over, chances are one in ten that you have a neurodegenerative condition called *mild cognitive impairment* (MCI).

You're diagnosed with MCI when a standard memory test shows that your memory is subpar compared with other people your age. You're starting to forget things you used to routinely remember, such as a dentist's appointment. And your family and friends also have noticed your memory is deteriorating. Worst of all, you're at high risk for dementia—each year, 5 to 10% of people with MCI develop Alzheimer's disease.

"There is no remedy for dementia," says Robert Krikorian, PhD, associate professor in the Department of Psychiatry at the University of Cincinnati. "And it's not clear when or if an effective therapy will be developed. But interventions started in individuals with pre-dementia conditions such as MCI might delay the progression of cognitive decline—and MCI might be the last point at which such an intervention is effective."

That's why Dr. Krikorian and his colleagues from the USDA Human Nutrition Research Center on Aging at Tufts University decided to test a preventive intervention—a fruit that a decade of animal research has shown might protect brain cells and improve memory.

The blueberry.

Memory Improved by 30%

The researchers studied nine older people with an average age of 76—and with MCI. The participants took two standard memory tests at the beginning and end of the three-month study. And every day for three months, they drank three 6-ounce glasses of blueberry juice—one glass with breakfast, lunch and dinner.

At the end of the three months, the tests showed that their memory had improved a lot—30% on one test, and 25% on the other.

They were also less depressed—a result that "provides further corroboration of neurocognitive benefit associated with the blueberry intervention," write the researchers, in the *Journal of Agricultural and Food Chemistry*.

Good news: Drinking all that sweet juice every day didn't cause blood sugar (glucose) problems. Just the opposite. The participants' fasting glucose levels (a blood sugar measurement taken first thing in the morning after not eating overnight) were healthfully lower at the end of the study.

"These findings are encouraging, and suggest that consistent supplementation with blueberries may offer a way to delay or lessen neurodegeneration," says Dr. Krikorian.

How they work: A decade of animal research conducted by James Joseph, PhD—a study researcher at Tufts University, and coauthor of *The Color Code: A Revolutionary*

Eating Plan for Optimum Health (Hyperion)—shows that the color-giving anthocyanins and hundreds of other compounds in blueberries may help the brain in several ways...

• Increase signaling between brain cells (neurons), particularly in memory centers.

• Protect neurons from inflammation and oxidation, "the evil twins of aging," says Dr. Joseph.

• Help neurons manufacture compounds that protect against cellular stress.

• Spark neurogenesis, the production of new neurons.

One Cup, Three Times a Week

• **One cup, for a healthier brain.** Eating one cup of blueberries, three to four times a week, may be enough to help protect the brain, Dr. Krikorian says.

He favors frozen berries, even in the summer. "They're fresher than fresh," Dr. Krikorian says. With the freezing process, which usually occurs within 24 hours of picking the fruit, there's little or no loss of micronutrients such as anthocyanins. But "fresh" berries in stores are usually days old, with diminished levels of micronutrients. The same goes for bottled juice, which loses 20% of its anthocyanins.

Dr. Joseph isn't a big fan of blueberry juice or dried blueberries. "I'd rather eat the berries," he says. "If you're going to buy blueberry juice or dried blueberries, check the label to make sure there is no added sugar."

• **Buying and storing.**

Here are guidelines for buying and storing blueberries, from the US Highbush Blueberry Council:

Fresh: Look for fresh blueberries that are firm, dry, plump, smooth-skinned and deep purple–blue to blue–black. Avoid soft or shriveled fruit and any signs of mold. Containers with juice stains indicate that the fruit may be bruised.

Refrigerate the blueberries as soon as you get them home, in their original pack or in a covered bowl or storage container, and use them within 10 days. Wash the berries right before using.

Frozen: You can find frozen, unsweetened blueberries in the frozen-food section of your supermarket. They should feel loose in the bag, not clumped together.

Frozen blueberries are individually quick frozen—you can remove as few or as many as you need. (Commercially frozen berries are washed before being frozen, so you don't need to wash them again.) Return the unused portion to the freezer. If berries thaw but aren't used, cover and refrigerate, and use within three days.

• **Ideas for intake.** "Eating a cup of fresh or frozen blueberries is so good, there's really no need for special recipes," says Dr. Joseph.

But here are some ideas for adding more blueberries to your diet:

• Whirl fresh or frozen blueberries in a smoothie.

Recipe: A blueberry-banana smoothie recipe, courtesy of Daniel Nadeau, MD, coauthor of *The Color Code*, includes 1 cup soy milk, 1 cup unsweetened fresh or frozen blueberries, 1 large banana, and 1 teaspoon dried flaxseed/linseed. Blend until smooth.

• Sprinkle them on cereal.

• Add blueberries to yogurt.

• Add blueberries to a peanut butter sandwich.

• Stir blueberry juice into iced tea or lemonade.

Resource: For dozens of blueberry recipes, visit the Web site *www.blueberrycouncil.com* or *www.wildblueberries.com*.

Robert Krikorian, PhD, associate professor, Department of Psychiatry at the University of Cincinnati.

James Joseph, PhD, researcher at Tufts University, and Daniel Nadeau, MD, clinical director of the Diabetes Endocrine Nutrition Center at Tufts University, coauthors of *The Color Code: A Revolutionary Eating Plans for Optimum Health* (Hyperion).

DASH Away From Dementia

The DASH diet—the Dietary Approaches to Stop Hypertension diet—is scientifically proven to protect the heart.

Rich in fruits, vegetables, whole grains, beans, nuts and low-fat dairy products, and emphasizing fish and chicken over red meat, the DASH diet can lower *systolic blood pressure* (the top number in a blood pressure reading) by up to 12 mmHg and *diastolic blood pressure* (the bottom number) by up to 6 mmHg.

Now: Research shows the DASH diet may also protect the brain. In fact, it might even help prevent Alzheimer's disease.

Whole Foods, Whole Brain

Researchers at Utah State University studied nearly 4,000 people aged 65 and older.

First, they gave them a food questionnaire that asked them what they ate and how often they ate it.

Next, they took their answers and divided the study participants into five levels—the top level had the greatest adherence to the DASH diet pattern; the bottom level had the lowest adherence.

Then, four times over the following 11 years, they gave the participants a Modified Mini-Mental State examination (3MS)—a standard test that measures mental prowess, such as memory, problem-solving and attention span, and that is also used to help diagnose memory problems and Alzheimer's disease.

Result: At the beginning of the study, those at the highest level of DASH adherence scored 1.42 points higher on 3MS. After 11 years, the high DASH-adherers scored 1.81 points higher than the lowest.

And in an analysis focusing on four food groups in the DASH diet—vegetables, whole grains, nuts/legumes and low-fat dairy products—the researchers found those with the highest adherence had a 3MS score 3.73 points higher than those with the lowest, and were 39% less likely to develop dementia.

"Adhering to the DASH eating pattern—and especially focusing on consuming recommended amounts of vegetables, whole grains, nuts/ legumes, and low-fat dairy products—may help to attenuate age-related cognitive decline and decrease risk for dementia among the elderly," said the researchers, at the Alzheimer's Association International Conference on Alzheimer's Disease.

Latest development: Researchers at Duke University Medical Center put 124 people with high blood pressure on the DASH diet—and found that after four months they had a number of "neurocognitive" improvements, such as better memory, better learning ability, clearer decision making and faster reflexes.

Servings of Health

"The DASH diet is a very healthy diet for anybody, whether you have high blood pressure or not," says Marla Heller, RD, a registered dietician in Northbrook, Illinois, and author of *The DASH Diet Action Plan* (Amidon) (*www.dashdiet.org*).

In terms of daily servings, a DASH diet might include…

- **4 servings of vegetables** (serving example: ½ cup cooked vegetables or 1 cup raw leafy green vegetables)

- **4 servings of fruit** (serving example: ½ cup fresh fruit or 4 ounces of fruit juice)

- **4 servings of whole grains** (serving example: 1 slice whole-wheat bread)

- **2 servings of low-fat or fat-free dairy foods** (serving example: 1 cup skim milk or 1 cup yogurt)

- **4 servings (a week) of beans, nuts or seeds** (serving example: ⅓ cup nuts, or ½ cup cooked beans)

- **3 to 6 servings of poultry, fish** (serving example: 1 ounce cooked skinless chicken)

- **2 to 3 servings of fats and oils** (serving example: 1 teaspoon low-fat mayonnaise or 1 teaspoon vegetable oil)

• **2 or fewer servings of sweets** (serving example: 1 tablespoon sugar)

"A typical day's DASH menu looks like a decadent feast," says Heller. "When you focus on the foods you include, rather than the foods you exclude, a diet becomes pleasurable and fun."

Here are Heller's top recommendations for easy ways to include more DASH-type foods in your diet...

• **Double up.** "The easiest way to make sure you get enough of the key DASH foods is to 'double up,'" says Heller. "Instead of one eight-ounce glass of low-fat or no-fat milk at breakfast, make it a 16-ounce glass—and you'll have consumed two servings of dairy. One cup of cooked vegetables makes two servings. One cup of green beans, one small salad, and one cup of potatoes gives you five servings of vegetables—at one meal."

Red flag: "Juices are one food item you don't want to double up on," says Heller. "A large glass of juice has 240 calories, little fiber, and won't keep you feeling full for very long. Limit juice to one serving per day."

• **Seek out DASH foods.** "It's almost like a treasure hunt," says Heller. "When you go out to dinner, think, 'How can I add extra fruits or vegetables?'"

Examples: Choose to have your pasta sauce on vegetables rather than pasta. Seasonal vegetables, salad or fresh fruit can be substituted for French fries.

• **Stockpile.** "Keep your refrigerator and freezer stocked with DASH delights," says Heller.

Example: Buy several bags of frozen vegetables at one time and keep them fresh after opening by using a clip-tight seal.

Buy convenience foods that are DASH foods. "Yogurt smoothies without added sugar, or skim milk in chuggable bottles, make refreshing health drinks," says Heller.

Marla Heller, RD, registered dietician in Northbrook, Illinois, and author of *The DASH Diet Action Plan* (Amidon). *www.dashdiet.org.*

Watch Out for Drug-Induced Dementia

When a doctor tells a patient that he/she has dementia, the diagnosis usually is correct. However, there are instances in which certain medications lead to reversible drug-induced cognitive impairment that can be confused with permanent dementia.

Older adults are especially susceptible because they metabolize drugs slowly and commonly take multiple drugs. Although a single medication might impair mental function, combining it with other drugs with similar side effects greatly increases the risk.

Mental impairments often are linked to tranquilizers, such as *diazepam* (Valium), and sleeping pills, such as *zolpidem* (Ambien).

Also risky: Opiate painkillers...some antidepressants...and antihistamines that contain *diphenhydramine* (such as Benadryl).

"If problems start after you begin taking one of these drugs, be very suspicious," says Sidney Wolfe, MD, director of Public Citizen's Health Research Group, a consumer advocacy organization. For more information, see *www.worstpills.org.* Dr. Wolfe's advice...

• **Assume that a drug may be causing a symptom** that begins after starting a new medication—or after the dosage of a drug you're already taking is increased.

• **Review all of the drugs you're taking** (including over-the-counter forms) and supplements whenever you see a new doctor.

• **Ask your doctor to prescribe the lowest possible dose if you're age 65 or older.** The dose can always be increased if needed.

Good news: Most drug-induced cognitive changes improve within a few days of stopping the medication.

Rebecca Shannonhouse, editor, *Bottom Line/Health,* Boardroom, Inc.

Sidney Wolfe, MD, director, Public Citizen's Health Research Group.

The Truth About Ginkgo For Dementia

Recent studies have cast doubt on the efficacy of ginkgo, an ancient Asian remedy and one of the best-selling herbs here in America, specifically with regard to its ability to fight dementia and sharpen cognitive function. According to Andrew L. Rubman, ND, one recent study (that received significant media attention) was a poor demonstration of ginkgo's medicinal effects and stands in stark contrast to prior research. Believing strongly that proper use of ginkgo is valuable for many medical challenges, including dementia prevention, Dr. Rubman continues to prescribe it for many of his patients and says they have experienced excellent results.

Flaws in the Research

In the *Ginkgo Evaluation of Memory* (GEM) study, research teams at five US medical academic centers followed 3,069 participants age 75 or older for approximately six years. At the beginning of the study, all either had normal cognition or mild cognitive impairment that did not interfere with their ability to live normal lives. Participants were randomly assigned to take either 120 milligrams (mg) of ginkgo twice daily or to take a similar-appearing placebo. Over time, 277 in the ginkgo group and 246 in the placebo group were diagnosed with dementia. Based on these summary numbers, the *Journal of the American Medical Association* study reported that ginkgo did not reduce the overall incidence of dementia or Alzheimer's disease in older people.

However, Dr. Rubman enumerated a variety of limitations in the study, which he believes wrongly influenced its conclusions. *For instance, he notes that...*

• While the study did use at least 240 mg/day in divided doses, as is recommended for a potent standardized material—in truth, older people need nearly twice this amount to achieve clinical effects, Dr. Rubman says. For such patients, he routinely prescribes doses approaching 500 mg/day of ginkgo.

• Not all ginkgo is created equal. The study utilized a standardized extract, EGb-761, which contains 24% flavone glycosides and 6% terpene lactones, but the research does not compare this to different formulations of ginkgo. Dr. Rubman generally prescribes whole leaf concentrates, which he finds to be more effective.

• Given that it is a "memory" study, the absence of verification that all of the participants consistently took the supplements raises questions.

• The study is in direct contrast to more than 50 other studies and reports published in respected journals, including the *Archives of Neurology* (1998) and JAMA (1997), demonstrating that ginkgo boosts cognitive function and fights dementia.

• The study failed to report other lifestyle factors that could nullify benefits of ginkgo. In addition, patients over age 75 might experience other aging-related physiological changes that may influence cognition.

How Ginkgo Boosts Brain Function

Ginkgo bolsters brain function through very specific biological processes, Dr. Rubman explains, which include antioxidant and anti-inflammatory effects on the nervous and circulatory systems. Helpful to all of us, this is especially beneficial to those who are experiencing early signs of dementia (confusion, agitation or mood swings, social withdrawal, memory loss, unclear thinking, etc.) because it may reduce the frequency or intensity of such disturbances. *In particular, says Dr. Rubman, ginkgo exerts a powerful neuroprotective effect on the brain by...*

• Acting as an antioxidant to wipe out free radicals that can otherwise lead to inflammation and disease and increase the symptoms associated with dementia.

• Stimulating the reception of important chemical messengers in the brain known as neurotransmitters. According to one study in

Neuropsychopharmacology, changes in serotonergic function may influence Alzheimer's disease and cognitive impairment.

● Keeping blood vessels and capillaries flexible, which improves the flow of blood and oxygen to the brain.

● Supporting healthy circulation by inhibiting the blood-clotting effects of platelet aggregation.

● According to the *Physician's Desk Reference for Herbal Medicines,* antioxidants in ginkgo prevent lipid peroxidation. Lipid peroxidation can cause vascular damage and neuronal loss.

Still a Valuable Treatment Option

Results of this study notwithstanding, Dr. Rubman remains convinced that ginkgo is a well-tolerated and effective supplement. Of course, it is always best to see a practitioner who is trained and experienced in botanical medicine to ensure you are receiving the proper type of ginkgo and dosage.

Andrew L. Rubman, ND, medical director, Southbury Clinic for Traditional Medicines, Southbury, Connecticut. *www.naturopath.org.*

Little-Known Ways to Keep Your Brain Healthy

Everybody wants as much brain power as possible. To achieve that goal, large numbers of Americans have started eating more omega-3-rich fish (or taking fish oil supplements) and begun daily exercise routines, such as walking, biking, swimming or aerobic dancing. But there are other lesser-known strategies that you also can adopt to maximize your brain power. *What Jamison Starbuck, ND, recommends to her patients in addition to fish consumption and exercise...*

1. Consider taking ginkgo biloba and bacopa monnieri. Ginkgo is widely recommended for its brain-boosting effects. However, a lesser-known herb—bacopa monnieri—is also an excellent choice. Both

herbs support cerebral circulation and mental focus. For patients who want to maximize their ability to retain new information, 120 mg of each herb daily is recommended.*

Also helpful: *Phosphatidylserine* (PS). Research has shown that this protein-derived nutrient is helpful in slowing the progression of dementia and improving focus and concentration. A typical dose is 300 mg per day. PS may be taken alone or in addition to the herbs described above. (See page 219 for more information on PS.)

Caution: People with a soy allergy should not take PS—most formulas are made from soy.

2. Watch out for anxiety. Many people fail to recognize the degree to which anxiety can interfere with focus and concentration. If you suspect that anxiety may be compromising your brain function, ask your doctor about taking *gamma amino butyric acid* (GABA), an amino acid that is naturally present in our brains. Optimal amounts of GABA allow the mind to both relax and focus, without causing sleepiness or sedation. A typical dose is 100 mg one to three times a day.

3. Try Kundalini yoga. All forms of yoga involve stretching and focused breathing, but *Kundalini* (the word refers to concentrated life force, according to Indian philosophy) is my favorite because it incorporates a variety of deep breathing exercises that simultaneously wake up and calm the brain. I recommend practicing this form of yoga for 45 minutes at least once weekly. To find a Kundalini yoga teacher near you, consult the International Kundalini Yoga Teachers Association, 505-629-1708, *www.kundaliniyoga.com.* As an alternative, you can improve your brain health by practicing deep breathing. Sit quietly in an erect position with a straight back and breathe in and out through your nose. Inhale as slowly and as deeply as you can, extending your abdomen outward...exhale as fully as possible, trying to push all

*Caution: If you are pregnant, breast-feeding or take any medication—especially for anxiety, depression, a mental disorder or dementia—consult your doctor before using the supplements described here or adding them to your treatment regimen. Ginkgo, in particular, should not be used with blood thinners, including aspirin.

of the air out of your lungs. Do this for five minutes daily, setting a timer if necessary. (For more information on the different forms of yoga, see appendix page 345.)

4. Keep your whistle wet. Adequate water intake is crucial for optimal brain health. Drink one-half ounce of water per pound of body weight daily.

Jamison Starbuck, ND, naturopathic physician in family practice, Missoula, Montana.

Are You Hurting Your Brain Without Even Knowing It?

Americans are increasingly at risk for a number of serious medical conditions that affect the brain. For example, it's estimated that 30 to 50% of Americans will develop Alzheimer's disease or other cognitive impairments by age 85, and one in four adults currently suffers from anxiety, depression or other psychiatric disorders.

What's going on? While researchers have identified a variety of factors, such as genetics, nutritional deficiencies and a sedentary lifestyle, a growing body of scientific evidence now implicates potentially brain-damaging substances (*neurotoxins*) that most people encounter in their day-to-day lives.

These so-called brain pollutants can impair the functioning of *mitochondria*, the energy-producing parts of cells. Mitochondrial damage has been linked to dementia as well as depression. The same neurotoxins also can produce inflammation, impair immunity and disrupt hormonal functions—all of which can hinder brain function.

Among the most dangerous…

●**Acetaminophen.** High doses of *acetaminophen* (Tylenol or Panadol, for example) deplete *glutathione,* an antioxidant that acts as a natural anti-inflammatory and protects the brain from oxidative injury and toxins. This medication generally is an issue only when used regularly (more than once or twice weekly)—for chronic joint pain, for example.

Advice: For joint pain, try nondrug methods, including eating three servings weekly of cold-water fish (such as wild salmon and sardines), which provide anti-inflammatory omega-3 fatty acids. Glucosamine and chondroitin supplements can help build cartilage and curb inflammation. If these approaches don't work, you may need tests to help identify an unsuspected cause of joint pain (such as allergens).

●**Antacids.** Antacids reduce the body's ability to fully digest protein and absorb minerals and vitamin B-12, which can lead to fatigue and cognitive declines. These effects can occur if you use antacids regularly (more than once or twice weekly).

Advice: Manage heartburn with natural methods—for example, do not eat within three hours of bedtime…and reduce consumption of foods and substances that tend to increase heartburn, such as caffeine, alcohol and spicy, citrus, fried or tomato-based foods. If you don't get relief, ask your doctor about testing for *Helicobacter pylori bacteria,* which can lead to heartburn-like symptoms.

●**Gluten.** A protein found in wheat, barley, rye and in some oats (which may be contaminated by wheat)—as well as in many processed foods, including some types of ice cream, soup, salad dressing and beer—gluten is one of the most common brain toxins. In some people, it triggers brain inflammation. Gluten also contains *glutamate*, a molecule that overstimulates neurons and causes premature cell death.

A review article published in *The New England Journal of Medicine* identified 55 conditions that have been linked to gluten, including dementia, neuropathy (nerve damage), anxiety and depression.

Self-test: Avoid all gluten for three months. Then, eat gluten-containing foods for several days. If you notice an increase in fatigue, depression or "brain fog" (inability to concentrate), you're probably sensitive to gluten and will need to avoid it altogether.

Advice: In addition to eliminating gluten from your diet, take zinc supplements (20 mg to 40 mg daily)*...glutamine (3 g to 5 g daily)...omega-3 fatty acids (2 g to 3 g daily)...gamma linolenic acid (1 g to 2 g daily)...and curcumin (500 mg twice a day). This regimen, followed for three to six months, will help repair damage to the gut caused by gluten.

●**Mercury.** It's an *endocrine* (hormone) disruptor that also increases mitochondrial death and reduces the brain's ability to respond to *dopamine,* a neurotransmitter involved in mood and cognitive functions.

Enormous amounts of mercury are released into the atmosphere as industrial byproducts. A diet high in large fish, such as tuna, swordfish and bluefish, causes significant levels of exposure. The mercury in amalgam dental fillings gradually vaporizes and gets into the body's tissues (although many people naturally excrete the mercury that is absorbed). There is no safe level of mercury.

Advice for all adults...

●**Don't eat large fish.** They have the highest concentration of mercury. Only eat seafood that is small enough to fit in a frying pan, such as sardines, flounder, trout, mackerel and herring.

●**Follow a daily metal-chelating regimen.** In addition to a daily multivitamin, take 500 mg to 1,000 mg of vitamin C...10 mg to 30 mg of zinc...and 100 micrograms (mcg) to 200 mcg of selenium.

If you have unexplained fatigue, memory loss or depression...

●**Get tested for mercury toxicity.** The test involves ingesting a *chelating* (binding) agent in pill form, then measuring the amount of mercury excreted in the urine over a 24-hour period.

If your mercury levels are high, your doctor may recommend a chelating agent, such as DMSA, that promotes mercury excretion from the body. Chelation therapy typically lasts three to 24 months, depending on the patient's mercury levels. Testing can be repeated every three to six months.

*Do not exceed 40 mg daily of zinc from supplements and diet without a doctor's supervision. Higher doses can cause gastrointestinal distress...or copper deficiency (if taken long term).

●**Processed sugar.** The average American consumes 158 pounds of sugar a year. Dietary sugars react with proteins and form plaques that damage brain cells. Some researchers refer to Alzheimer's disease as "type 3 diabetes" because elevated blood sugar greatly increases the risk for dementia. In fact, people with type 2 diabetes have four times the risk for Alzheimer's as those without diabetes. High fructose corn syrup, in particular, has been linked to increased risk for diabetes, heart disease and stroke.

Advice: Avoid processed foods. Most of these foods, including ketchup and salad dressings, contain added sugars, such as high fructose corn syrup. A little sugar (one to three teaspoons daily) usually is not a problem.

●**Dangerous mold.** Mold toxins (*mycotoxins*) are powerful neurotoxins. A 2003 study published in *Archives of Environmental Health* reported that 70% of people whose homes contained toxic molds showed symptoms of brain damage, including short-term memory loss. Molds can grow anywhere there is moisture, including on shower curtains, under appliances and in basements.

Red flags: A musty smell, discolored patches on walls or tiles or a greenish-black slime in damp areas.

Advice: Repair water leaks promptly. Maintain an indoor humidity level of no more than 50%. To monitor indoor humidity, buy a hygrometer, available at hardware stores.

If mold is present, clean the areas with a solution of one-half cup of bleach in a gallon of water. For extensive mold, call a contractor with experience in mold removal.

Also helpful: The prescription drug *cholestyramine* (Questran). Sometimes used to lower cholesterol levels, it helps remove toxins from the body. The drug is prescribed *off-label* (for a use that has not been FDA-approved) for mold toxicity and should be taken only under a doctor's supervision. Treatment usually lasts for one month.

Mark Hyman, MD, founder of The UltraWellness Center (*www.ultrawellness.com*) in Lenox, Massachusetts, and author of several books, including *The UltraMind Solution* (Scribner).

Don't Let Computer Use Harm Your Brain

The average American uses the Internet for 26 hours each month—writing e-mails, searching for facts or simply shopping online. But does all this online activity help—or harm—our brains?

Gary Small, MD, a leading authority on brain function, explains that computer use has both positive and negative effects.

Your Brain on the Internet

"Use it or lose it" has long been the motto for brain health. And according to new research, processing and responding to a shifting influx of information on the computer appears to dramatically increase mental activity.

Important new finding: When 24 adults with and without computer experience had their brain activity measured while they searched the Internet for information, the experienced users' brains were twice as lively as the others'. The increased activity was most striking in the brain's *prefrontal cortex* —the area that weighs complex information and makes decisions.

But the newcomers caught up fast. After spending just an hour a day on Internet searching for five days, their brains were just as active, when retested, as their more experienced counterparts'.

Online Social Skills

New technology means a world of new opportunities to socialize. For example, so-called social media outlets, such as Facebook (*www.facebook.com*), MySpace (*www.myspace. com*) and Twitter (*www.twitter.com*), make it possible to easily communicate with friends and acquaintances, including many you've never actually met.

The more you socialize online, the more adept at it you become, as brain circuits engaged by the activity grow stronger. This type of social activity engages the "thinking center" of the brain, as well as areas involved in language and memory functions.

The potential cost: When you spend long hours in front of the computer screen, you have less time for face-to-face conversations, which communicate a far richer stream of information than digital messages can. Facial expression, eye contact, tone of voice and body language convey subtleties of thought and feeling that are otherwise lost.

In fact, face-to-face conversation activates the brain more broadly and deeply than does computer communication—speaking, listening and interpreting nonverbal cues engage neurons in areas such as the *anterior cingulate*, the *insula* and parts of the frontal cortex that can weaken from disuse.

Self-defense: Become aware of the hours you spend online and be ready to set limits. Spend more physical time with people you care about—for example, schedule family dinners to reconnect with each other. To engage your brain even more fully, make special note of nonverbal communication when you are with people. For example, what do you think people are saying by the way they stand and gesture?

Too Much at Once?

Today's computer technology makes multitasking almost inevitable. Streams of information are constantly converging as e-mails and the lure of the Internet compete for our attention. Hopscotching back and forth grows easier with practice. Presumably it strengthens the part of the brain that lets us leave one task and focus on another—an area behind the forehead called the *anterior prefrontal cortex*.

The potential cost: Getting used to the staccato thinking style of dancing between tasks may make it more difficult to focus attention long enough to think through a problem. Some experts have suggested that symptoms of *attention deficit hyperactivity disorder* (ADHD) in adults—such as distractibility, impulsivity and inability to concentrate—may be due, in some cases, to brain shifts that occur in response to the continual bombardment of information delivered by technology.

You may think that you're getting more tasks done by multitasking, but in fact the brain is far more efficient when allowed to concentrate on one thing at a time. Studies have shown that mental efficiency declines during multitasking, and tasks take longer to complete than they do when done sequentially. (See page 221 for more on the hazards of multitasking.)

Self-defense: List your tasks in order of importance, and arrange your schedule accordingly. Set aside times when you focus on paying bills or returning phone calls—and turn off your e-mail if it distracts you.

Also helpful: When possible, take "power naps." A Harvard study found that a 30-minute nap renews the neural pathways depleted by multitasking and reduces overall fatigue.

Are You Addicted to Your Computer?

Many people have gotten hooked on online shopping, computer games, Internet porn and/or Internet gambling. Even mundane Internet searching—just looking for interesting Web sites—may be seriously habit forming.

The potential cost: Whether they are true addictions—not all experts think so—such activities apparently activate the same "reward circuits" in the brain that drugs and alcohol do.

As with substance abuse, dependence on computer stimulation can become an unhealthy preoccupation that persists even to the point where it puts jobs and personal relationships in jeopardy—and efforts to stop may trigger withdrawal-like discomfort.

Self-defense: Each day, substitute offline diversions that you enjoy, such as hobbies and sports, for computer activities. If certain Web sites prove hard to resist, use a program that filters content. (Have a family member or friend set up the filter and keep the password.)

Helpful: If the lure of toxic technology is truly interfering with your life, seek professional help. Contact the Center for Internet Addiction (814-451-2405, *www.netaddiction. com*).

Try Brain-Building Technology

Research shows that regular mental stimulation can spur new connections between neurons and improve memory.

Solving crossword puzzles in the newspaper, for example, and learning new subjects may slow brain aging—or even lower the risk for Alzheimer's disease.

Used wisely, your computer also can help promote brain health. For example, there are Web sites that feature games and puzzles specifically designed to challenge the brain at varying levels of difficulty.

Dr. Small's favorite Web sites: www.brain bashers.com (created by a math teacher in England, this free site offers puzzles, riddles, games and optical illusions)...and *www. braingle.com* (this site will e-mail you a free brain teaser each day and allows you to chat online with other brain teaser enthusiasts).

Gary Small, MD, professor of psychiatry and biobehavioral sciences and director of the Center on Aging, the Memory & Aging Center and the Geriatric Psychiatry Division at the Semel Institute for Neuroscience & Human Behavior at the University of California, Los Angeles. He is coauthor of *iBrain: Surviving the Technological Alteration of the Modern Mind* (HarperCollins).

Memory Robbers That Are Often Overlooked

Alzheimer's disease is such a dreaded diagnosis that you may be filled with panic if you experience occasional memory loss. But these worries may be unnecessary.

As people age, the brain undergoes changes that may lead to some decline in short-term memory. This is normal.

Of course memory loss that truly concerns you is another matter. *Ask your primary care physician to refer you to a neurologist or geriatrician for an evaluation if...*

• You have noticed a significant change in your everyday memory over the past six months.

● Friends or family members have expressed concern about your memory.

● You have begun forgetting recent conversations.

In the meantime, consider whether your occasional forgetfulness may be due to one of the following causes, all of which can be easily corrected...

Not Enough Sleep

Poor sleep is probably the most common cause of occasional memory lapses. The ability to concentrate suffers with insufficient rest. Sleep also appears to be essential for consolidating memory—whatever information you learn during the day, whether it's the name of a colleague or the street where a new restaurant opened, you need sleep to make it stick in your mind.

Self-defense: If you're not sleeping seven to eight hours nightly, make it a priority to get more sleep. If you are unable to improve your sleep on your own, talk to your doctor.

Widely Used Drugs

Impaired memory is a potential side effect of many medications. Obvious suspects include prescription sleeping pills...opiate painkillers, such as *meperidine* (Demerol)...and anti-anxiety drugs, such as *diazepam* (Valium) and *alprazolam* (Xanax).

Certain blood pressure–lowering medications, such as beta-blockers, and antidepressants also cause memory problems in some people. Even over-the-counter antihistamines, such as *diphenhydramine* (Benadryl), can have this effect.

If you're taking multiple medications, more than one may cause impaired memory, making it even more difficult to identify the culprit.

Timing is often a tip-off: When impaired memory is an adverse drug effect, it's most likely to appear when you start taking a new medication or increase the dose. But not always.

As we grow older, our bodies become less efficient at clearing medications from the body, so the same dose you've been taking safely for years may cause problems you never had before.

Self-defense: If you think medication might be affecting your memory, do not stop taking the drug or reduce the dosage on your own. Talk to your doctor or pharmacist for advice.

Emotional Upset

When you're anxious, stressed or depressed, your ability to concentrate suffers. Whatever it is that worries or preoccupies you keeps your mind from focusing on facts, names, faces and places, so they aren't absorbed into memory.

Self-defense: To keep everyday tensions from undercutting your memory, practice some form of relaxation or stress reduction. Yoga, meditation, deep breathing—or something as simple as allowing yourself a soothing time-out to walk or chat with a friend—can relieve accumulated stress and bolster your recall.

True depression is something else: Even mild-to-moderate depression can sap your energy, take pleasure out of life and affect your memory. If you suspect that you may be depressed, be alert for other symptoms—such as difficulty sleeping, sadness, apathy and a negative outlook—and see your doctor or a mental-health professional.

Too Much Alcohol

Moderate red wine consumption has been shown to promote the health of your heart and arteries. Because of this cardiovascular health benefit, red wine also may reduce risk for dementia.

Excessive drinking, on the other hand, is harmful to the brain. Among its devastating toxic effects is a severe and often irreversible form of memory loss called *Korsakoff's syndrome,* a condition that occurs in alcoholics.

Alcohol's effect on memory can be subtle. Some people find that even a glass or two of wine daily is enough to interfere with learning facts and recalling information. Pay attention to how mentally sharp you feel after having a drink. If you think your alcohol intake may be causing forgetfulness, cut back. Remember, tolerance for alcohol generally declines with age, giving the same drink more impact.

Self-defense: There is more scientific evidence supporting red wine's brain-protective effect than for any other form of alcohol. If you are a man, do not exceed two glasses of red wine daily, and if you are a woman, limit yourself to one glass daily.

Illness

A simple cold or headache is enough to interfere with your concentration and recall.

Illnesses that commonly go undiagnosed also may play a role. For example, when the thyroid gland (which regulates metabolism) is underactive, the mind slows down along with the body. (Other signs of an underactive thyroid include weight gain, constipation, thin or brittle hair and depression.) An overactive thyroid can affect your memory by making you anxious, "wired" and easily distracted.

Memory impairment also may be a symptom of other disorders, such as Parkinson's disease, multiple sclerosis or Lyme disease.

Nutritional Deficiency

An easily overlooked memory robber is a vitamin B-12 deficiency, often marked by general fatigue and slowed thinking. Older people are especially at risk—as we age, our ability to absorb vitamin B-12 from foods diminishes.

Self-defense: If you have occasional memory lapses, ask your doctor for a blood test to check your vitamin B-12 level.

Safeguarding Your Memory

Even if you've identified a relatively harmless cause for occasional forgetfulness, it's still wise to take steps to guard against cognitive decline in the future. *My advice...*

• **Get enough exercise.** Exercise helps prevent a wide range of serious health problems, including heart disease, diabetes and some types of cancer. The evidence also is strong that exercise protects against dementia—and enhances everyday memory performance by improving overall circulation and lowering risk for disorders that can affect memory, such as high blood pressure and obesity.

Self-defense: A leisurely stroll around the block may be relaxing, but you must get 30 minutes of moderate exertion (such as brisk walking or swimming), three to four days a week, to keep your memory intact.

• **Stay on top of chronic health problems.** Studies have shown repeatedly that people with high blood pressure, atherosclerosis (fatty buildup in the arteries), obesity and/or diabetes are at dramatically increased risk of developing dementia in their later years.

The effect of these chronic medical conditions on day-to-day memory is less clear. Research shows that memory declines when blood sugar rises in people with diabetes and improves when they take dietary steps to stabilize it.

Self-defense: If you have a chronic health problem, work with your doctor to keep your symptoms under control.

• **Give your brain a timed workout.** A growing body of research shows that mental exercise helps fend off everyday age-related cognitive changes that contribute to occasional forgetfulness.

Self-defense: Crossword puzzles and the number game Sudoku have gotten a lot of attention as "brain" workouts, but I prefer timed games, such as the word game Boggle or the card game Set (both available online or at discount stores). Racing against the clock gives your mental muscles a real workout by challenging such intellectual skills as attention, speed and decision making.

Cynthia R. Green, PhD, assistant clinical professor of psychiatry at Mount Sinai School of Medicine in New York City and president of Memory Arts, LLC. *www.memoryarts.com*. She is the author of *Total Memory Workout* (Bantam).

B-12 Blocks Brain Shrinkage

Brain degeneration is associated with Alzheimer's disease and is used as a marker for the disease's progression. Researchers from England, Norway and Australia examined 107 men and women, ages 61 to 87, without cognitive impairment at the beginning of the five-year study. Blood tests to assess vitamin B-12 status and *magnetic resonance imaging* (MRI) scans of the brain were performed annually.

Result: Those with the highest levels of vitamin B-12 were six times less likely to lose brain volume as those with the lowest levels.

Vitamin B-12 is required for the metabolism of *homocysteine,* an amino acid that, at elevated levels, is known to cause brain shrinkage and dementia. It is known that B-12 deficiency is rampant in the elderly because they often lose the ability to absorb the vitamin effectively. People over age 60 should take at least 100 micrograms daily of sublingual (under-the-tongue) vitamin B-12, which is absorbed more readily than other forms.

Mark A. Stengler, NMD, naturopathic medical doctor in private practice, La Jolla, California, and author of the *Bottom Line/Natural Healing* newsletter. *www.drstengler.com.*

Age-Proof Your Brain

Slowed learning. Misplaced glasses. A sudden blank where a good friend's name used to be. These brain glitches, or "senior moments" are all too common as we age. But with proper care, your brain can carry on its marvelous work, ensuring that you feel alert and active.

Mark Stengler, NMD, says one of the best substances for boosting memory and brain power is *phosphatidylserine* (pronounced fos-fa-TIdal-sare-een) or simply PS. Derived from soy, it is a type of *phospholipid,* a molecule containing both the amino acid *serine* and essential fatty acids found in all cell membranes. When we are young, we have all the PS we need in our cells. As we age, our PS level decreases. Studies have shown that PS is beneficial for cognition in general, but in particular for the parts of the brain affected by age-related decline in memory, ability to learn, vocabulary skills and concentration. In addition, PS can relieve symptoms of depression...dementia, including Alzheimer's disease (AD)...and the negative effects of stress.

PS Can Help in Many Ways

• **Boosts motivation.** Many studies have found that PS seems to improve overall brain function in older people. In a study of elderly patients without dementia, those who took PS showed improvement in motivation, initiative and interest in the world around them. They also were more social and had boosts in memory and learning compared with the placebo group.

• **Depression.** Studies on the effect of PS on depression in elderly patients have had positive results. An Italian study of older women with major depressive disorder found improvement in both behavior and cognitive performance in the PS group, compared with the placebo group. There are no known drug interactions with PS, and some patients take both PS and an antidepressant medication. If you are on an antidepressant medication, tell your doctor that you also are taking PS.

• **Alzheimer's disease.** Studies have shown that PS improves AD patients' memory, motivation and cognition. It also reduces anxiety, a problem in patients with AD. In a study of 425 people with moderate-to-severe cognitive loss, the PS group showed significant improvement.

Note: PS is not a cure for AD (none exists), and these patients' improvements did not last indefinitely. When Dr. Stengler's patients take both PS and an AD medication, he consults with their neurologists.

• **Stress.** PS appears to relieve the negative effects of stress on the body because of its effect on levels of *cortisol,* a hormone that is elevated during times of stress. After measuring cortisol levels of healthy volunteers following exercise, researchers found that PS modulated release of the hormone. Cortisol levels increase in depressed people, which is why PS also seems to help with depression. PS can be prescribed to alleviate the effects of stress in people of all ages.

In his practice, Dr. Stengler sees many patients with age-related cognitive impairment ranging from mild cognitive decline to dementia. After taking 300 mg of PS for two months, the majority shows a noticeable improvement in cognitive functioning. Because PS is not a blood thinner, it is particularly beneficial for people who take blood-thinning medication, such as *warfarin* (Coumadin). PS supplements are safe for almost everyone except those who are allergic to soy.

Some foods, such as Atlantic herring and white beans, contain a considerable amount of PS, but no food has the amount that can provide the therapeutic benefit found in supplements.

For patients with age-related cognitive decline and for those who simply want to improve their memory, Dr. Stengler recommends supplementing with two 200-mg doses of PS during the day and 100 mg each evening, for a total of 500 mg daily. He also prescribes this amount of PS for older people who are depressed, overly stressed or who lack motivation. PS can be taken with or without food. There are no reported side effects. Look for products with 100 mg of PS per capsule. He doesn't recommend the 100-mg formulas that contain a PS complex in which PS is only a percentage of the 100 mg. Products he does recommend include those made by KAL (800-669-8877, *www.nutraceutical.com*) and Natural Factors (800-322-8704, *www.natural factors.com*).

●**PS for children.** PS is safe for children as young as four years old. Dr. Stengler prescribes 300 mg to 500 mg daily for children with attention deficit hyperactivity disorder (ADHD). Preliminary studies show it to be effective, especially when used in combination with fish oil. In addition, Dr. Stengler regularly uses PS with children who have problems with focus, attention and learning. He recommends 300 mg daily of PS. When it continues to help, his patients are kept on it indefinitely.

●**Another memory-boosting supplement.** *Phosphatidylcholine* (pronounced fos-fa-TIdal-ko-lean), or PC, is another brain-boosting phospholipid. It provides the body with *choline,* a chemical similar to B vitamins and the precursor to the neurotransmitter acetylcholine. PC is a major component of lecithin, a fat found naturally in animal and plant tissues and isolated for supplement use from either soy or egg yolks. Lecithin is a good source of PC, which studies have associated with improved memory. (Lecithin and PC often are referred to interchangeably.) A study with 61 healthy volunteers showed that ingesting two tablespoons of lecithin daily improved memory test scores compared with the placebo group.

To prevent memory loss, you can boost your lecithin levels by consuming foods such as sunflower seeds, mustard, oatmeal and cauliflower. Dr. Stengler also recommends lecithin supplements for those who already have memory decline. For memory improvement, add two tablespoons of lecithin granules daily to a fruit smoothie or juice.

For patients who have early-stage dementia who have tried PS and lecithin and need a more aggressive approach, Dr. Stengler recommends both PS and lecithin.

Mark A. Stengler, NMD, naturopathic medical doctor in private practice, La Jolla, California, and author of the Bottom Line/Natural Healing newsletter. www.drstengler.com.

Rapid Weight Loss Linked to Dementia

In an eight-year study of 1,836 men and women (average age 72), those who unintentionally lost weight at a "fast" rate were nearly three times more likely to develop dementia than those who lost weight more slowly. Fast weight loss was defined as dropping more than one *body mass index* (BMI) point per year.

Theory: Weight loss in older adults may be an early physical sign of dementia that occurs before the disease affects memory function.

If you are an older adult who has experienced unexplained rapid weight loss: See your doctor for an evaluation.

Tiffany Hughes, PhD, MPH, researcher, Department of Psychiatry, University of Pittsburgh School of Medicine.

More Ways to Boost Brain Power

●**Exercise.** We have known for many years that regular exercise contributes to improved cognitive function in older adults. Recently, a study showed that exercise increases blood circulation to the brain, which seems to be the reason for the cognitive benefit. This is yet another reason to go for a long walk… take a bike ride…or go to the gym for a workout.

●**Try something new.** Studies have shown that taking on a new challenge, such as a ballroom dancing class, or having a new experience, perhaps volunteering in a school, boosts brain power.

●**Play video games.** A new study from the University of Illinois, Urbana-Champaign, found that certain types of video games improved the brain's "executive function" skills, such as planning, decision making and impulse control, in men and women in their late 60s.

The best brain-boosting games: Turn-taking strategy games that involve task switching, memory, visual short-term recall and reasoning.

Are Multitaskers Mini-Thinkers?

Picture the superior modern brain. Conditioned by the speed of twenty-first-century technology—by computers, cell phones and iEverything…by texting, chatting and twittering—it instantly and effortlessly switches from task to task, Mental Master of Media, prodigiously productive.

Surprising: A new study shows that people who do a lot of media multitasking have the weakest memories, the poorest ability to separate relevant from irrelevant information—and are the worst at switching from task to task!

Below Par Filtering and Focus

Led by Clifford Nass, PhD, professor of communication at Stanford University, researchers recruited 100 students, evaluated their level of multitasking and split them into two groups—those who regularly did a lot of media multitasking (heavy media multitaskers) and those who didn't (light media multitaskers).

Example: A heavy multitasker might have the computer on…with two screens open… one of which he's chatting in…while text-messaging on his cell phone…while sending an e-mail…while listening to his iPod…and writing a term paper.

"I was jealous of my undergraduate students who seemed to be able to so gracefully multitask," says Dr. Nass. "What was their secret skill?"

He and his team theorized that the heavy multitaskers must be uniquely skilled in filtering out relevant from irrelevant information—how else could they manage to multitask so much? So the researchers evaluated all 100 students in that skill, using a standard psychological test that required focusing on the position of two blue triangles while ignoring the position of several red ones. The heavy multitaskers performed…horribly.

Well, theorized the researchers, maybe the heavy multitaskers were better able to quickly organize and manage information—

221

what psychologists call "managing working memory." So they tested that skill, with a test that required remembering the sequences of alphabetical letters. The heavy multitaskers performed the worse.

Finally, they tested the students' ability to switch from task to task, figuring that surely the multitaskers would be better at...multitasking. The heavy multitaskers were (you guessed it) the worst.

"We kept looking for what they were better at, and we didn't find it," says Eyal Ophir, a study researcher at Stanford.

"When they're in situations where there are multiple sources of information coming from the external world or emerging out of memory, they're not able to filter out what's not relevant to their current goal," says Anthony D. Wagner, PhD, another study researcher.

Learn How to Uni-Task

Why do some people multitask so much? "One possibility is that they have faith in the new," says Dr. Nass. "They believe and trust that the new is going to be much more valuable than what they already have—that the informational grass is greener on the other side."

But that faith has a price.

"If you're a heavy multitasker, you're probably making yourself worse at all the abilities we tested—at sorting out relevant from irrelevant information, at storing and using information in working memory and at task-switching. In short, you're weakening your brain."

His conclusion: "There is no justification for multitasking—especially among people who like doing it the most."

But how can multitaskers stop?

"I have encountered the multitasking problem in people of all ages," says Margaret Lukens, a productivity trainer and organizing consultant. "Though the behavior seems addictive, it's really just habitual."

Changing the behavior requires replacing the bad habit of multitasking with the good

habit of "uni-tasking," she says. Her recommendations...

● **Understand the negative effect of multitasking—and the positive effect of breaking the habit.** "As the Stanford researchers showed, multitasking may cause substantial damage to your cognitive abilities," says Lukens. "But by not multitasking—by having greater focus and concentration—you'll enjoy greater productivity, less feeling of being overwhelmed, and more time for things that matter to you the most."

● **End the day by establishing priorities.** Lukens encourages clients who are habitual multitaskers to end the day by choosing the top three things they need to do the following day—and establishing the order in which to do them.

● **Start the day by focusing.** Then, she counsels them to begin the next day by working on their first priority—and only their first priority—for 90 minutes.

"I've never encountered a client who, having experienced the calm productivity that comes with focusing on one thing at a time—with uni-tasking—doesn't choose to stop multitasking to the greatest extent possible."

Helpful: "Sometimes it's not possible to avoid all interruptions," says Lukens. "If that's the case, I council clients to minimize the time they take to return to their main task after an unavoidable interruption."

● **Tame your e-mail.** The multitasking trap that snares most of us is constantly checking and rechecking e-mail when we're in the midst of doing other tasks, says Lukens.

"When you check and recheck e-mail, you're essentially saying to yourself, 'Let's see what I can respond to,'" says Lukens. "Now, if your job is customer service, that's perfectly reasonable. But if you have objectives that you want to move forward, being responsive is not what you want to spend most of your time on." *She recommends...*

● Commit to checking e-mail only twice a day. "Perhaps you'll decide to check it from 11 a.m. to 12 noon, and from 4 p.m. to 5 p.m.—

that would be sufficient for someone who gets a lot of e-mail."

●Limit the amount of time checking e-mail. "Another option is to set aside only 1 hour or so to go through your email, get done whatever you can get done—and then move on to another task."

●Include e-mail checking times in your e-mail signature. "Some of my clients include a line in their email signature that says, for example, 'I check e-mail at 11 a.m., 2 p.m. and 4 p.m.' That lets other people know not to expect an immediate response. If something does require an immediate response, a colleague can be told it's okay to call you."

Clifford Nass, PhD, professor of communication, Stanford University.

Eyal Ophir, researcher, Department of Psychology, Stanford University.

Anthony D. Wagner, PhD, associate professor of psychology and neuroscience, Stanford University.

Margaret Lukens, productivity trainer and organizing consultant. *www.newleafandcompany.com.*

Why You Should Take Your Neurons for a Walk

While exercise is toning your arteries, hardening your bones and building your muscles, it's also strengthening your brain cells, and thereby buffing up your memory.

How it works: Exercise strengthens brain cells in a number of ways, explains John Ratey, MD, an associate clinical professor of psychiatry at Harvard Medical School, and author of *Spark: The Revolutionary New Science of Exercise and the Brain* (Little, Brown). *Exercise can...*

●**Increase levels of the neurotransmitters serotonin, norepinephrine and dopamine,** brain chemicals that help neurons communicate;

●**Build new capillaries in the brain,** improving blood flow;

●**Spark neurogenesis,** the creation of new brain cells;

●**Produce proteins such as insulin-like growth factor** that activate genes in brain cells;

●**Generate brain-derived neurotrophic factor (BDNF),** which Dr. Ratey describes as "fertilizer" for neurons;

●**Decrease inflammation,** which damages brain cells and

●**Reduce levels of amyloid,** a toxic protein in the brain linked to Alzheimer's disease.

Important New Findings

And recent research shows that healthier brain cells lead to better mental performance—in all kinds of ways.

Slowing mental decline. Researchers at the University of Washington School of Medicine studied 33 people, average age 70, with *mild cognitive impairment* (MCI)—a type of mental decline that puts you at increased risk for dementia. Half participated in aerobic exercise and half didn't.

After six months, those who exercised regularly had significant improvements in a wide range of mental capabilities, including *executive function*—the mental ability to prioritize, plan, organize and implement.

"When people think about mild cognitive impairment, they often think about the deterioration of short-term memory," says Laura Baker, PhD, the study leader. "Well, that's the cognitive function that everyone notices. But research is showing that people with mild cognitive impairment may also have an impairment in executive function that probably precedes the memory loss."

The study also showed improvements among the exercisers in cognitive flexibility (the ability to shift from one task to another), and in search efficiency (not repeating the same action over and over again, such as looking for lost keys where you've already looked for them).

"The degree of cognitive benefit from exercise shown by this study—particularly in people who already had significant mental decline—was amazing," says Dr. Baker.

Dr. Baker thinks that exercise is a must for anyone experiencing age-related memory loss or mild cognitive impairment.

Resistance training works too. Researchers in the Brain Research Centre at the University of British Columbia found that women aged 65 to 75 who participated in only one session of resistance training (also called strength training and weight lifting) per week for one year had a 12% improvement in executive function. "For improving cognitive function in older adults, some exercise is better than none," says Teresa Liu-Ambrose, PhD, the study leader.

Better acumen behind the wheel. Researchers in Portugal found that regular exercise improved driving ability in older adults. "Exercise is capable of enhancing several abilities relevant to driving performance and safety in older adults," such as the ability to pay attention, reaction time and executive function, they conclude, in *Accident Analysis & Prevention.*

Fitter body, sharper mind. Researchers at Howard University in Washington, DC, analyzed the health habits of more than 7,000 adults over age 60 who had undergone mental testing. They found that higher levels of aerobic activity were linked to better cognitive performance. "Physical activity may reduce or prevent memory loss and other symptoms of mental decline," says Thomas O. Obisesan, MD, the study leader.

Fit Brain, Resilient Brain

"Exercise is the single most powerful tool you have to optimize your brain function," says Dr. Ratey. "When people ask me how much exercise they should do for their brain, I tell them that my best advice is to get fit—and then continue challenging yourself. The more fit you are, the more resilient your brain becomes and the better it functions, both mentally and emotionally. If you get your body in shape, your mind will follow." But, he adds, any level of activity will help tune up your brain.

Best: "Based on everything I've read and seen, the best type and level of exercise for the brain is some form of aerobic activity—walking, jogging, cycling—for 45 minutes to an hour, six days a week," says Dr Ratey. Adding resistance training to that routine is ideal.

"For four of those days, the amount of aerobic exercise should be on the longer side, at moderate intensity. On two of those days, it should be on the shorter side, at high intensity. On the shorter, high-intensity days, include some form of resistance training. In total, I'm talking about committing six hours a week to your brain. That works out to 5% of your waking hours."

Moderate intensity exercise is 65 to 75% of your maximum heart rate, and high intensity is 75 to 90%, he explains. Your maximum heart rate is approximately 220 minus your age.

Smart idea: "The only way to accurately gauge your level of intensity during exercise is to buy a heart monitor," says Dr. Ratey. "It consists of a chest-strap sensor that picks up your heartbeat, and a digital watch that receives the signal and displays the number of beats per minute on a screen.

"Let's say your regimen today calls for a high-intensity run. If you're forty-five years old, your maximum heart rate would be about 175, based on the formula of 220 minus your age. If you calculate 75% and 90% of your maximum, the lower and upper limits for a high-intensity workout are 131 and 158. This is your target heart rate zone for the workout. All you have to do is punch in these limits on the watch, which is no more difficult than setting the time, and then adjust your pace according to what the monitor tells you. It's a reasonably accurate way to listen to your body."

What most people don't realize: It's almost impossible to do too much exercise, says Vik Khanna, a clinical exercise specialist certified by the *American College of Sports Medicine* (ACSM), and chief "exercise" officer at Galileo Health Partners near Baltimore, Maryland. "The signs of too much exercise are excessive fatigue, disturbed sleep and not recovering from exercise activity within 24 hours. Until you get to that point—and almost no one gets to that point—there's room for improvement in fitness and health. So go ahead and fill it!"

John Ratey, MD, associate clinical professor of psychiatry, Harvard Medical School and author of *Spark* (Little, Brown).

Laura D. Baker, PhD, assistant professor, Department of Psychiatry and Behavioral Sciences, University of Washington.

Teresa Liu-Ambrose, PhD, assistant professor, Department of Physical Therapy, University of British Columbia.

Thomas Obisesan, MD, associate professor and chief of geriatrics, director, Washington Center for Aging Howard University.

Vik Khanna, clinical exercise specialist and chief "exercise" officer at Galileo Health Partners, Baltimore. *www. galileohealth.net.*

Powerful as Drugs for Slowing Alzheimer's— A Spouse's Love

Top experts in the study of Alzheimer's disease (AD) suggest a variety of ways to delay the disease after a person has first been diagnosed—ways that can "slow its forward march and ease its symptoms," according to P. Murali Doraiswamy, MD, author of *The Alzheimer's Action Plan* (St. Martin's).

● **Take a cholinesterase inhibitor,** such as *donepezil* (Aricept), a drug that boosts levels of *acetylcholine,* a compound that improves communication between brain cells.

● **Stimulate your mind with activities such as crossword puzzles or computer games** designed to improve brainpower.

● **Eat a brain-nourishing diet** that minimizes saturated fat, refined sugars and processed foods, and maximizes whole foods such as fish, poultry, fruits, vegetables, wholegrains, beans and low-fat dairy products.

● **Exercise regularly,** such as taking a brisk walk a few times a week.

● **Reduce stress,** by breathing deeply or meditating.

Now: Scientists have added a new item to that disease-slowing list: have a close relationship with your spouse!

Closer Feelings, Clearer Minds

Researchers from several institutions (including Johns Hopkins University School of Medicine, Duke University Medical Center, and Utah State University) studied 167 "pairs"—people who had had AD for an average of four years, and their main caregivers, either a spouse or an adult child.

Every six months during the study, for about two years, the caregivers were given a survey to measure their "closeness" with the person with AD.

In the survey, they rated the following statements from 1 (strongly disagree) to 4 (strongly agree):

● My relationship with care recipient (CR) is close.

● CR always understands what I value in life.

● CR makes me feel like a special person.

● CR and I can always discuss things together.

● CR is often critical of me.

● CR always makes me feel that whatever I do for him/her, it is not enough.

The overall score produced a "closeness" rating.

And every six months, those with AD were given a Mini-Mental State Exam (MMSE), which measures cognitive functions such as memory, concentration and learning ability. (On average, MMSE scores decline three points per year in a person with AD.)

Result: Among the 167 pairs, the spouses and their care receivers with the highest closeness scores had the slowest decline in MMSE scores.

Specifically, every 6-point increase in closeness was matched by a 0.72 slower yearly decline in MMSE. Put another way, those who were closest lost less than half as many points on their MMSE during the study.

The slowed decline in MMSE was similar to that achieved in studies of acetylcholine-boosting drugs, the researchers point out.

AD patients in pairs with greater closeness also scored better on a Clinical Dementia Rating test, which measures "functional decline"—the loss of personal abilities such as paying bills or remembering to take medications. (A close relationship with an adult child caregiver also slowed mental and functional decline, but not as much.)

"We've shown that the benefits of having a close caregiver, especially a spouse, can mean the difference between someone with Alzheimer's disease staying at home or going to a nursing facility," says Constantine Lyketsos, MD, one of the researchers in the study.

There are many reasons why a close relationship between a person with AD and a caregiver might delay the progression of the disease, says Kathleen Piercy, PhD, associate professor of family, consumer and human development at Utah State University, and author of *Working with Aging Families: Therapeutic Solutions for Caregivers, Spouses, and Adult Children* (W.W. Norton). A caregiver with a closer relationship might provide more mental and social stimulation. There might be less stress. And a loving spouse might give the care receiver more choice and autonomy in his or her daily routines, preserving the care receiver's dignity—and memory.

Promoting Closeness

"There are a lot of activities that can promote intimacy between the caregiver and the care receiver, irrespective of the stage of Alzheimer's" says Jamie Huysman, PsyD, LCSW, a spokesperson for the National Association of Social Workers (NASW), and coauthor of *Take Your Oxygen First: Protecting Your Health and Happiness While Caring for a Loved One with Memory Loss* (LaChance). *Some of his recommendations…*

● **Make music together.** "Music is one of the most powerful ways to connect someone with their positive emotions, and musical memory is one of the last types of memory to disappear in Alzheimer's disease," he says. If you can play the piano, play for your spouse. Or sing together.

"My husband became re-interested in music after developing Alzheimer's disease," says Eileen Haight, author of *Alzheimer's Caregivers: The Choice of Love*. "So I played CDs of John Philip Sousa marches, because I know he'd played the saxophone in a marching band in high school. He drummed to the beat with his fingers, and even sang along with the music. I also put on dance music, and we'd dance together—although he never danced with me before he had Alzheimer's!"

● **Reminisce.** "A strong intimate relationship involves communication and trust, and there is great communication and trust in talking about shared memories," says Dr. Huysman. "And people with AD often have more a command of distant memories of the past than they do of recent memories." Page through photo albums and scrapbooks with the care receiver, talking about the past.

● **Touch one another.** "I really believe touch is a human need—for the caregiver and the their loved one," says Dr. Huysman. He recommends taking the care receiver for a manicure or a massage, or having his/her hair styled—and doing the same for you!

"I've seen with my own eyes how closeness, intimacy and sexuality can slow the progression of Alzheimer's disease," says Katherine Forsythe, MSW, a social worker in San Francisco and an expert in sexuality for older individuals. "With touch—with intimacy and sexuality—there is an upsurge in endorphins and other brain-energizing chemicals."

Smart idea: Write down everything you know about care receiver's likes and dislikes in physical intimacy, says Forsythe—and then regularly do things on the list that they like, whether it's rubbing their ears, massaging their back, holding hands, or a particular type of sexual play.

She emphasizes that while intercourse and orgasm are wonderful, they're not required. "Closeness, intimacy and sexuality are about the pleasure, not the performance," she says. "Make pleasurable physical connection part of everything you do."

● **Take care of yourself.** "My mantra for personal and interpersonal well-being is, 'Peace begins with me,'" says Dr. Huysman. "It's hard to feel connected with your loved one unless you're connected with yourself. Self-care—through meditation, or deep breathing, or regularly attending a support group or psychological counseling—can lessen your anxiety and allow the care receiver to feel less anxious and safer around you."

"I highly recommend joining a local caregivers association," says Haight. "They can look after the care receiver for a few hours, giving you respite from non-stop caregiving, and they can help you organize all the practical and sometimes overwhelming details of caregiving. And a support group of friends or other caregivers can give you courage and humor about your difficult situation."

Resource: Dr. Huysman is the cofounder of The Leeza Gibbons Memory Foundation, which has created Leeza's Place, local, home-based centers through the US, where caregivers and their loved ones with memory disorders can receive "energy, empowerment and education." For more information, visit the Web site *www.leezasplace.org*, call 888-655-3392 or e-mail info@leezasplace.org.

P. Murali Doraiswamy, MD, author of *The Alzheimer's Action Plan* (St. Martin's).

Constantine Lyketsos, chairman, Department of Psychiatry, Johns Hopkins Bayview Medical Center, Baltimore.

Kathleen Piercy, PhD, asssociate professor of family, consumer and human development, Utah State University and author of *Working with Aging Families* (W.W. Norton).

Jamie Huysman, PsyD, LCSW, coauthor of *Take Your Oxygen First* (LaChance). *www.drjamie.com.*

Eileen Haight, author of *Alzheimer's Caregivers: The Choice of Love. www.alzheimer-caregiver.com.*

Katherine Forsythe, MSW, social worker in San Francisco. *www.getasecondwind.com.*

Soy Isoflavones— Improving Memory in Women and Men

In both women and men, there are *beta-estrogen* receptors in the parts of the brain that play a key role in memory and learning, and scientists theorize that estrogen is a must for optimal mental functioning. In fact, studies show that treating estrogen-depleted, postmenopausal women with estrogen (*hormone replacement therapy*, or HRT) improves memory.

However: HRT also increases the risk of heart disease, stroke and breast cancer.

That's why scientists around the world have conducted studies to find out whether a high intake of *isoflavones* (estrogen-like plant compounds, or phytoestrogens, found in soybeans) could improve memory and mental prowess after menopause.

Not every study produced positive results. But most did.

"Isoflavones may have positive effects on postmenopausal women, improving cognitive performance," said Italian researchers.

"Soy phytoestrogens may improve working memory in women through estrogen-dependent mechanisms," wrote researchers in Australia. (*Working memory* is the technical term for one aspect of short-term memory, which you use to store and manage recently acquired information you need to comprehend, reason and learn.)

"Significant cognitive improvements in postmenopausal women can be gained from consumption of a supplement containing soy isoflavones," say UK researchers, after women in their study took a daily supplement of 60 milligrams (mg) of isoflavones for 12 weeks.

"Soy isoflavones may mimic the actions and functions of estrogens on the brain, and they have been shown to have positive effects on the cognitive function of females," concluded Korean scientists, reviewing all the studies on isoflavones, postmenopausal women and memory.

Now: Hey, males—join the party! Two new studies show that increasing the intake of soy isoflavones can improve memory in women *and* men.

Exciting Development

Noting that none of the nine studies on estrogen and memory "included older men," researchers from the University of Wisconsin tested the power of soy isoflavones to improve mental functioning in 30 women and men, aged 62 to 89.

At the beginning of the study, the researchers conducted 11 cognitive tests designed to measure memory, learning and other mental abilities. Then they divided the study participants into two groups—half took a supplement containing 100 mg of isoflavones, and half didn't. After six months, they conducted the cognitive tests again.

Result: Those taking isoflavones improved on eight of the 11 tests. (There was little improvement in the placebo group.)

• Memory was stronger.

• Thinking was clearer.

• The use of everyday language was more fluent.

• Reaction times were faster.

"Isoflavones," concluded the researchers in *Age and Ageing,* "may offer a combination of cognitive effects for older men and women."

In another study, Australia researchers gave either a daily supplement of 116 mg isoflavones or a placebo to 34 men, ages 30 to 80.

After 12 weeks, those taking isoflavones had about a 20% greater improvement in working memory. The placebo-takers didn't have a similar improvement.

"Isoflavone supplementation in healthy males may enhance cognitive processes," say the researchers, in the *British Journal of Nutrition.*

"The improvement," they theorize, "may be due to increased binding of isoflavones to beta-estrogen receptors in the prefrontal cortex, a part of the brain which plays a critical role in working memory."

Two Servings a Day of Soy

"I suggest eating two servings of soy food a day, which would deliver approximately 100 mg of isoflavones," says Mark Messina, PhD, adjunct associate professor in the Department of Nutrition at Loma Linda University. "Three is ideal."

Getting two servings a day isn't difficult, considering all the soy foods on the market, he points out. "You can have soymilk with cereal, snack on soynuts or eat edamame—green soybeans harvested in the pod—as a vegetable. The choices of soy foods are virtually endless. I've eaten two servings of soy foods a day just about every day for 40 years, and I'm 57," he adds.

And men shouldn't worry that the phytoestrogens in soy will deliver more estrogen than they need. "Scientific data show that isoflavones don't have feminizing effects on men," says Dr. Messina. In fact, he says, studies show their effects in men are very positive—they slightly lower cholesterol and reduce the risk of prostate cancer.

If you don't think you'll reliably eat two servings of soy a day, isoflavone supplements are a good "secondary choice," he says.

What to look for: "When choosing a supplement, make sure all three isoflavones—*genistein, daidzein* and *glycitein*—are on the label, and that genistein is listed first," says Dr. Messina. (Genistein is the isoflavone with the strongest effect.)

One way to guarantee you're getting that combination is to look for a "Novasoy" logo (a small green leaf) on the supplement label, says Dr. Messina. It indicates the product contains a mixture of isoflavones standardized for genistein. (A Novasoy supplement was the type used by the researchers at the University of Wisconsin.)

Mark Messina, PhD, adjunct associate professor, Department of Nutrition at Loma Linda University, California.

The Common Food Additive That Can Addle Your Brain

What if the increasingly common use of an everyday food additive and fertilizer—found in ground beef, bacon, bologna, beer and cheese…and in agricultural runoff that ends up in drinking water—was the unsuspected cause of the striking rise in the number of people with Alzheimer's disease?

That's the shocking (but well-substantiated) theory of a team of researchers from Brown University in Rhode Island, detailed in a recent issue of the *Journal of Alzheimer's Disease.*

Nitrites and Nitrates

The researchers looked at the yearly death rates from diseases of aging, such as stroke, Alzheimer's disease (AD) and type 2 diabetes *mellitus* (T2DM). Then they matched those rates against exposure to *nitrites* (used as food additives) and *nitrates* (used as food additives and in fertilizer).

Result: They found a surprising parallel between increasingly high death rates from AD and increasingly high exposure to nitrites and nitrates.

Between 1968 and 2005, the death rates from AD among 75- to 84-year-olds increased 150-fold, while death rates from stroke in the same age group declined.

"These data show that trends in death rates from AD are not due to an aging population," says Suzanne de la Monte, MD, the study leader. "Such a dramatic increase in death rates in a relatively short interval of time is more consistent with exposure-related causes."

Exposure to what?

As death rates from AD were skyrocketing, so was the use of nitrate-containing fertilizer, which increased by 230% between 1955 and 2005.

And between 1970 and 2005, sales from fast-food chains and meat processing companies (processed meat is a major source of nitrites and nitrates in the diet) increased by more than eightfold.

"It is conceivable that chronic exposure to relatively low levels of nitrites, nitrates and *nitrosamines* [formed by the body from nitrites and nitrates] through processed foods, fertilizers and water is responsible for the current epidemic of AD, and for the increasing mortality rates associated with it," says Dr. de la Monte.

Theory: "We have become a 'nitrosamine' generation, she says. "We now eat a diet rich in amines from protein, and rich in nitrites and nitrates from additives, a combination that leads to increased nitrosamine production in the body. And not only do we consume nitrites and nitrates in processed foods, but nitrates get into our food supply by leeching from the soil and contaminating water supplies used for crop irrigation, food processing and drinking."

Surprising: That increased exposure to nitrates and nitrites might not only be causing the epidemic of Alzheimer's—it might also be causing the epidemic of type 2 diabetes mellitus (T2DM).

Nitrosamines can spark biochemical factors that create the chronic low-grade inflammation and oxidation underlying both AD and T2DM, explains Dr. de la Monte.

In her research, Dr. de la Monte found that the nitrosamine-like drug *streptozotocin*—used in animal experiments to induce diabetes—also causes AD-type neurodegeneration and cognitive impairment.

And studies now show that having T2DM nearly doubles your risk of developing AD.

"In essence, at the core of the development of AD and T2DM is insulin resistance with associated deficits in glucose utilization and energy metabolism, and increased levels of chronic inflammation and oxidative stress," she says.

"The prevalence rates of these two diseases have increased sharply over the past several decades and show no sign of plateau. Because there has been a relatively short time interval for this dramatic shift in disease incidence and prevalence rates, we believe the increase is caused by environmental exposures."

Minimize and Avoid

To stop the flood of nitrites and nitrates, Dr. de la Monte advocates reforms in public health policies. "Eliminating the use of nitrites and nitrates in food processing, preservation and agriculture...taking steps to prevent the formation of nitrosamines...and employing safe and effective means to detoxify food and water before human consumption."

But while you're waiting for industry and government to protect you from nitrates, nitrites and nitrosamines, here's how you can protect yourself:

Minimize or avoid foods high in nitrites. "Just about everybody in my lab changed what they ate after the results of this study," says Dr. de la Monte. "They stopped or minimized eating foods with added nitrites and nitrates."

Look at the label of any processed or preserved food, she advises. If it lists nitrites or nitrates—additives used for coloring (to make red meat redder), flavoring and as preservatives—don't buy it. "This is the easiest lifestyle change I can recommend."

Examples: processed meats (such as bacon, sausage, hot dogs and luncheon meats), cheese and cheese products, beer, nonfat dry milk.

Minimize or avoid cooking methods that form nitrosamines. These include frying and flame broiling, she says.

Eat more fruits and vegetables. "They help prevent the formation of nitrosamines in the stomach," says nutritionist Bronwyn Schweigerdt, in Oakland, California.

Suzanne de la Monte, MD, study leader and associate professor of pathology and medicine, Brown University, Providence, Rhode Island.

Bronwyn Schweigerdt, nutrition instructor and author of *The Undiet: Painless Baby Steps to Permanent Weight Loss* (ACW).

Chapter 11

MEN'S HEALTH

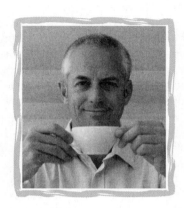

Five Things Men Can Do To Live Longer

These are difficult times for everyone, but especially men. Compared with women, men have lost more jobs in this recession and are struggling to get back on track in an increasingly competitive work environment while balancing ever-mounting pressures and responsibilities at home. Compounding these stresses are the inherent health disadvantages men face that have wedged five years in life expectancy between the sexes. The average woman lives to 80—the average man lives to age 75. Moreover, in every age group, men are more likely than women to die from heart disease, cancer, injuries, chronic obstructive pulmonary disease, infections such as flu and pneumonia, and suicide.

How Men Can Lengthen Their Lives

According to Marianne J. Legato, MD, professor of clinical medicine at Columbia Uni-

versity and author of *Why Men Die First: How to Lengthen Your Lifespan* (Palgrave MacMillan), the combination of genetics, physiology and the way our society conditions and trains men to behave has resulted in "unique fragilities" that include a weaker immune system, earlier onset of coronary artery disease (CAD) and a tendency to tough it out and not admit to pain or emotional difficulties. Consequently men are less proactive than women when it comes to their physical and mental health, resulting in missed opportunities to catch illnesses in their earlier stages, when they can be effectively treated. Moreover, in these stressful times, many men are not admitting to or recognizing their own feelings of depression, which itself is a risk for serious illness.

Dr. Legato offers some suggestions on what specific steps men can take to lengthen their lives...

1. Bolster Your Immune System

Generally speaking, the male immune system has a less vigorous response to diseases

231

and infections, leaving men more vulnerable to heart disease; colorectal, lung and liver cancers, melanoma and infectious diseases such as influenza and pneumonia. Because this somewhat weaker immune system is hardwired, Dr. Legato stresses that it becomes even more important for men to make lifestyle choices that help them stay strong and healthy.

2. Prevent Early Onset of Heart Disease

Men tend to develop CAD about 10 to 20 years before women, often in the prime of their lives—in fact, the symptoms can appear in men as early as the mid-30s and they are also likely to die from it at younger ages. Blame hormones—estrogen helps protect women from CAD until they are well into midlife by elevating levels of high-density lipoprotein (HDL) and keeping blood vessel walls relaxed, whereas in men, testosterone is thought to increase low-density lipoprotein (LDL—the so-called bad cholesterol), which, if it oxidizes, raises risk of heart disease and stroke.

Dr. Legato advises men to get an annual screening for CAD, which should include a careful assessment of their risk factors, starting with a baseline in their 20s. Tests should include an electrocardiogram...a test for inflammatory markers identifying factors that can contribute to serum cholesterol damage of vessel walls...and a cholesterol panel, paying particular attention to the ratio of good HDL to triglycerides and HDL to LDL.

Also important: Follow an anti-inflammatory lifestyle, eating nutritious foods (including plenty of fruits and vegetables and not too much animal protein), exercising regularly and getting sufficient omega-3 fatty acids, either by eating fish twice weekly or taking fish oil supplements.

3. Get Early Cancer Screenings

Cancer is the other main killer of men in middle and older age, says Dr. Legato. Early detection is the key to surviving the three most common (and lethal) cancers in men—prostate, lung and colon. To screen for prostate cancer, Dr. Legato recommends digital rectal exams beginning at age 45, followed by an ultrasound of the prostate when necessary. For lung cancer, those at high risk (smokers, men with a history of exposure to radon) should have annual or biannual chest X-rays. All men should begin colon cancer screening at age 50 and even earlier for those with family history of the disease.

4. Recognize and Treat Depression

Unlike women, who tend to express their emotions and have broader social networks to get help, men often struggle silently, holding in their feelings. The result, says Dr. Legato, is an "under-recognized epidemic of depression, which leaches the color out of men's lives." Depressed men tend to neglect their health, smoke more, self-medicate with alcohol and other drugs and exercise less. Heart disease is three times higher among men who are clinically depressed. Finally, depression sometimes leads to suicide, which is four times more likely in men compared with women.

One step that men who suspect they're suffering from depression can take is to ask their doctor to check testosterone levels, as both high and low levels can cause symptoms of depression. Low testosterone negatively affects energy, muscle mass, ability to perform prolonged exercise, memory, concentration and libido. High testosterone can cause restlessness, aggressive behavior and a general sense of dispiritedness. There are several different forms of treatment, including gels, patches and injections, to help restore testosterone to clinically functional levels.

It's also important to talk about your feelings and concerns with friends or family and, if that's not very helpful, seek professional counseling.

5. Reduce Stress

While stress can be motivating and challenging, it can also be physically and mentally exhausting. Strategies for stress management recommended by Dr. Legato include making a list of the factors that cause stress in your life, prioritizing those you can work on and crossing out the ones that you can't control. She says it is important to steal a few hours away from your busy day for just yourself. Figure out what helps you decompress—

maybe the aromatherapy or morning walk with friends through the neighborhood that your wife finds helpful isn't your style—but here's your excuse to go fishing...take the dog for a spirit-boosting run...or find a men-only yoga class or martial arts program that incorporates meditative exercise (such as ha-tha yoga, tae kwon do or tai chi). Anything you can do to make life better will likely help make it longer, too.

Marianne J. Legato, MD, founder of Partnership for Gen-der-Specific Medicine, professor of clinical medicine at Co-lumbia University College of Physicians and Surgeons and author of *Why Men Die First: How to Lengthen Your Life-span* (Palgrave Macmillan).

Best Holistic Cures For Men's Urological Problems

If you've ever had an acute infection of the prostate, you may know that antibiotics often clear up the problem in just a few days.

But as the antibiotics eliminate infection-causing bacteria, these powerful drugs also wipe out "healthy" organisms that aid diges-tion and help fortify the immune system. You may experience diarrhea, upset stomach or a yeast infection while taking the medication.

What's the answer? Holistic medicine uses alternative therapies, such as dietary supple-ments, nutritional advice and acupuncture, to complement—or replace—conventional med-ical treatments, including prescription drugs.

For example, probiotic "good" bacteria supplements help replenish the beneficial intestinal bacteria killed by antibiotics. Ask your doctor about taking 10 billion to 20 bil-lion colony forming units (CFUs) of probiot-ics, such as lactobacillus or acidophilus, two to three hours after each dose of antibiotics.*

Holistic treatments for other urological problems that affect men...**

Enlarged Prostate

Prescription drugs, such as *finasteride* (Pros-car) and *doxazosin* (Cardura), can relieve the urgent need to urinate and other symptoms caused by benign *prostatic hyperplasia* (BPH). But the drugs' side effects often in-clude reduced libido, fatigue and potentially harmful drops in blood pressure. *Holistic approach...*

● **Beta-sitosterol** is a plant compound that is found in saw palmetto, a popular herbal remedy for BPH. Men who do not improve with saw palmetto may want to combine it with beta-sitosterol (125 mg daily).

● **Pygeum africanum,** an herb derived from an evergreen tree native to Africa, has anti-inflammatory effects that interfere with the formation of prostaglandins, hormone-like substances that tend to accumulate in the prostate of men with BPH. Take 100 mg two times daily with or without saw palmet-to and/or beta-sitosterol.

● **Acupuncture also may help ease BPH symptoms.** It can be used in addition to the remedies described above. The typical regimen is one to two treatments weekly for about four weeks.

Whether you're taking medication or herbs, lifestyle changes—such as drinking less cof-fee (which acts as a diuretic)...avoiding spicy foods and alcohol (which can irritate the bladder)...and cutting down on fluids—are a key part of managing BPH symptoms.

Impotence

For stronger, more reliable erections, conven-tional medicine offers several medications, such as *sildenafil* (Viagra) and *vardenafil* (Levitra). But these drugs can have side ef-fects, including painful, prolonged erections and sudden vision loss. *Holistic approach...*

● **Maca is a root vegetable from South America.** In supplement form, it has been shown to increase libido in healthy men.

Recommended dosage: 500 mg to 1,000 mg three times daily.

●**Asian ginseng,** a well-studied herb from China and Korea, can improve erections. Take 900 mg three times daily.

●**Ginkgo biloba,** derived from a tree native to China, may improve erections by boosting circulation. Take 120 mg to 240 mg daily. Maca, Asian ginseng and ginkgo biloba can all be combined.

●**Niacin,** a B vitamin, widens blood vessels when taken in high doses (500 mg to 1,000 mg daily) and may help promote erections in some men who do not improve with the three impotence remedies described above. A doctor should monitor high-dose courses of niacin.

●**Vigorous exercise** (such as weight lifting, jogging or cycling) promotes healthy circulation and boosts testosterone.

Important: Erectile dysfunction may be an early warning of heart problems, so consult a doctor before starting an exercise program. Erectile dysfunction also may be a symptom of diabetes or other systemic illness—or stress and relationship issues. For this reason, men who experience erectile dysfunction should see a doctor for a full evaluation before trying holistic therapies.

Chronic Prostatitis

Pain and swelling of the prostate (*prostatitis*) may be caused by inflammation that develops for unknown reasons or by an infection. The prostate enlargement that characterizes BPH, on the other hand, is likely due to hormonal changes that occur as men age. Symptoms of chronic prostatitis, such as pelvic pain and pain when urinating, can linger for months. Conventional medicine has little to offer other than antibiotics. *Holistic approach...*

●**Fish oil and quercetin** (a plant-based supplement) are both anti-inflammatories. The fish oil supplements should contain a daily total of about 1,440 mg of *eicosapentaenoic acid* (EPA) and 960 mg of *docosahexaenoic acid* (DHA). Take 500 mg of quercetin twice daily. Fish oil and quercetin can be combined.

Incontinence

Because incontinence can be caused by various underlying problems, including an infection, a neurological disorder (such as multiple sclerosis) or an enlarged prostate, any man who suffers from incontinence should first be evaluated by a urologist. *Holistic approach...*

●**Buchu, cleavers and cornsilk** are herbal remedies that often help when overactive bladder (marked by a sudden, intense need to urinate) causes incontinence. Some products contain all three herbs. For dosages, follow label instructions.

●**Bromelain,** an enzyme derived from pineapple, acts as an anti-inflammatory to help treat incontinence caused by an inflamed prostate. Take 500 mg to 2,000 mg daily in two divided doses.

●**Pumpkin seed oil extract** may ease incontinence in men when overactive bladder is related to an enlarged prostate.

Typical dosage: 160 mg of pumpkin seed oil extract, taken three times daily with meals. Pumpkin seed oil extract can be combined with saw palmetto. Ask your doctor for advice on combining pumpkin seed oil extract with any of the other incontinence remedies described above.

*To find a doctor near you who offers holistic therapies, consult the American Holistic Medical Association, 216-292-6644, *www.holisticmedicine.org*. Holistic doctors can help you choose high-quality supplements—these products may contain impurities.

**Because some supplements can interact with prescription drugs, raise blood sugar and cause other adverse effects, check with your doctor before trying any of the therapies mentioned in this article.

Geovanni Espinosa, ND, MS.Ac, director of clinical trials, clinician and co-investigator at the Center for Holistic Urology at Columbia University Medical Center in New York City (*www.holisticurology.columbia.edu*). He is author of the naturopathic section in *1,000 Cures for 200 Ailments* (Harper-Collins).

Why Drugs Don't Work For Prostatitis—and What Does

As men age, many begin to suffer problems with the prostate gland. Prostate enlargement is the condition that is most widely recognized, but there can be another culprit.

Often-overlooked condition: At some point in their lives, about one in 10 men will be diagnosed with *chronic prostatitis*, pain and swelling of the prostate due to inflammation that results from unknown causes or an infection.

Like an enlarged prostate, chronic prostatitis causes urinary difficulties, such as urinary frequency (urinating more than once every two hours)...urinary urgency (urination is hard to delay once the urge occurs)...and reduced stream (slow urinary flow).

Chronic prostatitis also can lead to symptoms that do not typically occur with an enlarged prostate—for example, pain in the *perineum* (the area between the anus and the scrotum)...the tip of the penis...the testicles...the bladder area...and the rectum. Men with prostatitis may even suffer pain during urination or orgasm.

Symptoms, which last for three months or more, are intermittent or constant. In severe, untreated cases, the condition may interfere with a man's sleep, desire for sex and overall enjoyment of life—indefinitely.

Lessons Learned

When chronic prostatitis is diagnosed, more than 70% of primary care physicians prescribe an antibiotic such as *ciprofloxacin* (Cipro), according to a recent survey. About half of the surveyed doctors prescribe an alpha-blocker drug, such as *alfuzosin* (Uroxatral) or *tamsulosin* (Flomax), which is typically used for prostate enlargement (benign prostatic hyperplasia).

Antibiotics are prescribed because many doctors believe that chronic prostatitis is an infectious disease—but, in fact, bacteria are present in only about 5% of cases. Alpha-blockers are used in the hope they might relax the prostate and the perineum. But recent studies show that these approaches don't work.

New thinking: Because the symptoms are real, but no biochemical or mechanical cause has yet been found, nonbacterial chronic prostatitis is now considered to be a pain syndrome, called *chronic prostatitis/chronic pelvic pain syndrome* (CP/CPPS).

Diagnosing the Problem

If you think you have CP/CPPS, see a urologist for a standard urological evaluation. Urinary and prostate fluid cultures should be ordered to look for infection. Urodynamic testing (to measure the functioning of the bladder and prostate) and cystoscopy (an examination of the urethra and bladder) also may be performed. These and other tests will help rule out other diseases, such as prostate cancer or bladder cancer.

Treatments Worth Trying

If you are suffering from CP/CPPS, there are several effective therapies to consider...

●**Quercetin.** This antioxidant/anti-inflammatory is found in red wine, onions and green tea. By reducing inflammation, it may help curb the pain and urinary difficulties of CP/CPPS.

Scientific evidence: When researchers at the Harbor-UCLA Medical Center in Los Angeles asked 28 men with CP/CPPS to take either a quercetin supplement or a placebo twice daily for one month, those taking quercetin had a 35% decrease in pain, while the placebo group experienced only a 7.2% reduction.

Resource: Most reputable brands of quercetin should have this effect. In one part of the study described above, men took the quercetin-containing product Prosta-Q, available from the manufacturer, Farr Laboratories (877-284-3976, *www.farrlabs.com*).

Caution: Don't take any quercetin product along with a quinolone antibiotic—such as *ciprofloxacin...levofloxacin* (Levaquin)...

norfloxacin (Noroxin)…or *ofloxacin* (Floxin). The supplement can interfere with the antibiotic's action.

●**Relaxation and trigger point therapy.** Some scientists theorize that CP/CPPS is caused by chronic tension in the pelvis. This, in turn, creates knots (trigger points) in the muscles, reduces blood flow and irritates pelvic nerves. If you consciously learn to relax those muscles, even when you're in pain…and a physical therapist locates and releases the trigger points with pressure and stretching—symptoms can be reduced.

Scientific evidence: When 138 men whose CP/CPPS symptoms did not respond to any treatment underwent a relaxation and trigger point therapy called the Stanford Protocol, 72% said their symptoms were moderately or markedly improved in one month.

Resource: The Stanford Protocol is offered in a six-day program in northern California. To learn more, call 707-874-2225 or consult *www.pelvicpainhelp.com.*

●**Acupuncture.** Researchers believe that pain occurs in CP/CPPS patients when stimulation, such as that caused by sitting or sexual activity, travels up the spinal cord and becomes magnified in the brain. Introducing a different stimulus, such as acupuncture, in the area where the pain originates can interrupt the cycle.

Scientific evidence: When 10 men whose CP/CPPS symptoms did not respond to at least one conventional medical treatment received acupuncture twice a week, their pain and urinary symptom scores dropped by more than 70%.

Resource: To find an acupuncturist near you, consult the National Certification Commission for Acupuncture and Oriental Medicine (904-598-1005, *www.nccaom.org*).

●**Biofeedback.** A biofeedback machine monitors a specific bodily function that we typically are not conscious of, such as muscular tension. When the function is abnormal, the machine gives feedback, such as a beep or flashing light.

Scientific evidence: When 31 men with CP/CPPS underwent a "pelvic floor biofeedback re-education program"—a series of biofeedback treatments that showed them when pelvic muscles were tense and how to relax them—the men had a 52% decrease, on average, in pain and urinary symptom scores

Resource: To find a biofeedback practitioner near you, consult the Association for Applied Psychophysiology and Biofeedback, Inc., 800-477-8892, *www.aapb.org.*

(For more information on biofeedback, see appendix page 358.)

Rodney Anderson, MD, professor of urology (emeritus) at Stanford University School of Medicine in Stanford, California. He is coauthor of *A Headache in the Pelvis* (National Center for Pelvic Pain).

Erectile Dysfunction Supplements—Help Or Hype?

The market for products that treat erectile dysfunction (ED) is flooded with choices.

Many commonly prescribed drugs, such as *sildenafil* (Viagra), help men achieve and maintain erections by enhancing blood circulation to the penis. But these drugs also can cause serious side effects, such as digestive disturbances, headaches and vision loss. Natural ED remedies also help men achieve and maintain erections by boosting circulation. In addition, they enhance libido, genital sensation and orgasm intensity. But not all natural ED supplements do what their makers claim.

Buyer Beware

Perhaps the best-known natural ED supplement is Enzyte. Ads for the product feature "Smilin' Bob," a man with a constant grin—the result of taking Enzyte, of course. The company owner was sentenced to prison for bank fraud, conspiracy and other crimes. Enzyte is still on the market. There is nothing dangerous about its ingredients, but there are no studies proving that the product works.

Reputable ED Supplements

If you experience ED, see your doctor to determine the cause. ED can result from clogged blood vessels, a sign of heart disease. If you have heart disease, you need to treat this problem first.

Ask your physician to annually test both your total testosterone level and free testosterone level, the amount available in the bloodstream (not bound to protein). A low total or free testosterone level can cause ED, or it can indicate another problem. Note: ED supplements may not be safe for men with prostate cancer.

Mark Stengler, NMD, recommends the following natural supplements. Try one product or the other. *Do not take both at the same time...*

● **112 Degrees.** The ingredients in 112 Degrees have been shown to support long-term sexual health. *Tribulus terrestris*, a fruit extract regarded in China and Tibet as an aphrodisiac, is thought to enhance sexual desire. *Butea superba*, from the roots of a vine that grows in Thailand, improved erectile function and sexual performance in 82% of men with ED who took 250 milligrams (mg) of the herb daily for three months. *Panax ginseng* is known to increase sexual desire and improve erectile function.

Take two tablets of 112 Degrees once daily—or one tablet twice daily—on an empty stomach. If you have hypertension, have your blood pressure closely monitored. 112 Degrees is available only from the manufacturer ($59.95 per one-month supply, 800-901-5526, *www.112degrees.com*).

● **TestoPlex.** This blend of green oat extract, nettle extract, sea buckthorn and oat bran fiber is for men with low levels of free testosterone. Ten clinical trials looked at the effect of green oat extract and found that it increased levels of free testosterone in the body. In one of the studies, men experienced improvement in erectile function and frequency as their free testosterone levels increased.

Take four capsules for a total of 2,000 mg once a day in the morning with a full glass of water ($39.95 per one-month supply, available only through health-care professionals, 800-647-6100, *www.xymogen.com*).

Mark A. Stengler, NMD, naturopathic medical doctor in private practice, La Jolla, California, and author of the *Bottom Line/Natural Healing* newsletter. *www.drstengler.com.*

Help for Peyronie's Disease

Peyronie's disease is a condition in which scar tissue builds up along the length of the penis, causing the penis to bend. There are several possible causes, including microinjuries to the penis or a genetic predisposition. Some doctors suggest watching the condition for one to two years because it often heals on its own. Sometimes, *tamoxifen*, a cancer drug, is prescribed.

Mark Stengler, NMD, recommends oral treatment with the nutrient acetyl-L-carnitine (ALC), which counteracts inflammation and the development of fibrous tissue. An Italian study of men with acute or chronic Peyronie's disease found that taking 1,000 mg twice daily for three months reduced penile curvature significantly when compared with those who took tamoxifen. ALC, taken at 2,000 mg daily, is safe for everyone. If the condition doesn't improve after taking ALC for three months, return to your urologist for more aggressive treatment.

Mark A. Stengler, NMD, naturopathic medical doctor in private practice, La Jolla, California, and author of the *Bottom Line/Natural Healing* newsletter. *www.drstengler.com.*

Can the Penis Predict a Heart Attack?

Scientists have been asking that surprising but serious question for the past five years, since a study of nearly 10,000 men showed that erectile dysfunction was as important a risk factor for having a heart attack as a family history of heart disease, high cholesterol or smoking.

Now: A new study shows the answer is yes—at least in men aged 40 to 49.

The Link Between ED and CAD

Researchers from the Duke University Medical Center and the Mayo Clinic studied 1,402 men, aged 40 to 79, who didn't have heart disease.

At the beginning of the 10-year study, the researchers found out who did and didn't have erectile dysfunction (ED)—the consistent inability to achieve and maintain an erection sufficient for intercourse.

Among age groups, the percentages of ED were...

- 40 to 49—2.4%
- 50 to 59—5.6%
- 60 to 69—17%
- 70 and up—38.8%

Every other year for the next ten years, the men were screened for the development of heart disease (coronary artery disease, or CAD).

Results: Men with ED at the start of the study were 80% more likely to develop CAD, compared with men without ED.

And when the researchers matched ED and CAD by age group, they found the youngest men with ED at the start of the study also had the weakest hearts...

- Men aged 40 to 49 with ED at the start of the study were 50 times more likely (5,000%) to develop CAD in the next ten years.
- Men aged 50 to 59 with ED at the start of the study were five times more likely (500%) to develop CAD.
- Men aged 60 to 69 with ED at the start of the study were twice as likely (200%) to develop CAD.
- Men aged 70 and up with ED at the start of the study were 21% more likely to develop CAD.

ED in young men may be an early manifestation of systemic arterial disease, preceding the development of coronary disease by decades, say the researchers, in *Mayo Clinic Proceedings*.

Theory: ED and CAD are different manifestations of the same disease—arterial disease, or atherosclerosis.

Arterial disease clogs the arteries of the heart—but may clog the smaller arteries of the penis first. (The arteries of the heart are 3 to 4 millimeters [mm] in diameter, while the arteries of the penis are 1 to 2 mm.)

Arterial disease also robs arteries of their flexibility and strength—and may weaken smaller penile arteries first.

"It's very possible that a common, underlying problem explains both of these seemingly different conditions," says Brant Inman, MD, the study leader and an assistant professor of urology.

See Your Doctor

An estimated 5 to 10% of men aged 40 to 49 have ED. If you're one of those men, it's crucial that you see your doctor—about ED and CAD, says Dr. Inman. (The same advice is prudent for any man with ED.)

"The doctor should look for factors that increase your risk for heart disease, such as high blood pressure, high cholesterol, overweight and high blood sugar levels," he says.

"Along with taking medications to control those conditions, you should seriously consider making lifestyle changes that are beneficial to the health of the heart—such as losing weight; eating a balanced diet without excessive amounts of fat, sugar and other refined carbohydrates; exercising regularly and quitting smoking.

"ED can be a strong motivating factor for you to make these changes—because you may protect your heart and improve your sexuality, as arterial health improves," says Dr. Inman.

(For more ideas on preventing and controlling heart disease, please see the chapter "Heart Disease" on page 176.)

Brant Inman, MD, assistant professor of urology, Duke University Medical Center, Durham, North Carolina.

Boost Testosterone

That's Mr. Testosterone to you.

This testes-produced hormone is what makes a man, well, manly.

Like a miracle drug, testosterone interacts with every cell in the body and bestows upon guys their muscles and strength...their sperm, sex drive and erections...their deep voice and daily growth of beard...and their "desire to take charge and take on the world," says Shafiq Qaadri, MD, a physician in Toronto and author of *The Testosterone Factor* (Da Capo).

Problem: "There's a steady but accelerating decline in a man's testosterone level, starting around age 30 and getting steeper with time, particularly at midlife," says Dr. Qaadri.

And as testosterone goes, so goes the guy.

"Even though you might not have testosterone levels so depleted a doctor would diagnosis you with a condition called *late-onset hypogonadism,* you might very well have low testosterone levels," says Dr. Qaadri. And you might have some or all of the symptoms that go with low testosterone, he says. You're easily fatigued and irritated...you lack enthusiasm and ambition...you don't sleep well... your concentration and memory are dulled... you have vague aches and pain...your spare tire is inflated...and your sex drive (not to mention your sex organ) is deflated.

In fact, a recent 12-year study of nearly 800 men aged 51 to 90 showed that those with the lowest testosterone levels were 40% more likely to die than men with the highest levels.

Well, if you think the testosterone in your tank is low, just pull up to your doctor's office and ask for a prescription of the hormone, which could take the form of a testosterone patch you wear, testosterone gel you smear on every day, a testosterone pill, a testosterone injection or a testosterone implant. You'll be feeling like a teenager again in no time.

Red flag: Even though supplemental testosterone has been on the market for many years, new research shows that using it is not without risk.

The Risks of Testosterone Therapy

Evaluating all the studies to date on testosterone replacement therapy (TRT), a team of gerontologists from the Saint Louis University School of Medicine said that TRT has downsides that could include...

• **Increased risk of prostate and breast cancer**

• **Worsened benign prostatic hypertrophy,** the swollen prostate condition that is a common cause of urinary problems in older men

• **Damaged liver or liver cancer**

• **Thickened blood (*hyperviscosity*),** possibly causing vision problems and headaches

• *Gynecomastia,* the development of breasts in a man

• **Caused or worsened obstructive sleep apnea,** the nightlong snoring, breathing difficulties and fitful sleep common in older men

• *Erythrocytosis,* an increase in red blood cells, which might increase the risk of heart attack and stroke (as well as causing symptoms such as easy bruising, and red, painful skin)

• **Worsened congestive heart failure**

• **Infertility**

• **Water retention**

• **Skin problems such as itchiness (from the patch)**

Important: And somewhat mirroring the downfall of hormone replacement therapy (HRT) for women (a major study showed that it increased the risk of breast cancer, heart disease and stroke), the researchers note that "studies conducted to date have been too small to address potential long-term adverse effects" of TRT. In other words, nobody knows what might happen to you if you take the hormone for many years.

239

Natural Testosterone Boosters

"If you're a middle-aged or older man, you can refuse to just let your testosterone fade away," says Dr. Qaadri. "You can learn how to naturally increase your body's testosterone production capacity—and enjoy your newly enhanced vitality and virility."

His recommendations for boosting the hormone he calls "T" for short...

●**Be a deeper sleeper.** "Sleep is T-time," says Dr. Qaadri. "The more refreshing your sleep, the more your body will produce T and build a better production capacity for testosterone."

●Just say no. For at least two to three hours before you sleep, don't have caffeine, a large meal, alcohol, nicotine, strenuous exercise or liquids.

●Wear earplugs. To optimize sleep, sleep in complete silence. Make sure your alarm clock is loud enough to hear through earplugs.

●Wear a sleep mask. Sleep in complete darkness, by wearing an opaque sleep mask over your eyes to block out all light, which can play havoc with your natural rhythms.

●Sleep half-naked. "Give the testes what you've deprived them of all day—freedom," says Dr. Qaadri. "Then they will be able to set their own desired temperature without interference." Wear a long shirt, a sports jersey or an oversized T-shirt.

●Cool the room slightly. By cooling the room, you can focus the blood flow to your vital organs, including the testes.

●**Get enough sex.** The testosterone concentration in the testes is 100 times the concentration of testosterone in the blood. "Sex is the force that accesses this storage vault," says Dr. Qaadri. "The blast that releases some of this T into circulation. Even anticipating sex increases T."

●Extend foreplay. "The longer you engage in foreplay, the more your testosterone percolates, boils, rises and builds in anticipation," he says.

●Cultivate variety. Try different positions, locations and lingerie. "T doesn't spike as intensely when you have settled into a routine that no longer excites you," says Dr. Qaadri.

●Have an orgasm. "That's the major event that releases T throughout the body."

●Self-service when necessary. Men report that when they self-pleasure their orgasm is more intense than when they have intercourse, he says. "Biochemically, that means their T-rush is greater."

●**Exercise your pelvis.** Exercise enhances the production, release and distribution of testosterone—it even increases the number of testosterone receptors in the part of the body being exercised, he says.

●Do pelvic cardio exercise. Along with a regular heart-pumping exercise such as brisk walking, vigorously exercise your pelvis to boost T production. Pelvic cardio exercise pumps T out of the testes to the rest of the body. *Do each of the following three exercise for about three minutes a day, he instructs...*

1. While standing in a slight squat, hands on hips, thrust your pelvis back and forth, in your best heave-ho, isolating your pelvis as much as possible from your torso.

2. Stand with one foot forward, one foot back, as if you're about to lunge like a fencing champion. Thrust back and forth as before.

3. While standing, slightly squatting down, hands on hips, move your pelvis in wide circles. Remember the hula hoop—same type of movement.

●**Make testosterone-smart food choices.** "A typical high-fat, high-sugar, high-salt diet is toxic to many body systems, including the testosterone-production system," says Dr. Qaadri.

●**Choose foods that maximize testosterone.** Excessive estrogen levels in men can decrease testosterone. *To reduce estrogen...*

● Broccoli, cauliflower and shellfish speed up liver enzymes that metabolize estrogen.

● Red grapes diminish the activity of *aromatase*, an enzyme that converts T into estrogen.

● Garlic, onion and cayenne help the liver metabolize environmental estrogens (xenoestrogens).

● Celery helps the T-production cycle.

● Oysters are rich in zinc, which enhances T production.

● **Take T-enhancing supplements.** Certain supplements enhance testosterone production and effects, he says.

● Zinc. The enzyme aromatase steals circulating testosterone out of the blood and turns it into the female hormone estrogen. Zinc lowers the amount of this enzyme.

Suggested intake: 50 mg daily.

● Calcium. "By taking adequate calcium, you relieve testosterone from its bone-repairing duty, and T is freer to work elsewhere," says Dr. Qaadri.

Suggested intake: 1,000 mg daily; over age 50, 1,500 mg daily.

● Vitamin C. "Vitamin C helps to reduce and neutralize one of T's major opponents, the stress hormone cortisol," he says.

Suggested intake: 1,000 mg daily.

● Selenium. This trace mineral helps in the testosterone manufacturing process, says Dr. Qaadri.

Suggested intake: 200 micrograms (mcg) daily.

● Vitamin D. "In men, vitamin D helps to soften estrogenic effects," he says.

Suggested intake: 800 IU daily.

Best: Take a high-quality multivitamin-mineral that supplies these and other nutrients.

Shafiq Qaadri, MD, a physician in Toronto and author of *The Testosterone Factor* (Da Capo). *www.doctorq.ca.*

For Male Infertility— Natural Ways to Strengthen Your Sperm

Every year, six million American men and women—about one out of every seven couples—have a fertility problem," says Harry Fisch, MD, director of the Male Reproductive Center at Columbia University Medical Center, and author of *The Male Biological Clock* (Free Press).

Surprising: In 40% of these couples, the problem lies with the man.

Specifically, with the man's sperm—too few sperm (low sperm count), sperm that are inactive (low sperm motility), or abnormally shaped sperm (poor sperm morphology).

And if you're aging, your sperm are aging right along with you. "Men older than 35 are twice as likely to be infertile as men 25 or younger," says Dr. Fisch.

Good news: Several recent studies show that there are natural (and pleasurable) ways to boost sperm count and motility, and improve morphology.

Surprising Finding

● **Omega-3.** Researchers in Iran found that infertile men had blood and sperm levels of omega-3 fatty acids (found in fatty fish such as salmon, mackerel, herring and sardines) that were nearly two times lower than those of fertile men.

Theory: Omega-3 fatty acids are crucial for the flexibility and fluidity of spermatozoa, and for successful fertilization," says Mohammad Reza Safarinejad, MD, the study leader.

Recommendation: "Since omega-3 fatty acids are widely available and have an excellent safety profile, they can be taken as a supplement to improve semen quality," says Dr. Safarinejad. "The recommended dosage for male infertility is 1.12 grams per day of EPA, and 0.72 grams per day of DHA."

● **Coenzyme Q10.** In other, recent research, Dr. Safarinejad studied 212 infertile men, dividing them into two groups—one received a daily supplement of 300 mg of the antioxidant Coenzyme Q10 (CoQ10), while the other took a placebo. After six months, those taking CoQ10 had a higher sperm count, better sperm motililty, and better sperm morphology.

Theory: "The spermatozoa is highly sensitive to oxidative stress and can be easily oxidized," says Dr. Safarinejad. "CoQ10 acts as an essential antioxidant, protecting the sperm from oxidation. In addition, it is able to recycle and regenerate other antioxidants, such as vitamin E and vitamin C."

Recommended: "CoQ10 has an excellent safety profile and at 300 mg a day is a worthwhile supplement for male infertility," he says.

• **Daily sex.** Australian researchers studied 118 men and found that daily sex (or ejaculating daily) for seven days reduced DNA damage in sperm.

"Further research is required to see whether improvement in these men's sperm quality translates into better pregnancy rates," says David Greening, MD, the study leader. "But previous studies have linked lower levels of sperm DNA damage with higher pregnancy rates."

Theory: Sperm that spends less time in the body is less likely to be oxidized, the main cause of DNA damage.

Important: "Although frequent ejaculation decreased semen volume and sperm concentrations, it did not compromise sperm motility, and in fact this rose slightly," says Dr. Greening.

Recommended: "Couples with relatively normal semen parameters should have sex daily for up to a week before the ovulation date," says Dr. Greening. "This simple treatment may assist in improving sperm quality and ultimately achieving a pregnancy."

Improving Sperm Count

"There are several other actions a man can take to markedly improve his sperm count and motility," says Jacob Teitelbaum, MD, a naturally oriented physician in Hawaii. *His recommendations...*

• **Vitamin C.** "Increasing your dosage to 500 to 1,000 milligrams (mg) a day has a marked effect on increasing sperm count and motility," he says. "Taking 500 mg twice a day, for example, can cure infertility in 20% of infertile males."

Important: Vitamin C also protects the sperm from genetic damage that can cause inherited diseases or cancer in the child.

• **Selenium.** 200 micrograms (mcg) a day.

Caution: Don't take more than 200 mcg. Higher levels can be toxic.

• **Vitamin E.** 400 IU a day. This antioxidant can also increase male fertility.

• **Zinc.** 50 mg a day of this antioxidant is also helpful.

• **Factors to avoid.** *Dr. Teitelbaum counsels infertile men to avoid the following...*

• Soy products. "Foods such as soy milk, tofu, miso and tempeh can increase estrogen production and may significantly decrease sperm counts," he says.

• Conventionally grown meat. "Using meat from animals that have not been raised and fattened using estrogen is important for any man who is infertile," he says.

• Toxins and chemicals. "Research suggests that sperm counts have fallen by 40% over the past 50 years throughout the industrialized world," says Dr. Teitelbaum. "There's a good possibility that this is being caused by industrial chemicals, especially pesticides, which mimic estrogen effects in the body. Eating organic foods and otherwise minimizing exposure to chemicals and other toxins could be helpful."

Harry Fisch, MD, director of the Male Reproductive Center at Columbia University Medical Center, and author of *The Male Biological Clock* (Free Press).

Mohammad Reza Safarinejad, professor of urology, Aja University of Medical Sciences, Iran.

David Greening, MD, reproductive medicine, Sydney, Australia.

Jacob Teitelbaum, MD, author of *Pain-Free 1-2-3!* (McGraw-Hill) and *From Fatigued to Fantastic!* (Avery). *www.endfatigue.com.*

Chapter 12

OSTEOPOROSIS

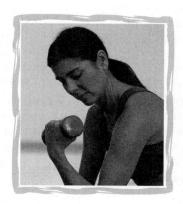

Yoga—A Great Way to Strengthen Bones

When you think of bone-strengthening exercises to prevent, slow or reverse osteoporosis, you probably picture weight lifting, walking, running, aerobic dancing—the weight-bearing exercises (where your bones support your weight) typically recommended by experts to battle bone loss.

New approach: Several new studies show that there's another (and surprisingly effective) exercise for osteoporosis.

Yoga.

Reversing Bone Loss

Researchers studied 26 older women (average age 68) who had undergone a DEXA (*dual energy x-ray absorptiometry*) scan to measure *bone mineral density* (BMD) and had been diagnosed with either osteopenia or osteoporosis. (A so-called T-score of -1 to -2.5 points below the normal BMD for healthy women in their twenties is osteopenia; a T-score under -2.5 is osteoporosis.)

Two years later—after two years of regular yoga practice for 18 of the women—the 26 women had another DEXA scan.

On average, the yoga practitioners had gained 0.76 points in the spine and 0.94 points in the hip.

"Five women with osteopenia were reclassified as normal, and two women with osteoporosis are now osteopenic," says Loren Fishman, MD, the study leader, medical director of Manhattan Physical Medicine and Rehabilitation and coauthor of *Yoga for Osteoporosis* (Norton). "These were very impressive results. The women practicing yoga gained a lot of bone."

Meanwhile, the women not practicing yoga lost an average of 0.10 points.

"Yoga appears to be an effective way to build bone mineral density after menopause," concludes Dr. Fishman in the quarterly publication *Topics in Geriatric Rehabilitation.*

243

In other recent research on yoga and bone health, doctors at the University of Pittsburgh studied seven osteopenic, postmenopausal women who took a weekly, one-hour yoga class and also practiced yoga at home. After 12 weeks, the women had high blood levels of several compounds that play a key role in bone formation—and the more hours of yoga, the higher the levels.

"Yoga may have beneficial effects on bone turnover in osteopenic postmenopausal women," conclude the researchers, in the *International Journal of Yoga Therapy*.

And researchers at the University of California, Los Angeles, studied the effect of yoga on people with *hyperkyphosis*—the medical term for dowager's hump, the bent-over posture caused by osteoporotic fractures of the spine.

The researchers divided the study's 118 participants—81% women, average age 75, most with daily or frequent back pain—into two groups. One group practiced yoga three days a week and one group didn't.

After six months, the spines of the yoga group were, on average, nearly 5% less curved, their average height had slightly increased and they had less upper back pain. There was little improvement in the non-yoga group.

The study shows that "hyperkyphosis is remediable," say the researchers, in the *Journal of the American Geriatric Society*, and that yoga might be a "critical first step in the pathway to treating or preventing this condition."

Why it works: When a bone cell is compressed during exercise, it produces *osteon*, a protein that forms a structure on which minerals build new bone.

"Yoga puts muscular pressure on bones—much greater than gravity alone—and the bones get stronger in exactly the areas of pressure," says Dr. Fishman.

"Yoga stimulates many parts of the body simultaneously and in many different directions, providing a variety of beneficial stresses on the bone," agrees Ellen Saltonstall, a yoga teacher in New York City and coauthor of *Yoga for Osteoporosis*.

Why Yoga Works

Dr. Fishman thinks yoga is an ideal bone-building exercise because…

• Unlike weight lifting, the movements of yoga are "regulated and smooth," and don't create the same risk for injuries (approximately one out of every 10 people are injured lifting weights, says Dr. Fishman);

• Unlike impact exercises such as running and jumping rope, the movements of yoga don't increase the risk for arthritis;

• Unlike the gentle movements of tai chi, yoga provides sufficient muscular pressure to build bone;

• Unlike core exercises such as Pilates, yoga for osteoporosis is designed to avoid forward-bending movements, a major risk for fractures in those with osteopenia and osteoporosis;

• Unlike many exercises, it doesn't require specialized equipment and you can do it at home;

• Unlike almost any other exercise, yoga has been time-tested over thousands of years and

• Unlike medicines for bone-building, the "side effects" of yoga are positive—better balance, greater range of motion, increased strength and greater calm.

Find the Right Yoga for You

Dr. Fishman and Saltonstall have these recommendations for people who want to use yoga to slow, stop or reverse bone loss:

• **Choose a style of yoga with enough force and precision to build bone.** They recommend either Iyengar yoga or Anusara yoga, the style taught by Saltonstall. "These are the most anatomically sophisticated and therapeutically oriented styles of yoga," says Dr. Fishman.

"Practicing yoga for osteoporosis isn't just about stretching and relaxing," says Saltonstall. "What's important is an active and vigorous use of muscles so that bone is stimulated; precision, so that maximum benefit is derived from each posture and duration, holding the pose for long enough to produce a positive effect."

(For more information on different forms of yoga, see appendix page 345.)

Resource: You can find a teacher of Anusara Yoga by visiting the Web site *www.anusarayoga.com* and using the "Teacher Directory" on the home page.

● **Find a good teacher.** Dr. Fishman says that individuals with osteopenia or osteoporosis should look for a teacher who has at least ten years of experience and is a member of the Yoga Alliance (which has fairly rigorous standards of admission), and has taught yoga to people with osteoporosis. A good teacher asks if you have any physical problems that need to be taken into account, pays close attention to you during class and doesn't verbally or physically abuse students (for example, by berating them for not "achieving" a posture or asking them to move into postures that hurt).

Best: Ask the teacher for an initial one-on-one lesson, and then join the class.

● **Don't hurt yourself.** "I've been teaching yoga for 35 years, and none of my students has ever had a fracture," says Dr. Fishman. However, as already mentioned, those with osteopenia or osteoporosis should avoid forward-bending poses, which might fracture a vertebrae in the spine.

The biggest cause of injury in yoga is overdoing it, says Dr. Fishman. "Don't embrace the pose at first—flirt with it. Initially doing one-third of the pose or halfway is fine." And never cross your "threshold of pain," he says. And use whatever support you need (such as a wall) so that you don't fall while in a standing pose.

Resource: Audio downloads of "Yoga and Osteoporosis," instructional material by Dr. Fishman and Saltonstall, are available at *www.sciatica.org.*

Loren Fishman, MD, medical director of Manhattan Physical Medicine and Rehabilitation (*www.manhattanphysicalmedicine.com*).

Ellen Saltonstall, yoga teacher in New York City (*www.mohiniyoga.com*). She is coauthor with Dr. Fishman of *Yoga for Osteoporosis* (Norton).

The Best Bone-Building Exercises

Women whose bones are fragile and porous—due to the severe loss of bone density that characterizes osteoporosis—often avoid exercise for fear that jarring or twisting motions could cause fractures.

Done properly, however, exercise is not only safe for people with osteoporosis or its milder form, osteopenia, it actually can reduce or even reverse bone loss. For people whose bones are still healthy, exercise helps ensure that osteoporosis never develops.

Reason: When a muscle exerts tension on a bone, it stimulates specialized cells that increase new bone formation. Also, when muscles that contribute to balance are strengthened, falls (and resulting fractures) are less likely.

Keys: Doing the types of workouts that build bone most effectively...and modifying techniques as necessary to avoid overstressing already weakened bones.

What to do: Start by exercising for 10 to 20 minutes several times a week, gradually building up to 30 minutes a day six days per week. Alternate between a strength-training workout one day and an aerobic activity the next.

Important: Before beginning the exercise program below, ask your doctor which instructions you should follow—the ones labeled "If you have healthy bones" or the ones labeled "If you already have bone loss."

Strength Training for Bones

The only equipment you need are hand weights (dumbbells) and ankle weights (pads that strap around the ankles), $20 and up per pair at sports equipment stores.

For each exercise, begin with one set of eight repetitions ("reps"). If you cannot do eight reps using the suggested starting weights, use lighter weights. Over several weeks, gradually increase to 10, then 12, then 15 reps. Then try two sets of eight reps, resting for one minute between sets...and again gradually increase the reps. When you can do two sets of 15 reps, increase the weight by one to two pounds and start again with one set of eight reps.

Keep your shoulders back and abdominal muscles pulled in. With each rep, exhale during the initial move...hold the position for two seconds...inhale as you return to the starting position. Move slowly, using muscles rather than momentum. Do not lock elbow or knee joints.

● **Upper body.** These exercises build bone density in the shoulders, arms and spine.

If you have healthy bones: Stand during the exercises. Start by holding a five-pound weight in each hand...over time, try to work up to eight, then 10, then 12 pounds.

If you already have bone loss: To guard against falls, sit in a straight-backed chair while exercising. At first, use no weights or use one- or two-pound weights...gradually work up to three-, then five-, then a maximum of eight-pound weights if you can. Avoid heavier weights—they could increase the risk for vertebral compression fractures.

●**Arms forward.**

To start: Bend elbows, arms close to your body, hands at chest-height, palms facing each other. *One rep:* Straighten elbows until both arms are extended in front of you, parallel to the floor...hold...return to starting position.

●**Arm overhead.**

To start: Raise right arm straight overhead, palm facing forward. *One rep:* Bend right elbow, bringing right hand down behind your head... hold...return to starting position. Do a set with the right arm, then with the left.

●**Arms up-and-down.**

To start: Have arms down at your sides, palms forward. *One rep:* Keeping elbows close to your

sides, bend arms to raise hands toward shoulders until palms face you...hold...lower to starting position.

●**Midbody.** This strengthens and stabilizes "core" muscles (abdomen, back, pelvic area). By improving body alignment, it helps prevent falls and reduces pressure on the vertebrae, protecting against compression fractures of the spine. No weights are used.

If you have healthy bones: Do this exercise while standing...or try it while lying on your back, with knees bent and feet flat on the floor.

If you already have bone loss: Done while standing, this is a good option for osteoporosis patients who are uncomfortable exercising on the floor. If you have balance problems, hold onto a counter...or sit in a chair.

● **Tummy tuck/pelvic tilt.**

To start: Have arms at sides, feet hip-width apart. *One rep:* Simultaneously contract abdominal muscles to draw your tummy toward your spine, tighten buttocks muscles, and tilt the bottom of your pelvis forward to flatten the arch of your back...hold...return to starting position.

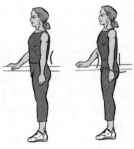

Start   **Tuck/Tilt**

● **Lower body.** These moves increase bone density in the legs and feet. For each rep, raise the leg as high as possible without leaning...hold for two seconds...return to starting position.

Advanced option: Try not to touch your foot to the ground between reps.

If you have healthy bones: Start by wearing a two-pound ankle weight on each leg... gradually increase to 10 pounds per ankle.

If you already have bone loss: Hold onto a counter for balance. To begin, use no weights…build up, one pound at a time, to five pounds per ankle.

- **Leg forward-and-back.**

To start: Stand on your right foot. *One rep:* Keeping both legs straight, slowly swing left leg forward and up…hold…swing leg down through the starting position and up behind you…hold…return to starting position. After one set, repeat with the other leg.

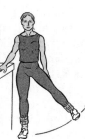

- **Leg out.**

To start: Stand on your right foot. *One rep:* Keeping both legs straight, slowly lift left leg out to the side…hold…return to starting position. After one set, repeat with the other leg.

Bone-Benefiting Aerobics

Biking, stationary cycling, swimming and rowing are good for heart health—but they do not protect against osteoporosis.

Better: Weight-bearing aerobic activities in which you're on your feet, bones working against gravity, build bone mass in the hips and legs.

If you have healthy bones: Good choices include jogging, dancing, stair climbing, step aerobics, jumping rope, racket sports and interactive video games, such as Wii Fit and Dance Dance Revolution. Pick whatever activity you enjoy the most and will do on a regular basis. If you enjoy walking, you can boost intensity by wearing a two- to 20-pound weighted vest ($50 and up at sports equipment stores).

Warning: Do not wear ankle weights during aerobic workouts—this could stress your joints.

If you already have bone loss: Refrain from high-impact activities (running, jumping) and those that require twisting or bending (racket sports, golf). Do not wear a weighted vest.

Safe low-impact options: Walking, using an elliptical machine (available at most gyms), qigong and tai chi.

Illustrations by Shawn Banner.

Raymond E. Cole, DO, clinical assistant professor, Department of Internal Medicine, Michigan State University College of Osteopathic Medicine, East Lansing. He is author of *Best Body, Best Bones: Your Doctor's Exercise Rx for Lifelong Fitness* (Wellpower). *www.drraymondcole.com.*

Run for Better Bones

Running is more effective for building bones and lowering risk for osteoporosis than weight lifting or cycling.

Reason: The impact of a runner's feet hitting the ground stimulates bones to grow stronger.

Running is convenient and inexpensive. The only "equipment" needed are good running sneakers. You can start with a walk/jog routine and work up to a faster pace.

Pam Hinton, PhD, associate professor, Department of Nutrition and Exercise Physiology, University of Missouri, Columbia.

Vitamin C for Healthier Hips

In a four-year study of 606 men and women, researchers found that men with the highest intake of vitamin C (314 mg daily) from food and supplements had the lowest levels of bone loss in the hip. Vitamin C is required for the formation of collagen, the main protein in bone. There was no similar finding in women, possibly because they already had adequate vitamin C levels.

For strong bones: Strive to eat five to nine servings daily of vitamin C–rich fruits and vegetables (such as strawberries and red peppers).

Katherine L. Tucker, PhD, director, Dietary Assessment and Epidemiology Research Program, Human Nutrition Research Center on Aging, Tufts University, Boston.

Another Benefit of Moderate Drinking— Stronger Bones

Moderate drinking—which is usually considered one drink (4 ounces wine, 12 ounces beer, 1½ ounces hard liquor) a day for women, two for men—is associated with greater bone density, and thus could fight osteoporosis and reduce the risk for fractures.

Recent finding: Postmenopausal women who consumed two or more alcoholic drinks a day had 5 to 8.3% better bone mineral density in the hip and spine than nondrinkers. For men who had one or two drinks a day, the improvement was 3.4 to 4.5%.

Caution: Other studies have suggested that women should have no more than one drink a day.

Self-defense: Ask your doctor what is best for you.

Katherine L. Tucker, PhD, director, Dietary Assessment and Epidemiology Research Program, Jean Mayer USDA Human Nutrition Research Center on Aging, Tufts University, Boston.

DHEA Supplements Build Better Bones

Older women (not men) who supplemented daily with the *hormone dehydroepiandrosterone* (DHEA) plus calcium and vitamin D had a 4% average increase in spinal bone density after two years—enough to reduce spinal fracture risk by up to 50%.

Women who took only calcium and vitamin D had no bone density increase. Ask your doctor about taking 50 milligrams of DHEA daily. Avoid DHEA if you have a history of breast or endometrial cancer.

Edward Weiss, PhD, associate professor of nutrition and dietetics, Doisy College of Health Sciences, Saint Louis University.

Millions of Men Have "Silent" Osteoporosis

Virtually every woman knows about osteoporosis, the main cause of weakened bones and fractures as women age. Few men, however, realize that they face similar risks.

Fact: About 30% of men 50 years and older will suffer an osteoporosis-related bone fracture at some time in their lives. Yet only about 10% of men with osteoporosis ever get diagnosed.

According to the National Osteoporosis Foundation, more than two million men have osteoporosis. Nearly 12 million more have osteopenia, a precursor condition that commonly leads to full-fledged osteoporosis.

Few doctors take the time to investigate bone loss in men. They, too, tend to think of osteoporosis as a "woman's disease," even though men are twice as likely as women to die following a hip fracture or hip-replacement procedure due to osteoporosis.

Who Gets It?

The strength and density of bones largely depend on the amount of calcium and other minerals that are present. The body is constantly creating and breaking down bone, a process called *remodeling*. For both men and women, the formation of new bone exceeds bone breakdown until about age 35. After age 35, the reverse happens. Men and women lose more bone than they create, leading to an overall loss of bone strength.

Women experience a precipitous loss of bone mass when estrogen declines after menopause. They also have smaller bones to begin with, which means they have fewer bone reserves. It's not unusual for women in their 70s to have lost up to 50% of their total bone mass.

Men experience a similar process, but without the rapid "bone drain" caused by declining estrogen. They lose bone more slowly than women—and because they start out with more bone mass, it takes them longer to start getting fractures. But once a man reaches his mid-70s, his risk for getting osteoporosis is about the same as a woman's.

Men with osteoporosis often are diagnosed only when they suffer a low-impact fracture. This is when even a minor impact or movement—falling down or bumping into something—causes a bone to break. Most fractures occur in the wrists or hips. Spinal fractures also are common, although they're typically asymptomatic and thus less likely to be diagnosed.

Male Risks

A sedentary lifestyle and nutritional deficiencies—mainly of calcium and vitamin D—are among the main causes of osteoporosis in men as well as women. Also, people who have taken oral steroids for a six-month period over their lifetime (for severe asthma, rheumatoid arthritis or some other condition) are at increased risk. *Additional risk factors for men...*

- **Low body weight.** Older men who weigh less than 154 pounds are more than 20 times more likely to get osteoporosis than heavier men—partly because they have smaller bones and possibly because men with other osteoporosis risk factors, such as smoking and heavy alcohol consumption, tend to be thinner.

- **Prostate cancer.** The disease itself doesn't increase a man's risk of osteoporosis but some of the treatments do. For example, the drug *leuprolide* (Lupron) reduces levels of androgens, male hormones that play a protective role in bone strength. Men who are given antihormone drugs for prostate cancer—or who have undergone actual castration—are now assumed to be at high risk for osteoporosis.

- **COPD.** Men with *chronic obstructive pulmonary disease* (COPD) often develop osteoporosis. Smoking, the main cause of COPD, weakens bones. Also, COPD is commonly treated with steroids, drugs that decrease bone strength.

Diagnosis

The *dual-energy X-ray absorptiometry* (DEXA) test measures bone density at the hip and spine, and sometimes at the wrist. The test gives a T-score—your bone density compared with what normally is expected in a healthy young adult with peak bone mass. *Any reading with a minus sign indicates that bone density is lower than average...*

- -1 indicates some bone loss.

- -2.5 is a borderline reading that indicates a significant problem.

- Below -2.5 is diagnosed as osteoporosis. It's not unusual for older men to have a T-score of −4, which indicates their bones are almost like paper.

Who should get tested? Men over age 60 with low weight and/or COPD should get a bone-density test—as should anyone who has taken steroids for six months.

Treatment and Prevention

In February 2008, the National Osteoporosis Foundation issued official guidelines for treating and preventing osteoporosis in women and men age 50 and older. *These include...*

- **Get regular exercise.** It's among the best ways to increase bone mass during peak bone-building years. It also can increase bone density and strength in men who already have osteoporosis.

Bonus: Exercise increases balance and muscle strength—important for avoiding falls.

Any exercise is beneficial, but weight-bearing aerobic workouts, such as walking or lifting weights, may be superior to swimming or biking for stimulating bone growth.

- **Supplement with calcium and vitamin D.** Both are essential for bone strength. Dietary sources probably aren't enough. The body's ability to absorb calcium declines with age. There's also an age-related decline in vitamin D synthesis from sunshine.

Men need 1,000 milligrams (mg) to 1,200 mg of calcium daily until age 65 and 1,500 mg thereafter. After age 40, men should take

200 international units (IU) of vitamin D daily...400 IU after age 50...and 600 IU at age 71 and older.

●**Ask your doctor about bone-building drugs.** Many drugs that treat osteoporosis in women also are effective in men. These include the *bisphosphonates* (such as Fosamax and Actonel), *calcitonin* (Miacalcin) and *parathyroid hormone* (Forteo). Each of these drugs slows bone loss, and some increase the body's ability to build new bone. Your doctor can tell you if you need drugs and, if so, which one is right for you.

A T-score of –2.5 or worse may warrant drug intervention, and many doctors think a score of –2.0 is reason for a "drug discussion" with patients.

●**Don't smoke.** Nicotine is toxic to bone marrow. Also, men who smoke tend to weigh less than those who don't.

●**Limit alcohol.** Heavy alcohol use in men is one of the main risk factors for osteoporosis. Excessive alcohol inhibits the body's ability to form new bone, and men who are alcoholics often eat poorly.

●**Deal with depression.** People who are depressed tend to have lower-than-normal bone density, possibly because they exercise less and eat less.

Caution: Some research has linked SSRI antidepressants, such as Prozac, Paxil and Zoloft, with lower bone density. People should not stop taking these drugs because of concerns about osteoporosis—but they should ask their doctors if they need to be screened for osteoporosis.

Angela J. Shepherd, MD, associate professor, Department of Family Medicine at University of Texas Medical Branch, Galveston. She specializes in osteoporosis screening and prevention.

Want Stronger Bones? Vibrate Them

The tennis champion Serena Williams vibrates. The Green Bay Packers, Indianapolis Colts and San Diego Chargers vibrate.

Even Martha Stewart vibrates.

And experts in the study of osteoporosis are saying maybe you should vibrate, too—using a whole-body vibration machine.

The machine (a platform large enough to comfortably stand on, and a bar or other type of grip to hold on to) vibrates very slightly, 20 to 50 times a second, causing the muscles of a person standing on the machine to reflexively contract, as the body automatically compensates for the slight shaking.

Athletes like to use whole-body vibration because benefits include improved muscular strength and flexibility, and faster recovery from muscle strain and injury.

Now: Research shows whole-body vibration can also increase *bone mineral density* (BMD), a must for preventing, slowing or reversing osteoporosis, the bone-fracturing disease that afflicts 52 million Americans.

Positive Stress

Australian researchers studied 51 women, dividing them into three groups. Group one used *whole-body vibration* (WBV) machines two times a week. Group two used whole-body vibration and also participated in resistance training (working out with weights to strengthen muscles). Group three didn't do either.

After four months, group one had an increased hip BMD of 2.7%. Group two had an increased hip BMD of 2% and an increased spinal BMD of 1%. Group three didn't have increased BMD in either area.

"Whole-body vibration may provide an efficient stratagem to achieve peak bone mass and help stave off osteoporosis," say the researchers.

Also, as you increase bone mass, you may decrease fat mass. Recently, doctors in Belgium put overweight people on a diet and one of two activity regimens—WBV or conventional exercise. Those using WBV lost 37% more weight and 64% more belly fat.

How it works: The vibration applies positive stress to the bone, which responds by adding thickness and strength, says Clinton

T. Rubin, MD, professor, chair of the Department of biomedical engineering at the State University of New York at Stony Brook.

Start Slowly and Build Up

"I use a whole-body vibration machine for my clients with osteoporosis, because it's incredibly effective for the problem—far more effective than drugs or any other natural method," says Becky Chambers, a naturopath in Lexington, Massachusetts.

If you decide to use a whole-body vibration machine, start off with a very brief session, such as 15 seconds, and build up over weeks or months to five to 10 minutes a session, two to three times a week, says Debra Bemben, PhD, an expert in whole-body vibration. She is an associate professor in the Department of Health and Exercise Science and director of the Bone Density Research Laboratory at the University of Oklahoma-Norman.

"The postmenopausal women in my scientific studies on whole-body vibration have loved using the machines—far more than they enjoyed weight lifting," she says. "They told me a session of whole-body vibration was relaxing and enjoyable. And because they started off at a very low level and gradually built up, they didn't have any problems using the machines."

Caution: Don't use a whole-body vibration machine if you're pregnant or if you have one or more of the following conditions, says Dr. Bemben: kidney stones, epilepsy, bone cancer, postural hypotension, acute rheumatoid arthritis, severe diabetes, migraines, arrhythmia or serious heart disease. Do not use if you have a pacemaker or if you recently had surgery or joint implants (such as knee or hip).

Resource: To find a local fitness or wellness facility near you that has a whole-body vibration machine, visit the Web site of Power Plate (*www.powerplate.com*), a manufacturer of the device, and use the state-by-state "Plate Locator."

You can also find whole-body vibration machines at Lady of America Fitness Centers, which has hundreds of locations in the US. To find a center near you, visit the Web site *www.ladyofamerica.com*, go to the "Club Information" page, and use the "Find a Club Near You" function.

Whole-body vibration machines for the home are expensive, ranging from around $2,000 to $5,000. If you decide to purchase a home machine, Chambers recommends the Body Vibe machine, available at *www.body vibeusa.com*.

Clinton T. Rubin, MD, chair, Department of Biomedical Engineering, State University of New York.

Becky Chambers, naturopath in Lexington, Massachusetts (*www.bcvibranthealth.com*).

Debra Bemben, PhD, associate professor, Department of Health and Exercise Science, and director, Bone Density Research Laboratory, University of Oklahoma–Norman.

Your Body May Be Missing the Best Nutrient for Your Bones (It's Not Calcium)

Adequate calcium is essential for the development of bone, says Susan Brown, PhD, director of The Osteoporosis Project and author of *Better Bones, Better Body—Beyond Estrogen and Calcium: A Comprehensive Self-Help Program for Preventing, Halting and Overcoming Osteoporosis* (McGraw-Hill). But what is "adequate" depends on many other factors. They include the intake of calcium-depleting nutritional factors, such as excess protein, salt, fat, sugar or alcohol…tobacco use…lack of physical activity…excess stress…and, perhaps most important, the intake of another bone building nutrient—vitamin D.

"Calcium is not the most important nutrient for bones—vitamin D is," says Dr. Brown. "Several researchers have estimated that up to 60% of all osteoporotic fractures are due to insufficient vitamin D, not to insufficient calcium."

Vitamin D is the body's most important regulator of calcium absorption, she explains.

People low in vitamin D absorb 65% less calcium than those with adequate levels.

"The whole calcium story will be revisited and we'll realize that we're recommending way too much calcium for people—and nowhere near enough vitamin D."

Several recent studies from an international team of researchers provide strongest evidence that Dr. Brown is right.

Striking Research Finding

The researchers—from the Centre on Aging and Mobility in Switzerland, Tufts University and the Harvard School of Public Health—conducted several analyses of data on vitamin D, calcium and the risk of fractures and falls.

● **Vitamin D outperforms calcium.** To figure out the importance of the two nutrients, researchers analyzed health data from 10,000 people, matching calcium intake and blood levels of vitamin D to bone mineral density (BMD).

The only consistent relationship they found was with blood levels of vitamin D— the higher the level, the lower the risk of fracture.

"Vitamin D status seems to be the dominant predictor of BMD," say the researchers.

● **Vitamin D works—but only if you take enough.** The researchers noted that several recent studies had shown no reduction in fracture risk from taking vitamin D, but that there were two problems with those studies—they used low doses of vitamin D and they used vitamin D-2 rather than vitamin D-3, the more effective form of the nutrient.

In their analysis, they found no reduction in fractures among people who took 400 IU of vitamin D or less.

But in people who took 500 IU of vitamin D or more, they found a 20% reduction in all non-spinal fractures (hip, wrist, rib, etc.) and a 18% reduction in hip fractures.

Analyzing data from two subgroups—older people living independently and institutionalized older people—they found that if a high enough dose of vitamin D-3 was used, the nutrient reduced the risk of hip and other nonspinal fractures by 29% in those living independently, and by 15% in those institutionalized. And the effect of vitamin D was "independent of additional calcium supplementation," they add.

"A higher dose of vitamin D should reduce non-spinal fractures by at least 20% for individuals 65 and older," the researchers conclude, in *Archives of Internal Medicine.*

● **Vitamin D prevents falls, too—but only in higher doses.** The researchers also analyzed data from eight studies on vitamin D and falls, a common cause of osteoporotic fractures in older people.

Supplementing with sufficient vitamin D-3 reduced falls by 23%.

"Falls were notably not reduced by low dose supplemental vitamin D (less than 700 IU a day) or by an achieved blood vitamin D levels of less than 24 nanograms per milliliter (ng/ml)," say the researchers, in *BMJ* (*British Medical Journal*).

The protective amount of vitamin D is more than the current recommendation. "Current intake recommendations of 200 to 600 IU vitamin D may be insufficient for important disease outcomes reduced by vitamin D," say the researchers, in *Osteoporosis International.* They reached that conclusion after analyzing the results of 20 studies on vitamin D and fractures and falls.

"Vitamin D blood levels of 35 to 44 ng/ml provide optimal benefits…without increasing health risks," they say, and "these levels can be best obtained with oral doses in the range of 1,800 to 4,000 IU vitamin D per day."

Getting Enough Vitamin D

"Vitamin D is not so much a 'vitamin' as it is a 'pre-hormone' produced in skin that is exposed to sunlight," explains Dr. Brown.

Problem: "Throughout our evolution, we humans have obtained the vast majority of our vitamin D from exposure to sunlight—and very few human foods, aside from fish oil, contain significant amounts of vitamin D," she says.

"If a healthy adult regularly avoids sunlight exposure, research indicates a necessity to supplement the diet with at least 5,000 IU of vitamin D daily," says John Cannell, MD, executive director of The Vitamin D Council. "To obtain this amount from milk, you'd need to consume 50 glasses. With a multivitamin, more than 10 tablets would be necessary."

His recommendation: "Take 5,000 IU per day, for two to three months, then obtain a 25-hydroxyvitamin D test for blood levels of vitamin D. Adjust your dosage so that blood levels are between 50–80 ng/mL year-round.

Resource: You can find a link to an in-home vitamin D blood test from ZRT Laboratory at the Web site of the Vitamin D Council or go to *www.zrtlab.com* (866-600-1636).

Best: "I believe cholecalciferol (vitamin D-3) is the preferred oral form of vitamin D, as it is the compound your skin makes naturally when you go into the sun," says Dr. Cannell.

Important: "When scientists first became aware of vitamin D, they also became aware that is was fat-soluble and stored in the body, and thus had the potential for toxic accumulation," says Dr. Brown. "For various reasons, vitamin D toxicity became an issue of exaggerated concern. Scientists now realize vitamin D toxicity is rare and generally occurs from extremely high oral intake."

Also helpful: You also can boost your blood levels of vitamin D by spending more time in the sun, says Dr. Brown.

"The skin produces approximately 10,000 IU vitamin D in response to 20 to 30 minutes of summer sun exposure—50 times more than the US government's recommendation of 200 IU per day," adds Dr. Cannell.

Dr. Brown's guidelines for safe sun exposure…

• **Short periods, 15–20 minutes daily, of near full-body exposure are best** for light-skinned people (without sunscreen).

• **Use sunscreen after this initial period to avoid a sunburn.**

• **The useful ultraviolet rays are strongest between 10 a.m and 2 p.m.**

• **Very dark-skinned people require four to six times more sunlight exposure than light-skinned people.**

• **In northern or southern latitudes, longer exposure is needed,** especially during the spring and fall.

• **In climates of the northern or southern latitudes distant from the equator, very little or no vitamin D is produced** in the skin during winter months.

Susan Brown, PhD, director of The Osteoporosis Project and author of *Better Bones, Better Body: A Comprehensive Self-Help Program for Preventing, Halting and Overcoming Osteoporosis* (McGraw-Hill). *www.betterbones.com*.

John Cannell, MD, executive director of the Vitamin D Council. *www.vitamindcouncil.org*.

Treat Your Heartburn, Break Your Hip

If you're an older person worried about osteoporosis, you're probably aware of the major risk factors for the disease, such as too little calcium and vitamin D, or a sedentary lifestyle. But there's one risk factor you probably don't know about.

Surprising new risk factor: Recent research confirms what medical experts have suspected for years—regular use of popular acid-reducing heartburn drugs can raise your risk of osteoporotic fractures.

41% More Broken Hips

Researchers from Kaiser Permanente Medical Center in San Francisco tracked the use of two types of heartburn drugs—*proton pump inhibitors* (PPIs) and *histamine-2 receptor antagonists* (H2RAs)—in more than 163,000 people, 33,000 who had broken their hips and 130,00 who hadn't.

PPIs include: *lansoprazole* (Prevacid) *esomeprazole* (Nexium), *omeprazole* (Prilosec), *pantoprazole* (Protonix) and *rabeprazole* (Aciphex).

H2RAs include: *cimetidine* (Tagamet), *ranitidine* (Zantac), *famotidine* (Pepcid) and *nizatidine* (Axid).

Results: Those who took acid-blocking PPIs for two years or longer were 30% more likely to have broken a hip.

Those who took acid-reducing H2RAs for two years or longer were 18% more likely to have broken a hip.

When the researchers analyzed the data by number of pills taken per day, they found that higher doses led to higher risk for hip fracture. Those who took an average of 1.5 or more pills a day had an increased risk of 41% and those who took ¾ or less per day had an increased risk of 12%.

And those who had taken a heartburn drug and then stopped—who hadn't had a prescription for the drug in the last three to five years—saw their risk drop from 30 to 9%.

The findings were in *Gastroenterology*.

In another recent study, Canadian researchers found that taking PPIs for seven years or more increased the risk of any osteoporotic fracture by 92%...taking the drug for five years or more increased the risk of hip fractures by 62%...and taking the drug for seven years or more increased the risk of hip fractures by 455%.

Theory: According to Douglas Corley, MD, PhD, leader of the Kaiser Permanente study, heartburn drugs can hurt bones by...

• Blocking or reducing stomach acid, which can hinder the absorption of bone-building calcium;

• Increasing the excretion of calcium via the urine;

• Altering hormones that regulate bone building and

• Damaging bone enzymes that spark bone-building.

Minimize Your Risk

• **Lower the dose.** Take the lowest dose possible of a heartburn drug, advises Dr. Corley.

Osteoporosis Risks

You're at increased risk for osteoporosis if you are...

• **Diagnosed with osteopenia,** a pre-osteoporotic level of low bone mineral density

• **A woman**

• **Postmenopausal**

• **Caucasian**

• **Very thin**

• **The child or sibling of someone with osteoporosis**

• **Not getting enough calcium or vitamin D**

• **Not exercising regularly**

• **Consuming two or more alcoholic drinks a day**

• **Taking corticosteroid medications regularly**

• **Taking other bone-harming medications regularly,** such as an aromatase inhibitor for breast cancer, an antidepressant or an antiseizure medication

• **Suffering from an eating disorder,** Crohn's disease or have had weight-loss surgery

• **Take calcium and vitamin D with a heartburn drug.** This strategy might decrease the risk of hip fracture, he says.

If you're already at risk for osteoporosis, stop the drug. If you already have one or more risk factors for osteoporosis (see sidebar), Dr. Corley recommends talking to your doctor about possibly discontinuing the medication, and finding other ways to manage heartburn.

Manage heartburn without drugs. Most people can control heartburn without drugs, says Elaina George, MD, an otolaryngologist in Atlanta, Georgia. *Her recommendations...*

• **Lose weight.** Taking off five to 15 pounds often solves the problem.

• **Minimize intake of heartburn-causing foods.** Common culprits are those that relax the muscular valve between the esophagus and stomach, allowing acid to "reflux" out of the stomach and into the esophagus.

They include: fatty foods, fried foods, dairy products, caffeine-containing foods and beverages, spicy foods, peppermint and gum chewing after meals.

• **Take a probiotic supplement.** These "friendly" digestive bacteria help speed digestion, cutting the production of acid.

• **Take a digestive enzyme supplement with meals.** This type of supplement also aids digestion, reducing acid.

"These lifestyle changes control heartburn in about four out of five people," says Dr. George.

However: Some people with severe esophageal or stomach problems—such as those with a history of gastritis, peptic ulcer disease or Barrett's esophagus—do need to take an acid-controlling medication, she says.

Elaina George, MD, otolaryngologist in Atlanta, Georgia. *www.drelainageorge.com.*

Douglas Corley, MD, PhD, gastroenterologist, assistant clinical professor, University of California, San Francisco.

Your Bones Love Carrots And Tomatoes

Your list of reasons to eat vegetables may not include bone health—but perhaps it should, now that there's new evidence demonstrating that antioxidant pigments in fresh produce protect against bone loss and hip fractures in older people.

At Tufts University, Boston University and Hebrew SeniorLife in Boston, Tufts professor Katherine L. Tucker, PhD, and her colleagues examined data from 370 men and 576 women, average age 75, enrolled in the long-term Framingham Osteoporosis Study. Over a 17-year period, the participants regularly filled out food questionnaires. A hundred of them reported hip fractures during this time.

Looking at total and individual carotenoid intake, investigators found that...

• **People who consumed the most total carotenoids from foods like tomatoes, carrots, sweet potatoes and cantaloupe** experienced a significantly lower risk of hip fractures.

• **Those who consumed the most *lycopene*—a carotenoid commonly found in tomatoes and watermelon**—likewise had a lower rate of hip fractures and nonvertebral fractures.

• **Beta-carotene—abundant in carrots, sweet potatoes, mangoes, papayas, etc.**—had a small, statistically insignificant protective effect, but only against hip fractures.

Alpha-carotene, beta-cryptoxanthin and *lutein* plus *zeaxanthin* did not demonstrate any independent protective effect.

Dr. Tucker believes that the protective impact of carotenoids is derived from their antioxidant activity, as antioxidant pigments block oxidative stress that contributes to bone loss. Study results were published in the *Journal of Bone and Mineral Research.*

Strengthen Bones Naturally Through Diet

According to Dr. Tucker, the carotenoids most strongly associated with both bone density and reduced fracture risk come from red, orange, yellow and dark green fruits and vegetables. Though some fruits and vegetables are more helpful than others, generally speaking, the more you eat, the better your bones will fare. To strengthen your bones and prevent fractures, Dr. Tucker advises eating more than the recommended "Five a Day." She prefers food over supplements, since it is most likely the synergistic impact of the various polyphenolic compounds and nutrients found in fruits and vegetables that confers the greatest bone protection.

Katherine L. Tucker, PhD, director, Dietary Assessment and Epidemiology Research Program, Jean Mayer USDA Human Nutrition Research Center on Aging, Tufts University, Boston.

Chapter 13

OVERWEIGHT

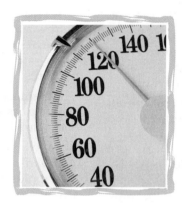

Can't Lose Weight? Here's How to Get The Results You Want

When an overweight or obese patient comes to Louis J. Aronne, MD, frustrated by his/her inability to lose weight, one of the first questions he asks is, "Do you feel full when you eat?" His patient's answer is often "No."

Why most people can't lose weight: When it comes to weight loss, biology often trumps willpower. If a person is obese, complicated metabolic issues almost always play a role, making it difficult—and in some cases impossible—for even the most diligent dieter to lose weight. (For those who are overweight but not obese, metabolic problems also may occur but are less common.)

Here's what happens: When you consume a fattening food (usually a high-calorie combination of sugar and fat), it interrupts the body's weight-regulating mechanisms,

causing resistance to a hormone called *leptin*. When functioning properly, this hormone signals the brain, indicating how much fat is being stored and promoting a sense of satiety (fullness).

When your brain can't tell how much fat is being stored, it's like driving a car without a functioning gas gauge. Fearful of running out of gas, you fill up at every stop along the highway, even storing extra gas cans in the trunk.

If the situation is compounded by a lack of exercise, the body's cells become increasingly resistant to leptin. The more the person eats, the hungrier he becomes, setting off a vicious cycle.

Simple but amazingly powerful solution: Enjoy filling, high-volume foods, including salad (such as mixed greens)...broth-based soup...and vegetables (such as steamed spinach, mushrooms and carrots) at the start of a meal to stimulate your body's fullness mechanisms. When it's time to eat the rest of the meal, which is likely to include more-fattening foods, you'll be more satisfied and less inclined to overeat.

Real-Life Success Stories

The following case studies are based on real patients Dr. Aronne has treated over the course of his 23-year career as a weight-loss specialist. Each of these patients reached his/her target of a 5 to 10% weight loss—and has maintained that loss. If you're overweight and can relate to any of their stories, discuss these strategies with your doctor.

● **Lack of sleep was to blame.** Jack, age 67, complained of weight gain, fatigue and constant hunger.* During the exam, Dr. Aronne noted that his neck was bigger than normal, which made him suspect *obstructive sleep apnea,* a disorder that results from a blockage of the upper airway that causes sufferers to stop breathing during sleep multiple times a night. Jack admitted that he snored or woke up in the middle of the night with a choking sensation (both signs of sleep apnea).

What is the sleep–weight gain connection? If you don't sleep enough, your body produces lower levels of the satiating hormone leptin and higher levels of the appetite-stimulating hormone *ghrelin.*

Solution: Jack began to use a special mask that assists with breathing—a treatment known as *continuous positive airway pressure* (CPAP)—during sleep.

Result: Jack dropped from 220 to 202 pounds. His sleep dramatically improved, his hormones leveled out and his fatigue disappeared.

● **Not eating enough.** For Stella, age 55, eating breakfast (typically toast or instant oatmeal) made her feel hungrier by mid-morning, so she began skipping the first meal of the day. As a result, she was ravenous by lunch and dinner, and she even ate a late-night "snack" of chicken pot pie.

For optimal performance, our bodies require at least three daily meals. Since Stel-

*Patients' names and some identifying characteristics have been changed to protect their privacy.

la skipped breakfast, her body viewed her lunch as breakfast and her dinner as lunch and wanted even more calories late at night. Stella then fell asleep with a full stomach, promoting weight gain and making it more difficult to remain asleep.

Solution: A high-protein, fiber-rich breakfast (such as an omelet and unlimited veggies—fresh or frozen)…for lunch and dinner, Dr. Aronne recommended cooked vegetables, salad, plus chicken, turkey or fish for protein and one-half cup of a carbohydrate (such as rice or pasta) if needed…and a small nighttime snack, such as sugar-free gelatin or yogurt.

Result: Stella dropped from 165 to 153 pounds, had more energy during the day and slept better. But the key change was that Stella got her appetite under control and no longer felt famished by lunchtime.

● **Medication was the culprit.** John, age 72, was obese and taking medications for elevated blood sugar (*glucose*) levels. Based in part on his primary care doctor's advice, he was following a high-carbohydrate, low-fat diet—a typical breakfast was cereal with a banana and juice…lunch was turkey on rye with lettuce, tomato and mustard…and dinner was pasta with chicken and a salad.

But the scale was inching up and John was hungry all the time, so he snacked. Unbeknownst to John, the medications he was taking were causing higher-than-normal levels of *insulin* (a hormone necessary to move sugar from food into cells). Elevated insulin levels are associated with excessive hunger and the storage of calories as fat, potentially leading to weight gain and obesity.

Solution: John switched to a combination of different diabetes drugs—*metformin* (Glucophage) and *exenatide* (Byetta)—both of which suppress production of glucose by the liver and often cause weight loss.

Dr. Aronne also prescribed a higher-protein diet with more carbohydrates coming from vegetables rather than the cereal, toast and bread that he had been eating.

Breakfast became a big bowl of plain yogurt with berries…lunch was salad, lots of veggies, lean turkey and one-half cup of brown rice toward the end of the meal (so he would be consuming the high-calorie rice when he was nearly full)…and salmon, steamed asparagus and a green salad for dinner.

Result: John dropped from 210 to 180 pounds, and his blood sugar levels stabilized.

What many people don't know: Certain medications can stimulate weight gain, including some sleep medications…antihistamines… heart drugs…migraine medication…and certain drugs prescribed for depression or bipolar disorder.

Louis J. Aronne, MD, founder and director of the Comprehensive Weight Control Program at New York–Presbyterian Hospital/Weill Cornell Medical College and author of *The Skinny on Losing Weight Without Being Hungry* (Broadway).

The Simple Secret to Keeping Off the Pounds You Lost

What's the easiest way to gain weight? Lose it first.

Fact: Within a year, most people regain more than 35% of the weight they've lost during a diet. Within five years, it's likely every pound has returned. Overall, about 90% of those who lose weight regain a big percentage of it.

"Weight regain is the biggest obstacle in our ability to curtail the obesity epidemic," says Paul S. MacLean, PhD, an assistant professor of medicine in the Center for Human Nutrition at the University of Colorado Denver.

What happens: The overweight body has built up energy stores over many years and adapts to the extra weight, he explains. When those stores are depleted by weight loss, the body has a biological imperative—an automatic metabolic response—to replete those energy stores. "If you look at weight loss from the body's perspective—the perspective of biology—the body 'wants' to regain the weight it lost," he says.

However: "If you recognize the body's unconscious biological imperative for what it is, you can make a conscious choice to change your actions and thwart the body's objective to regain weight."

And a new study by Dr. MacLean and his colleagues shows that the best (and maybe only) way to thwart your biology is with regular exercise.

Exercise Stops Weight Regain

Dr. MacLean decided that the most accurate way to study the biology of weight loss, weight regain and exercise was to study rats.

"For people, control of body weight is very complex, involving many behavioral and environmental variables," he says. "Using a rodent model of weight loss, weight regain and exercise allows us to remove all of those variables and focus on the biological control of weight."

The researchers fed mature, overweight rats on a high-fat food for four months, allowing them to eat as much as they wanted (and the rats pigged out). Then they put the rats on a low-fat, low-calorie "diet" until the animals lost about 15% of their weight.

For the next two months, they kept the rats on that low-fat, low-calorie diet—but half the rats were stimulated (in humane ways) to exercise regularly on a treadmill, while the other half were allowed to stay sedentary (which they were happy to do).

For two months after that, all the rats stopped "dieting"—they were allowed to eat as much low-fat food as they wanted to (low-fat, to simulate a post-diet, weight-maintenance regimen).

But the exercise rats kept exercising, and the sedentary rats stayed sedentary.

Well, if those two groups of rats had been contestants on *The Biggest Loser*, the exercising rats would have won, paws down.

• **Less weight regain.** After two months of not dieting, the exercising rats kept off about 20% of their weight. The sedentary rats regained all of theirs—and another 20%.

• **Burned more calories.** Needless to say, the exercising animals burned more calories

—a must for maintaining the "energy balance" (equal amounts of calories burned and ingested) that prevents weight regain, says Dr. MacLean.

●**Less appetite.** Both groups of animals overate when they stopped dieting, but the exercising animals to a much lesser extent. "That's a very significant sign that exercise may help us say 'no' to our biology," he says.

●**Lower set point.** *Set point* is the weight the body tends to automatically stay at or return to after weight loss. "The exercising rats ended up at a lower weight than their original weight at the start of the study," says Dr. MacLean. "Exercise lowered their set point."

●**Burned fat for energy, rather than carbohydrates.** The exercising rats burned more fat for fuel, while the sedentary rats burned more carbohydrates. "Burning more carbohydrates for energy may lead to greater between-meal hunger," says Dr. MacLean.

●**Fewer fat cells.** As they started to eat all they wanted, the sedentary rats created more new, small fat cells than the exercising rats. "Those small cells are like invitations for fat to fill them up, causing weight gain," he says.

●**Less abdominal fat.** Trimmer tummies are important in humans, not only for better looks, but for better health—extra stomach fat generates biological compounds linked to heart disease and type 2 diabetes.

More Activity Is Better

"I'm a believer in 'the more physical activity, the better,' as long as it's okay with your doctor," says Dr. MacLean. "But I don't think one-size-fits-all when it comes to exercise." *His recommendations...*

●**Set achievable goals.** Set achievable, sustainable physical activity goals that fit with your daily schedule, rather than setting unattainable goals that you can't maintain.

"Many people who try to exercise 60 minutes a day, six days a week, fail and conclude 'I tried exercise and I can't do it,'" he says. "It's better to make small changes in your daily routine—taking the stairs rather than the elevator, parking farther away from the entrance to the mall—and gradually work toward a more active lifestyle. Any increase in physical activity is positive."

●**Pick a physical activity you enjoy.** "Everyone likes different kinds of physical activity," says Dr. MacLean. "Some people like to go out and run five miles. For me, I have to be involved in a game with an objective, like soccer or roller hockey, to be physically active."

"Exercise only works if you do it," agrees James Hill, PhD, a study researcher, director of the Center for Human Nutrition at the University of Colorado Denver, and author of *The Step Diet: Count Steps, Not Calories, to Lose Weight and Keep It Off Forever* (Workman). "Find something you're going to do, day in and day out, every day, for the rest of your life—because the ability of exercise to prevent weight regain stops when you stop exercising."

●**Walking may work best.** "If you look at people who are successful in maintaining weight loss, the majority of them choose walking as their regular activity," says Dr. Hill.

Paul S. MacLean, PhD, assistant professor of medicine in the Center for Human Nutrition at the University of Colorado Denver.

James Hill, PhD, study researcher, director of the Center for Human Nutrition at the University of Colorado Denver, and author of *The Step Diet: Count Steps, Not Calories, to Lose Weight and Keep It Off Forever* (Workman).

Eat All You Want and Lose Weight! (Just Eat Every Other Day)

Imagine you're on a diet that lets you eat anything you want. That's right—anything. Scrambled eggs, bacon and buttered toast for breakfast—and don't forget the doughnut! Drive over to McDieters for lunch and order the hamburger, fries and milkshake. Ditto on unrestricted eating for dinner. And enjoy your snacks!

But daydreaming about a no-dieting diet isn't the same as dieting, right?

New approach: That daydream can be an every-other-day reality—when you're following an eating regimen that nutritional scientists call Alternate-Day Fasting (ADF), a new type of diet that recent research shows can help you lose a lot of weight—without minding so much!

Steady Weight Loss

A typical diet cuts calories anywhere from 15 to 40% per day, says Krista Varady, PhD, assistant professor in the Department of Kinesiology and Nutrition at the University of Illinois at Chicago, and a leading researcher on alternate-day fasting. That day-after-day caloric restriction is difficult to maintain, she says. (As you've no doubt noticed, if you've ever been on a diet).

Is there any way to achieve that same level of calorie restriction without the constant deprivation of dieting? researchers wondered.

Well, why not allow dieters to eat whatever they want one day (the "feed" day) and then cut calories by 75 to 80% the next day (the "fast day")? You're still cutting calories an average of 40% a day—but the restriction is confined to every other day.

In the only study testing the diet with overweight people, conducted several years ago, nine men and women followed the ADF regimen for two months.

On average, they lost 8% of their weight. They also had a 10% decrease in "bad" LDL cholesterol, a 40% decrease in *triglycerides* (a blood fat that can hurt the heart), and big decreases in biomarkers of oxidative stress and inflammation, cell-damaging processes that one researcher has called "the evil twins of chronic disease."

Dr. Varady and her colleagues decided to conduct another study. They recruited 16 people with a body mass index (BMI) of 30 to 39.9, a level researchers define as "obese." (A BMI of 24.9 or below is considered "normal," and a BMI of 25 to 29.9 is "overweight.")

First, the researchers figured out the daily energy needs (minimum healthy calorie intake) of the participants. Then, they asked them to consume about 25% of those calories

(about 500 to 600 calories) on the fast day, at one meal eaten between noon and 2 p.m.

For the first month of the two-month study, the researchers supplied the "fast day" foods to the participants. The participants were also asked to limit themselves a little bit on the "feed day," restricting fat to no more than 30% of their total calorie intake, and choosing low-fat meats and dairy products.

For the second month, the participants were on their own—they weren't given premade "fast day" meals, and they could eat whatever they wanted on the "feed day." (However, they met with a nutritionist, who guided them on how to follow the diet, and encouraged them to make healthy food choices on "feed day.")

The researchers wanted to see if the participants could actually stick with the ADF diet, without supervision.

And the participants did stick with the diet. They were adherent about 85% of the time—in the first, supervised month and in the second, on-your-own month.

"We wondered if the participants would eat twice as much food on the 'feed day,'" says Dr. Varady. "But they didn't—they ate about 90 to 110% of their caloric needs.

"Fasting has so many benefits, including regulating metabolism and appetite," she says. "At first, the study participants said that planned to eat a huge breakfast on the 'feed day.' But over time they lost interest in doing that, because fasting put their 'satiety signals'—their subjective feelings of hunger and fullness—back on the right track, and they weren't as interested in overeating."

The participants steadily lost weight during the first month and the second month of the study—losing an average of 5.8% of their body weight, or about 12 pounds. (Individual dieters lost anywhere from 7 to 30 pounds.)

They also had big drops in total cholesterol (21%), LDL cholesterol (25%), and triglycerides (32%). And they had a decrease in systolic blood pressure (the upper reading) and heart rate (both signs of a healthier heart).

"This study is the first to show that ADF is an effective dietary intervention to help obese individuals lose weight and lower cardiovascular disease risk," concludes Dr. Varady and her coworkers, in the *American Journal of Clinical Nutrition.*

And noting that the level of weight loss was the same as in most day-after-day diets, the researchers say ADF "may be considered a suitable alternative…to help obese individuals lose weight."

Implementing the Diet

As mentioned earlier, the people in Dr. Varady's study met with a nutritionist to help them figure out how to follow the diet. If you're thinking about giving ADF a try, she recommends that you see a nutritionist and get your physician's okay.

Or, with your doctor's approval, you can follow the ADF regimen in *The Alternate-Day Diet* (Putnam), by James Johnson, MD, a doctor who has conducted several studies on ADF.

"I had struggled most of my life to maintain a healthy weight," says Dr. Johnson. Then he read about some of the early research using ADF on mice and decided to try it himself.

"I became my own lab mouse and on alternate days began to restrict my calories to 20% of what I normally ate," he says. "On nonrestrictive days I ate whatever and as much as I wanted. I lost 35 pounds in the first 11 weeks—and have kept that weight off since.

"The goal of the 'down day'—when you eat less—is to simplify your food choices so that you won't have to think too much about what you're eating. This way you'll be less inclined to cheat. And you'll soon learn to differentiate between true hunger and the desire for a gratifying taste sensation or emotional hunger."

Example: A typical 'down day' of about 500 calories looks like this, says Dr. Johnson:

- **Breakfast**—1 slice, high-fiber whole grain bread, 1 tablespoon peanut butter (155 calories)

- **Lunch**—1 cup chicken noodle soup (165 calories)

- **Dinner**—1 bowl turkey and bean chili (210 calories)

"The 'up days' are up to you," says Dr. Johnson. "You'll be eating what you normally eat, without restriction, as long as you keep calories low on the down days."

Krista Varady, PhD, assistant professor, Department of Kinesiology and Nutrition at the University of Illinois, Chicago.

James Johnson, MD, author of *The Alternate-Day Diet* (Putnam).

Safe Slimming Supplements

"You're willing to lose weight—more than willing," says Harry Preuss, MD, professor of medicine at Georgetown University School of Medicine, and author of *The Natural Fat-Loss Pharmacy* (Broadway). "But dozens of trials and temptations stand in your way, from the all-you-can-eat buffet to the éclair on the dessert tray. You need some effective assistance—a helping hand—and that's what natural weight-loss supplements can provide."

Dr. Preuss says natural weight-loss supplements—made from food extracts and other naturally occurring compounds—have various mechanisms of action. *They can help you…*

- Reduce fat absorption from food,

- Burn more body fat,

- Stop the formation of new fat cells and

- Curb your appetite.

And when taken according to sensible dosage recommendations, natural weight-loss supplements are typically safer than drugs, he says.

But you can't sit back and watch a supplement power your weight-loss while you don't do anything to help out.

"Healthy eating, appropriate physical activity and stress management are the basics of weight control," says Pamela Peeke, MD, clinical assistant professor at the University of Maryland School of Medicine and author of *Fight Fat After Forty* (Penguin). "Once these basics are in place, a supplement can have a role."

Latest Findings

Here are some of the latest scientific developments in the world of safe, effective natural weight-loss supplements...

•**Conjugated linoleic acid (CLA).** Discovered in 1979, this *fatty acid* (a component in fat) is found in meat and dairy products. Studies show it is anti-inflammatory, anti-cancer—and, surprisingly, anti-fat.

Researchers in the Department of Human Nutrition at Ohio State University studied 35 overweight postmenopausal women, dividing them into two groups.

Both groups went on a low-calorie diet—but one group took a CLA supplement, while the other group took a safflower oil supplement. After four months, the women taking CLA had lost a few pounds and an average of 3.2% of their body fat—without losing any muscle. (People often lose fat and muscle on low-calorie diets. And that's unfortunate, says Dr. Preuss, because muscle is a calorie-burning engine, and maintaining muscle while dieting is key to not regaining the weight you've lost.) The women taking safflower oil didn't lose any weight.

How it works: There are several ways CLA might frustrate fat cells, says Michael Pariza, PhD, director of the Food Research Institute at the University of Wisconsin, and one of the discovers of CLA. It probably stops dietary fat from getting into fat cells by blocking the action of *lipase,* an enzyme that helps with the job, CLA may also limit the development of new fat cells.

Recommended intake: Dr. Preuss recommends 4 grams a day, in two, 2 gram doses, with meals. He favors Tonalin CLA, the type used in most weight-loss studies on the nutrient. It is found in many brands of CLA, including GNC, Natrol, Nature's Way, Now and Vitamin Shoppe.

•**Green tea extract.** Green tea is rich in *catechins,* antioxidant compounds. And a supplement of catechins—a "green tea extract"—might help you lose your double chin.

In a study in *Alternative Medicine Review*, a team of Italian researchers studied 50 people on a low-calorie diet, dividing them into two groups—one took a green tea extract and one didn't. After three months, those taking the extract had lost 31 pounds while those in the diet-only group had lost 11 pounds. The product studied was GreenSelect Phytosome.

Japanese researchers studied 107 overweight and obese adults involved in an exercise program (30 minutes a day of brisk walking, six days a week), dividing them into two groups. One group took a supplement containing 625 milligrams (mg) of green tea catechins and 39 mg of caffeine, and one took a caffeine supplement without catechins.

After three months, those taking the catechins/caffeine combo had lost nearly five pounds, while those taking caffeine had lost two pounds. The catechin group also lost 63% more abdominal fat.

Weight-loss supplements that contain both green tea catechins and caffeine (mirroring the content of green tea itself) are the most effective, says Margriet Westerterp-Plantenga, PhD, professor of Regulation of Food Intake in the Department of Human Biology, Maastricht University, the Netherlands.

How it works: Catechins boost calorie-burning, boost fat-burning and don't burn up muscle, says Abdul Dulloo, PhD, at the University of Fribourg in Switzerland, who has done extensive research on natural weight-loss compounds.

Recommended intake: The ideal green tea supplement for weight-loss and weight-maintenance is 575 mg of tea catechins (with 325 mg from *epigallocatechin gallate,* or EGCG, the most bioactive catechin) and 100 mg of caffeine, says Dr. Westerterp-Plantenga. A product that supplies close to that mixture and amount is Schiff Green Tea Diet.

- **Probiotics.** Probiotics such as *lactoba-cillus acidophilus* (the same bacteria that ferments yogurt) are "friendly," health-giving bacteria in your digestive tract. New research shows they're also pro-thinness.

Researchers at the Stanford University School of Medicine studied 44 people who had recently undergone gastric bypass surgery, giving half probiotics.

After three months, those taking probiotics had lost 48% of their presurgery weight—while those not taking probiotics had lost 39%.

The people taking probiotics also had 34% higher B-12 levels. (B-12 deficiency is a common side effect of weight-loss surgery).

"I now recommend probiotic supplements to all my gastric-bypass patients," says John Morton, MD, the study leader.

How they work: Bacteria might help people digest and absorb food that are otherwise indigestible, theorizes Jeffrey Gordon, MD, of the Washington University School of Medicine in St. Louis.

"Although how much you eat and how much you exercise are dominant drivers of your energy balance, it's possible that microbial communities and how they work also comprise a factor that determines your risk for obesity," he says.

Recommended amount: The gastric-bypass study participants took Acidophilus Complex from Puritan's Pride, which supplies 10 billion active bacteria per capsule.

Harry Preuss, MD, professor of medicine at Georgetown University School of Medicine, and author of *The Natural Fat-Loss Pharmacy* (Broadway).

Pamela Peeke, MD, clinial assistant professor at the University of Maryland and author of *Fight Fat After Forty* (Penguin).

Michael Pariza, director emeritus, Food Research Institute, University of Wisconsin-Madison.

Abdul Dulloo, PhD, research fellow, Department of Medicine/Physiology, University of Fribourg, Switzerland.

Margriet Westerterp-Plantenga, PhD, professor, Department of Human Biology, Maastricht University, Netherlands.

John Morton, MD, associate professor of surgery, Stanford University School of Medicine.

Jeffrey Gordon, MD, director, Center for Genome Sciences, Washington University School of Medicine, St. Louis.

The Extreme Dangers of Belly Fat

Everyone knows that it's unhealthy to be obese. What's surprising to many people, however, is just how serious it can be to have "belly fat."

Important recent finding: A study published in *The New England Journal of Medicine* that looked at more than 350,000 people found that a large waist can nearly double your risk of dying prematurely—even if your weight is "normal" (according to your body mass index, a measure of body fat based on height and weight).* Some people who don't exercise but generally keep their overall body weight under control, for example, may have dangerous fat deposits around the abdomen.

Why is belly fat, in particular, so dangerous?

Here's what you need to know...

What's Your Shape?

It's been widely reported that about one-third of Americans are considered obese—the highest percentage of any country in the world. Though estimates vary, obesity, which is strongly linked to diabetes, heart disease, stroke and even cancer, is blamed for at least 26,000 deaths in the US each year.

Most of the body's fat—known as subcutaneous (under the skin) fat—accumulates in the thighs, buttocks and hips. This fat distribution, which leads to a so-called pear body shape, applies to most women—and many men.

However, belly fat—generally associated with an apple body shape—presents the greatest risks. Also known as *visceral fat,* it is stored mostly inside the abdominal cavity, where it wraps around (and sometimes invades) the internal organs, including the heart.

*To calculate your body mass index, go to the National Heart, Lung and Blood Institute Web site, *www.nhlbisupport. com/bmi.*

Long known to damage blood vessel linings, belly fat is a metabolically active tissue that secretes harmful inflammatory substances that can contribute to a variety of health problems. People with an apple body type are far more likely to die of heart attacks than those with a pear shape.

The worst of the worst: Hard belly fat (commonly known as a "beer belly") is even more dangerous than soft belly fat—perhaps because many people with hard belly fat have high levels of C-reactive protein (CRP), an inflammation marker and risk factor for heart disease. Alcohol has been shown to slow fat metabolism by more than 30%, which is compounded by the fact that beer drinkers tend to eat high-calorie snack foods while drinking and beer itself is high in carbohydrate calories.

An increasing body of evidence is now linking belly fat to other serious health risks, such as...

• **Cancer.** Both men and women with higher percentages of belly fat are more likely to develop a variety of cancers, including malignancies of the colon, kidney and breast.

• **Dementia.** In a study of 6,583 adults, the bigger the belly, the greater the risk for dementia.

Surprising finding: Among those of normal weight who had excess belly fat, dementia risk was 1.89 times higher than for those of normal weight who did not have excess belly fat.

• **Lung problems.** Lung function is reduced in patients with higher stores of belly fat, possibly because of the higher secretion of lung-damaging inflammatory chemicals.

• **Diabetes.** An apple-shaped fat distribution greatly increases the risk for *insulin resistance* (a condition in which the body's cells don't use insulin properly) and diabetes.

The risks are even higher in those who are sedentary. People who have lost muscle mass, as a result, take in less blood sugar (glucose), which is used as fuel—further increasing diabetes risk.

• **Migraines.** Researchers at Drexel University College of Medicine found that women with large amounts of belly fat were up to 30% more likely than lean women to suffer from migraine headaches.

Inches That Really Count

Research has shown that waist size—even in people who aren't obviously overweight—is a key predictor of long-term health.

Important finding: In a study reported in *Circulation: Heart Failure*, researchers found that a four-inch increase in waist size raised the risk for heart disease by about 15%, even in people of normal weight. Other studies report that each five-centimeter increase in waist size (a little less than two inches) raises the risk for premature death by 13% in women and 17% in men.

Recommendation: A waist size of 35 inches or less in women and 40 inches or less in men. Even slight increases above these numbers significantly raise your health risks.

Best way to measure your waist: Place a tape measure just below your navel, exhale gently, then record the measurement.

Strategies for Waist Loss

There are no proven ways to selectively reduce accumulations of visceral fat. *Advice...*

• **Strive for healthy overall weight loss.** People who follow a sensible diet, such as the American Heart Association's No-Fat Diet (*www.americanheart.org*) or the Weight Watchers plan (*www.weightwatchers.com*), lose weight proportionally—that is, they lose more weight from areas where they have the most body fat. Someone with a high percentage of visceral fat will show the effects most in the abdomen.

Another advantage of such diets is that they include large amounts of natural, wholesome foods, such as vegetables and whole grains. A plant-based diet supplies large quantities of anti-inflammatory, disease-fighting compounds.

Important: When you're trying to lose weight, avoid or eliminate most dietary sugars

—not only from sweet snacks, but also from processed carbohydrates, such as white bread, snacks, beer and fruit juices. These foods have a high glycemic index—that is, they cause a rapid spike in blood sugar that may increase the accumulation of visceral fat.

● **Drink green tea.** A study in the *Journal of Nutrition* found that obese adults who drank green tea lost about twice as much weight over 12 weeks as a control group even though people in both groups followed similar diets and exercise patterns. It's thought that compounds known as *catechins* in green tea increase metabolism and accelerate the breakdown of fat.

● **Focus on aerobic exercise.** This is the best way to increase metabolism, burn calories and reduce fat. Aerobic exercise is more effective than resistance workouts (such as lifting weights) because it burns more calories per hour.

There's some evidence that overweight women who engage in sustained aerobic workouts—such as 20 minutes or more of brisk walking daily—can lose up to one inch of belly fat in just four weeks.

● **Turn down the thermostat.** Researchers have recently made exciting discoveries related to so-called "brown" fat, which has been shown to burn energy to generate body heat.

This type of fat was once thought to disappear after infancy, but new studies indicate that it's present in many adults and can be activated by exposure to cool temperatures—roughly 61°F.

People who are overweight or obese may have lower brown fat activity, which could be an underlying cause of weight gain. Spending a few hours in cool temperatures—say, at night when you sleep—could potentially increase the body's energy expenditure, which, over time, could result in weight loss. More research is needed, but in the meantime, set your thermostat as low as is comfortable year-round.

Bill Gavin, MD, an interventional cardiologist and medical director of the heart program at Providence St. Peter Hospital in Olympia, Washington. He is author of *No White at Night: The Three-Rule Diet* (Riverhead).

Your Taste Buds Are Being Fooled!

Take a moment and think of a food that is irresistible to you. You probably can see it vividly in your mind's eye…and you even may start to salivate.

Chances are that the food you imagined is not a vegetable or fruit but rather a processed food made with a precise combination of ingredients that trigger repeated cravings similar to those of addicts who can't resist a drug or alcohol.

Can our taste buds really be so easily tricked by food manufacturers?

Absolutely, says David Kessler, MD, former head of the Food and Drug Administration. Dr. Kessler, who has extensively researched the eating habits of Americans, recently answered questions about the ways the food industry is controlling our appetizers.

It's widely reported that about one-third of American adults weigh too much. Why has this occurred in the US?

There should be a balance between the food we consume and the energy we expend. All the evidence says that it's the amount we eat that's gotten out of hand.

It's useful to note that in 1960, the average 40- to 49-year-old American woman weighed 142 pounds. By 2000, the average weight in that age group had jumped to 169 pounds. Research shows that also during this period, American adults were gaining more from ages 20 to 40. Instead of just a few pounds, the average man gained more than 12 pounds during these ages.

Why are Americans now eating so much more?

While past generations ate most of their food at mealtimes, processed foods that are highly "palatable"—meaning that they stimulate the appetite and prompt us to eat more—are now available 24/7. With such ready access, it's become socially acceptable to eat these foods at any hour of the day. For many people, they're impossible to resist.

Can't a person use willpower to resist such foods?

Not necessarily. It's not a question of people lacking self-control or being lazy. What's really happening is that their brain circuitry has been "hijacked."

Considerable animal and human research shows that foods are made palatable by three ingredients—fat, sugar and salt. Sugar is the main driver of food appeal. Fat and salt work synergistically with sugar.

Get the proportions right, and you hit what might be called the "blisspoint." Candy bars, buffalo wings, Big Macs, cheese fries—they all combine fat, sugar and salt. The white chocolate mocha frappuccino served at Starbucks is coffee diluted with a mix of sugar, fat and salt.

How do these foods hijack our brain circuits?

Foods that taste good are reinforcing—that is, they keep us coming back for more. But highly palatable—or so-called "hyperpalatable"—foods do even more.

They stimulate brain circuits that release *dopamine,* the neurotransmitter that focuses attention and increases motivation. It can take only a single taste of a hyperpalatable food to set this process in motion.

After you've eaten such a food several times, you become more sensitive to cues surrounding the experience—for example, the sight of the wrapper and the name of the food arouses your memory of how it felt to eat the food and focuses your attention on getting it.

Each time you repeat the experience by eating the food, you strengthen the neural circuits involved, making yourself ever more sensitive to anticipation cues—literally rewiring your brain.

What is the food industry's role in all this?

The basic business plan of the typical modern food company is to sell foods loaded with fat, sugar and salt.

"The three points of the compass" is what one high-level food industry executive calls sugar, fat and salt. "They make food compel-

ling," he told me. "They make it indulgent. They make us want to eat more."

But it's easy for consumers to tell when a food is fatty, salty and sugary—it's not like the food industry can hide it.

Actually, experts in the food industry have found additional, sneakier ways to increase what they call the "craveability" of food products.

They've learned how to combine ingredients, including chemical enhancers (such as artificial sweeteners, hickory smoke flavor and cheese flavorings) to create a complex series of flavors and textures that magnify the sensory appeal.

Food manufacturers even have spent considerable effort making their creations easier to swallow. It used to be that the average bite of food in the American diet required 20 chews before swallowing—now it's only two or three chews.

As soon as that fleeting taste and oral stimulation fade, you reach for more. Through careful engineering by food companies, you're led to eat quickly enough to override your body's "I'm full" signals.

On top of that, incessant advertising adds pleasurable associations to the sensory experience—it pairs foods with images of parties, barbecues and friends having fun. The combined effect is very powerful.

People in the food industry would argue that they're just giving consumers what they want. But we now know this means excessively activating our brains to overeat—not what most consumers would want once they understood what was happening.

What can we do to defend ourselves?

Simply knowing that the food industry has created many of its products in a way that is calculated to take control of your eating behavior will go a long way toward helping you see hyperpalatable foods for what they are—which is not at all appealing.

When you're armed with this knowledge, you can take some concrete steps to replace one set of automatic behaviors with another set that is much more healthful.

For example, for people who are overweight and those who may not be overweight but want to avoid unhealthful processed foods, I suggest that they establish their own rules and enforce them ruthlessly. Identify the foods that you know are uncontrollably appealing and decide that they're absolutely off limits.

For a while at least, plan all your eating. Decide what you want to eat and when, and limit it to three meals a day, with a midmorning and midafternoon snack.

What if I start to lose my resolve?

If you feel yourself slipping into a mental dialogue of "This looks great, but I know I shouldn't have it...maybe just this once..." then reframe your thoughts and remind yourself of your goals. Tell yourself, for example, "If I don't give in to my desire for this food, I'll feel a lot better about myself tomorrow."

Many of us have gotten so caught up by the stimulation of food that we have lost touch with how much we really need to eat to feel satisfied. How much will it take to keep you from getting hungry until the next meal? Try increasingly smaller portions—you may be surprised by what you find out.

David A. Kessler, MD, former head of the Food and Drug Administration. A professor at the University of California, San Francisco, he is author of *The End of Overeating: Taking Control of the American Appetite* (Rodale).

Why Pine Nuts Help You Lose Weight—and Other Tricks to Drop Pounds

Most weight-loss diets are hard to stick to. That's because you have to eliminate 3,500 calories to lose just one pound a week and that comes to 500 calories a day. This degree of calorie restriction can make people feel hungry all the time—and reluctant to stick with any diet for very long. That's also why it is hard for people to maintain the weight that they do lose. Roughly 95% of those who lose weight are unable to maintain the weight loss longer than a year or two.

Better: Eat foods that curtail appetite and increase feelings of fullness. People who do this naturally take in fewer calories overall and are more likely to maintain their weight loss. *What to eat...*

● **Protein at every meal.** Protein is a natural appetite suppressant. People who often feel hungry probably aren't getting enough protein.

Self-test: Eat a regular meal or snack. If you're hungry again within two hours, the meal probably didn't include enough protein.

Protein should make up about 25% of every meal—three ounces to six ounces of protein is ideal. Good protein sources include chicken, seafood, lean red meats, egg whites, beans and low- or nonfat dairy.

Trap: Many traditional breakfast foods, such as a bagel or a Danish, are high in calories but low in protein. People who start the day with these foods invariably want to eat more within a few hours, adding unnecessary calories.

Always include protein with your morning meal—by spreading peanut butter on whole-wheat toast, for example.

Also helpful: High-protein snacks, such as string cheese or yogurt. They're more satisfying than carbohydrate snacks, such as pretzels or chips.

● **More fat.** Until recently, weight-loss experts advised people to eat less fat. This made intuitive sense because fat has about twice the calories as an equal amount of protein or carbohydrate. But today, after about 15 years of low-fat dieting, Americans are heavier than ever.

Reason: People who don't feel satisfied on a low-fat diet often eat excessive carbohydrates to make up the difference.

Fat is a satisfying nutrient. You may feel full after eating a lot of carbohydrates, such as pasta or bread, but you'll still want more. Fat, on the other hand, makes you crave less food, so you'll be less likely to fill up on calories from other sources.

●**Have a little fat with every meal.** If you're having a salad, for example, use full-fat dressing in moderation rather than fat-free. Add a tablespoon of olive oil when making pasta sauce. A slice of cheese or a serving of cottage cheese also provides satisfying amounts of fat.

Easy does it: Use fats only in small amounts to avoid excess calories. One tablespoon of olive oil, for example, has about 120 calories. Small amounts curtail your appetite without adding too many calories.

●**A handful of pine nuts.** A hormone called *cholecystokinin* (CCK) has been found to increase feelings of fullness. About one ounce or a small handful of pine nuts (which actually are seeds, not nuts) stimulates the body to release CCK. This reduces appetite and helps you feel fuller even when you take in fewer calories overall.

●**Fiber, especially early in the day.** High-fiber diets increase feelings of fullness and aid in weight loss. High-fiber foods also may stimulate the release of appetite-suppressing hormones.

Virtually all foods that are high in fiber, such as fruits, vegetables, legumes and whole grains, are relatively low in calories. People who eat a lot of these foods tend to feel full even when they take in fewer calories during the day.

Try to get 25 to 30 grams of fiber daily. Beans are high in fiber, with about six grams in one-half cup. Blackberries are another excellent source, with about eight grams of fiber per cup.

●**Spicy foods as often as possible.** Cayenne, jalapeños, curries and other spicy foods contain *capsaicin* and other compounds that may increase metabolism and cause the body to burn slightly more calories. More important, these foods appear to affect the "satiety center" in the brain, causing people to feel more satisfied and consume fewer calories.

●**Water before a meal.** Drink a full glass of water before you start eating, and keep sipping water throughout the meal. Water takes up space in the stomach. Or you can start your meal with a broth-based soup (not a cream soup, which is higher in calories). People who consume liquids before and during meals consume fewer calories than those who go straight to the main course.

Caution: Avoid high-calorie liquids. Americans consume about 20% more calories now than they did 20 years ago. Many of these calories come from soft drinks, sports drinks and coffee beverages that include sugar and cream. Some of these drinks contain 400 calories or more, which could result in almost one extra pound of weight a week if consumed daily.

Jodi Citrin Greebel, RD, CDN, registered dietitian and president of Citrition, LLC, a nutrition consulting company in New York City. She is coauthor of *The Little Black Apron: A Single Girl's Guide to Cooking with Style & Grace* (Polka Dot).

Can't Keep the Weight Off? You Could Have a Food Addiction

Most diets are guaranteed to fail. Popular diets focus on limiting calories, fat and/or carbohydrates. They don't address addiction, which is the underlying cause of both weight gain and repeated failures to lose weight.

Like other addictions, an addiction to food causes intense cravings, particularly during times of stress. People also experience withdrawal when they go without food for even a short time. The discomfort of cravings and withdrawal is so intense that people find themselves unable to reduce portion sizes, eat less often or avoid fattening foods. It hurts too much when they try.

Toxic Hunger

The American diet is loaded with fried foods, sugar-laden baked goods, soft drinks and other foods that stimulate the production of free radicals and other toxins. After eating, the body goes through a detoxification phase in order to break down and remove these toxins.

• **Detox is painful.** People who eat a lot of unhealthy foods invariably experience both physical and emotional discomfort, including feelings of anxiety, irritability and fatigue, in the hours between meals. In an effort to stop the discomfort, they eat again... and again. As long as the digestive tract is working, detoxification is delayed. Without knowing why, people find themselves eating all the time just to forestall these uncomfortable feelings.

Joel Fuhrman, MD, author of *Eat for Health* (Gift of Health) calls these feelings "toxic hunger" because they're produced by a toxin-producing (and fattening) diet—and because people often confuse the sensations of withdrawal with the sensation of hunger.

• **Detox takes a few weeks.** You may feel strange the first week, but during week two, the sensations will start to change and soon you will not be driven to overeat.

To break the cycle...

Eat High-Antioxidant Foods

These include beans, fresh vegetables, nuts, seeds and berries. The body experiences high levels of oxidative stress when it's detoxifying between meals. This is largely what fuels the symptoms of toxic hunger. People can reduce this discomfort by consuming foods high in disease-fighting antioxidants. These foods also make it easier for the liver to eliminate *metabolites* (chemical by-products that are produced during digestion and that intensify discomfort between meals).

Recognize True Hunger

Most people who struggle to lose weight complain that they're always hungry. What they're really experiencing is the discomfort of detoxification, which includes symptoms such as a growling stomach and irritability. They eat to feel better, not because they need to.

People should eat only when they feel true hunger, the body's call for nutrients. True hunger feels different from toxic hunger. *What to notice...*

• **A hard-to-describe sensation in your throat that only occurs when you're genuinely hungry.** It's like an itch that's relieved by eating.

• **A slight increase in salivation.**

• **A dramatically heightened taste sensation, in which anything you eat tastes wonderful.** If you notice that you're craving a specific food, you're not experiencing true hunger, because everything should taste wonderful at this point.

Dr. Fuhrman often advises patients to delay or skip meals so that they learn to distinguish true hunger from toxic hunger. The first step is to eat a high-antioxidant diet for two weeks. Then try eating a light breakfast and postponing lunch for perhaps six hours until you are sure that you feel hungry. This simple experiment can be revelatory for those who rarely go more than a few hours without eating. They discover that even ordinary foods taste great (and extraordinary foods taste amazing).

Eat More, Not Less

Food volume is critical for controlling hunger. Feelings of satiety are largely controlled by stomach stretch receptors. Eating large amounts of healthy, low-calorie foods activates these receptors and "turns off" hunger sensations to a degree that's not possible with snacks or high-fat or fried foods—unless you eat way too many calories.

Example: Imagine two different stomachs, each containing 400 calories of a single kind of food. The stomach with 400 calories of protein (such as beef) would be mainly empty space—all of the calories come from a small volume of food. A stomach filled with 400 calories of vegetables and legumes, on the other hand, would be filled to capacity, prompting the stomach to send "I'm full" signals to the brain.

This is why people who eat two to three servings of vegetables, fruits, legumes, whole grains or other wholesome foods at every meal are more likely to lose weight—and experience less discomfort—than those who diet.

Choose Nuts and Seeds

Even though these foods are high in fat, people who eat nuts and seeds regularly are more likely to lose weight than people who don't eat them. Nuts and seeds are high in plant sterols, which promote feelings of fullness and contain substances that suppress appetite.

Bonus: Clinical trials have shown that diets that include nuts can lower cholesterol and reduce the risk for diabetes. On average, people who eat one or more servings of nuts a day have a 59% lower risk of developing fatal heart disease than those who don't eat nuts.

Recommended: One ounce daily of unsalted nuts (all nuts are good) and/or seeds, such as pumpkin seeds and sunflower seeds.

Socialize More

Many people who are overweight use food for emotional comfort just as other addicts use drugs or alcohol. Eating temporarily increases *dopamine,* a brain chemical that elicits feelings of well-being, temporarily suppressing feelings of unworthiness or depression. This naturally encourages people to eat more.

Better: An active social life. People who engage in pleasurable activities with other people experience the same dopamine surge that they would otherwise get from eating. They also tend to have higher self-esteem and are more motivated to take care of themselves and improve their health.

Don't Overload on Caffeine

People who are trying to lose weight often use caffeinated beverages, such as coffee, tea and diet colas, in place of food to forestall between-meal discomfort. It doesn't work. People feel even worse when caffeine levels drop. At that point, they're even more tempted to "self-medicate" with food.

Dr. Fuhrman usually advises patients to give up caffeine initially because it will help them get through the detox phase more quickly. Once they've reached a satisfactory weight, they can start drinking caffeine again.

Joel Fuhrman, MD, family physician who specializes in natural and nutritional medicine, Flemington, New Jersey and author of *Eat for Health: Lose Weight, Keep It Off, Look Younger, Live Longer* (Gift of Health). *www.drfuhrman.com.*

The Easiest Way to Cut Calories—Chew Gum!

Obesity researchers emphasize that there's no magic bullet for weight loss—no one way to quickly and easily melt off extra pounds.

But there is a "magic stick" that might help you cut calories and feel less hungry—a stick of gum.

Newest Research

Kathleen Melanson, PhD, RD, assistant professor of nutrition and food science at the University of Rhode Island, studied 35 people to see what effect chewing sugar-free gum might have on calories—calories eaten and calories burned.

The study lasted two days. Participants chewed gum on one of the days but not the other.

On the gum-chewing day, they chewed sugar-free gum three times, in 20-minute sessions of relaxed, natural chewing—once before breakfast and two times between breakfast and lunch.

Result: On the gum-chewing day, they ate an average of 68 fewer calories at lunch—and didn't eat more calories later in the day. Many of the participants also said they felt less hungry on the day they chewed gum.

Theory: Gum-chewing might cut calorie intake and hunger two ways, says Dr. Melanson. The sensations in the mouth might send "I'm full" signals to the brain's appetite center. And nerves in the muscles of the jaw that are stimulated by gum chewing might send those signals, too.

The participants also burned about 5% more calories during gum-chewing sessions.

And they felt more upbeat on the day they chewed gum—they said they had more energy, and that it seemed to take less energy to accomplish tasks.

"Gum chewing may be a useful addition to a weight-management program," says Dr. Melanson, who reported her research at a recent annual meeting of The Obesity Society.

In another study on gum chewing and weight loss, reported at the same meeting, researchers from the University of Wisconsin School of Medicine, led by Leah Whigham, PhD, tested the effect of gum chewing on 13 overweight people.

They found that study participants who needed to exercise a lot of "cognitive restraint" in their eating habits—who would otherwise find themselves mindlessly snacking or eating even when they weren't hungry—ate fewer daily calories when they chewed gum six times a day, for 15 minutes each time.

Your Weight-Loss Toolbox

"If you're attempting to lose weight, give gum chewing a try to see if it works to help you cut calories and feel less hungry," says Dr. Melanson. "Use sugar-free gum as one tool in your weight-loss toolbox."

To use gum to help you lose weight, consider one or more of the following strategies, says Dr. Whigham. *Chew sugar-free gum...*

● In between meals, when you're craving a high-calorie snack;

● When watching TV, instead of snacking;

● For 15 minutes immediately after lunch and dinner;

● When you go out to eat, while waiting for the main course;

● In "high risk" situations for overeating, such as at parties, weddings, sporting events or the movies;

● When you're bored—since boredom is often a trigger for eating and overeating and

● When you're stressed—since stress is also trigger.

Kathleen Melanson, PhD, RD, assistant professor of nutrition and food science at the University of Rhode Island, Kingston.

Leah Whigham, PhD, research nutritionist, Grand Forks Human Nutrition Research Center, US Department of Agriculture.

Chapter 14

RESPIRATORY & IMMUNE PROBLEMS

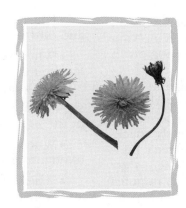

The B Vitamin That Banishes Allergies

Your nose is clogged and runny...your watery eyes itch...you're sneezing so often that nobody is even bothering to say *gesundheit* anymore...and you're bone-tired from the time you roll out of bed in the morning to the time you crawl back in at night, wondering why, oh why, you're among the one in six people with an allergy.

Yes, allergies are no fun. Your immune system has decided that an everyday substance (such as the pollen wafting from trees or the dander stirred up when you pat Fido's head) is an enemy, an allergen.

To fight back, it produces an antibody called *immunoglobulin E* (IgE), which teams up with a mast cell. The antibody is the navigator, on the lookout for the enemy-allergen; the mast cell is the warrior, bristling with weapons. And one of those weapons is an inflammatory chemical called *histamine*, released when the enemy is engaged.

Unfortunately, your allergic symptoms are the collateral damage.

And more and more people are being hit by bursts of histamine.

The rate of allergies has "increased dramatically" in the past 20 years, say researchers from Johns Hopkins University in Baltimore, writing in the *Journal of Allergy and Clinical Immunology*. Nobody really knows why, but there are plenty of theories—more allergens, more pollutants or sugary, fatty diets, to name a few.

Latest development: A new study by the Johns Hopkins researchers shows that low dietary levels of one nutrient may play an important role in the upsurge (and prevention!) of allergies. That nutrient is the B vitamin *folate* (also called *folic acid*).

The Folate Connection

The researchers analyzed two years of nutrition and health data from more than 8,000 Americans, aged 2 to 85.

Result: Compared with people with the most folate in their diets, those with the least dietary folate had…

- 30% greater risk of high IgE levels

- 31% greater risk of allergic symptoms

- 40% greater risk of wheeze, a symptom of asthma (asthma and allergies go hand in hand, with nearly 75% of asthmatics also having allergies)

- 16% greater risk of having asthma

And when the researchers divided the 8,000 people into five levels of folate intake, they found a "dose-response" relationship between folate and allergy/asthma symptoms—people at the lowest level had the most symptoms…there were fewer symptoms the next level up…even fewer at the level above that, and so on.

"Our findings are a clear indication that folate may help regulate immune response to allergens, and may reduce allergy and asthma symptoms," says Elizabeth Matsui, MD, the study leader.

Theory: A low folate intake has been linked to many diseases where inflammation plays a role, such as heart disease and rheumatoid arthritis, say the researchers. Allergic diseases are also "inflammation mediated," they say—and a higher folate intake might calm that inflammation and help prevent and control allergy.

The study researchers also note that folate is important in methyl donor metabolism—fundamental biochemical reactions in the body that "donate" or transfer molecules, helping to build DNA and repair cells. Low levels of folate lower the "methyl donor pool," they say—and other studies have linked a depleted "pool" to a higher risk of allergy symptoms.

Increasing Intake

Want to make sure you're getting enough folate in your diet?

- **Take a B vitamin supplement.** "Supplements appear to have the greatest effect on blood folate levels," say the researchers.

Take a daily B vitamin supplement that contains 800 micrograms of folate, says Robert Ivker, DO, author of *Asthma Survival* (Tarcher).

- **Take a digestive enzyme.** "If someone is low in folate—as well as vitamins B-2, B-6, and B-12—they will be 'under-methylators' and have higher histamine levels," says Ellen Cutler, DC, author of *Live Free from Asthma and Allergies* (Celestial Arts). But, she adds, many people with allergies and asthma have food sensitivities—including sensitivity to B vitamin supplements and many foods containing B vitamins! To counter this difficult-to-solve problem—to B or not to B—she recommends adding digestive enzyme supplements to your daily health routine, taking one right before or with each meal. The enzymes aid in the absorption and utilization of B vitamins (and other nutrients), helping to "desensitize" you.

Products: MicroMiracles, a chewable digestive enzyme, available at *www.drellencutler.com* or call 877-246-7381; OxiCellZyme or DigestZyme at *www.enzymessentials.com* or call 866-439-5014; Digest and Digest Gold at *www.enzymedica.com* or call 888-918-1118.

- **Eat folate-enriched foods.** Folate-enriched ready-to-eat breakfast cereals and folate-enriched cereal grain products (such as bread) are also excellent sources of the vitamin, say the researchers.

- **Eat fruits and vegetables.** "Good sources of folate also include fruits and vegetables, especially citrus fruits, tomatoes, leafy greens, spinach, lettuce and broccoli," says Dr. Cutler. "To retain folate, serve fruits and vegetables raw, or steam or simmer in a small amount of water."

Elizabeth Matsui, MD, associate professor, pediatrics, epidemiology, Johns Hopkins Children's Center, Baltimore.

Robert Ivker, DO, author of *Asthma Survival and Sinus Survival* (Tarcher).

Ellen Cutler, DC, author of *Live Free from Asthma and Allergies* (Celestial Arts) and *Micro Miracles* (Rodale).

The Superfoods That Relieve Allergies to Pollen, Dust, Mold...

The right foods can help relieve allergies to dust, pollen, mold and other spores in the air—easing symptoms that include sneezing, stuffy nose and wheezing.

Recent finding: Allergy symptoms are less common on the rural Greek island of Crete than elsewhere in Greece, even though there's no shortage of allergens blowing around. According to a study published in *Thorax*, the people of Crete can thank their diet. Researchers tested 690 island children for airborne allergies and asked their parents to answer questions about their children's diets and symptoms. Eighty percent of the children ate fruit at least twice a day, and 68% ate vegetables that often. Those who ate more nuts, grapes, oranges, apples and tomatoes—the main local products—had fewer allergy symptoms than those who ate less.

Allergy symptoms occur when an overactive immune system responds to harmless substances as if they could cause disease. Inflammation is an early step in the immune response. Most of the foods that relieve allergies are anti-inflammatory, modulating the immune system response.

Foods That Fight Allergies

The following foods help battle airborne allergies...

● **Fruits high in vitamin C,** an antioxidant, may help reduce inflammation. Year-round, eat two pieces of fruit daily. When you're especially congested, choose from these twice a day—an orange, one cup of strawberries, an apple, one cup of grapes or a medium-sized wedge of watermelon. Bonus: The skins of red grapes are loaded with the antioxidant resveratrol and were found to relieve wheezing in the Crete study.

● **Nuts,** especially almonds, hazelnuts and peanuts, are a good source of vitamin E, which helps minimize inflammation. Eat a single one-ounce serving of any of these nuts daily year-round to help prevent symptoms. If you do have symptoms, increase the servings—try two tablespoons of peanut butter and one ounce each of hazelnuts and almonds a day.

● **Cold-water fish** (wild salmon, mackerel, trout, herring and sardines), as well as walnuts and flaxseed, contain omega-3 fatty acids, which help fight inflammation. Eat at least two servings of cold-water fish each week year-round and three servings during the seasons when you experience airborne allergies. Also have 12 walnuts and one tablespoon of ground flaxseed a day.

● **Oysters, shrimp and crab, as well as legumes, whole grains and tofu,** are all high in zinc, which has antibacterial and antiviral effects that provide relief for immune systems overtaxed by fighting allergies. Have six oysters, six shrimp or a few crabs every week, and twice that when your allergies bother you. Also have one serving of whole grains and one of beans or tofu a day.

● **Tea,** whether green, white or black, is full of *flavonoids*, plant compounds that reduce inflammation. Tea also increases proteins in the body that fight infection, again relieving an overtaxed immune system. Enjoy one cup daily, and increase to two when your allergies are a problem.

Helpful: Drink your tea first thing in the morning with lemon and honey to stimulate the *cilia*—the tiny hairs in the nose that sweep pollen and dust out of the way.

● **Horseradish,** hot mustard, fennel, anise and sage also stimulate the cilia and act as natural decongestants. Add a dash to food whenever possible.

Foods to Avoid All Year

If you experience congestion or other symptoms year-round, ask an allergist to conduct a skin test to identify allergies to dust, mold and foods. *Then consider the following changes in your daily diet...*

• **Mold and yeast in food can aggravate an allergy to mold in the air.** If you're allergic to mold, avoid foods that contain yeast, such as bread and baked goods (unless they are labeled "yeast free")…wine, beer and spirits…fermented foods, such as sauerkraut and cider…foods that tend to get moldy, such as cheese and mushrooms…vinegar and sauces that contain vinegar, such as mayonnaise, barbecue sauce, mustard and salad dressing.

Helpful: Use lemon juice and spices in dressings instead.

• **Milk and dairy products,** such as yogurt, butter and ice cream, could be making you feel worse if you have a congested nose year-round, a symptom typically caused by an allergy to dust. One explanation is that *casein,* the protein in milk, can promote the formation of mucus. Although there isn't strong science showing that milk aggravates congestion, it's worth experimenting by cutting dairy from your diet for at least two weeks. If your allergies improve when you avoid dairy products, eliminate dairy year-round. You will then need to take a calcium supplement, usually 1,000 milligrams (mg) a day, to compensate for the decreased calcium intake that accompanies a dairy-free diet.

• **Soy, corn and wheat.** Soy, including soy milk, tofu, soybean oil, edamame and soy sauce, may aggravate chronic congestion, according to clinical observation. Even if you don't appear allergic to soy on a skin-prick test, experiment by eliminating soy from your diet for at least two weeks.

The same is true of corn (including cornflakes, corn chips and corn oil) and wheat (including all breads and baked goods unless they are marked "wheat-free" or "gluten-free"). If you find that your symptoms are alleviated when you stop eating any of these foods, eliminate them year-round.

Leo Galland, MD, founder of Foundation for Integrated Medicine in New York City. An internist, he treats many patients with chronic allergies and specializes in integrating nutrition and herbs with conventional medicine. *www.md heal.org.*

Chinese Herbs—Strong As Steroids for Asthma

To a practitioner of Traditional Chinese Medicine (TCM), if you have asthma, you don't just have asthma—you probably also have a deficiency of *qi* (pronounced chee) (life-energy) in the lung, and perhaps a chronic deficiency of chi in the kidney. The herbs used by a TCM practitioner to treat asthma (usually combined in a formula) are meant to stimulate and balance lung and kidney qi.

Well, the medicine may be traditional, but the scientific proof is up-to-date. A new study shows those herbs work.

Anti-Asthma Herbal Formula

Researchers from Mount Sinai School of Medicine in New York studied ASHMI (antiasthma herbal formula), a three-herb TCM formula that had already proven effective in a preliminary one-month study and in animal experiments.

In a "Phase I" study designed to test the formula's safety, 20 adults (average age 32, and diagnosed with asthma when they were 12 to 15 years old) took either ASHMI or an inhaled *corticosteroid* (prednisone), an anti-inflammatory drug. (Corticosteroids are also called *steroids,* but they're not the same drug as the anabolic steroids used illegally to build muscle.)

These individuals had moderate to severe allergic asthma. Their asthma was complicated by allergies and severe enough that they had to use a *bronchodilator*—an inhaled drug that opens airways—every day, often many times a day.

The one-week study showed ASHMI was "safe and well-tolerated," say the researchers, in the *Journal of Alternative and Complementary Medicine.*

And the earlier, one-month study showed that those taking ASHMI had an improvement in lung function. They also had fewer allergic and asthmatic symptoms, and required less bronchodilator. Those improvements were almost at the same level as in the study where participants took *prednisone*—a steroid taken in pill form and one of the most powerful drugs in the asthma arsenal.

The study also showed that people taking ASHMI had an increase in their blood levels of *cortisol*—the body's natural, anti-inflammatory hormone, produced by the adrenal gland—while those taking prednisone had a decrease in cortisol.

The fact that ASHMI might be able to reduce or replace steroids is a huge breakthrough for asthmatics.

Trap: Prednisone and other steroids control the inflammation of asthma that swells and shuts airways. Their short-term and long-term side effects range from the distressing to the devastating. Short-term side effects can include indigestion, bloating, insomnia and irritability. Long-term side effects can include osteoporosis, hip fractures, diabetes, high blood pressure, fragile skin, cataracts and shrinking adrenal glands (the very side effect that led to the decrease of cortisol in the ASHMI study).

"There's a great desire on the part of the medical profession and on the part of adults with asthma and parents of children with asthma to develop a safe alternative to steroids," says Xiu-Min Li, MD, a study researcher and a physician trained in both Western medicine and TCM. "Even if ASHMI is not as immediately powerful as steroids, it may have the same effect when taken over time, or it could be used in conjunction with steroids, reducing their dosage."

Important: Those taking ASHMI had a return to nearly normal cortisol levels, says Dr. Li—and these were folks who had taken steroids on and off for years. Which means that ASHMI might also help heal some of the damage to the cortisol-manufacturing adrenal gland from those drugs.

Finding the Formula

ASHMI isn't commercially available. The Phase I study was only the first step in FDA's possible approval of this "botanical prescription drug," says Dr. Li.

But ASHMI (and other Chinese herbal remedies) are available to patients at the Center for Chinese Herbal Therapy for Allergy and Asthma, Dr. Li's clinic at the Mount Sinai School of Medicine in New York.

Resource: To contact the Center for Chinese Herbal Therapy for Allergy and Asthma at Mount Sinai School of Medicine, call 212-241-5548.

Dr. Li has patients from all over the United States and the world. "Those living outside New York are asked to return every three to six months for a checkup," says Dr. Li. "Meanwhile, they work with their local pulmonologist, who can help them gradually reduce their current drug intake as they take ASHMI and other Chinese herbal remedies that I have developed."

Red flag: There have been several products advertised online that purport to be the same as the ASHMI formula—but they aren't. "The quality of the three herbs, and the exact amount of each herb, is very critical to the success of the formula—and that can't be duplicated without knowing the exact details, which are patented," says Dr. Li.

If a trip to New York isn't possible, you might want to see a certified practitioner of Traditional Chinese Medicine trained in Chinese herbology, and ask him/her to make the classic anti-asthma formula that was the basis of Dr. Li's ASHMI formula. (She derived her three-herb formula from a fourteen-herb TCM formula, after several years of rigorous and systematic testing.)

Here are the herbs in that TCM formula, says Jake Paul Fratkin, OMD, LAc, a TCM practitioner in Boulder, Colorado, and author of *Chinese Herbal Patent Medicines* (Shya Publications):

• Su zi (fructus perillae frutescentis), 9 grams (g)

• Ting li zi (semen lepidii), 9 g

• Xing ren (semen pruni armeniacae), 9 g

• Huang qin (radix scutellariae baicalensis), 9 g

• Ku shen (radix sophorae flavescentis), 9 g

- Dang gui (radix angelicae sinensis), 9 g
- Bai shao (radix paeoniae lactiflorae), 9 g
- Ge gen (radix puerariae), 9 g
- Jie geng (radix platycodi grandiflori), 6 g
- Zhen zhu mu (concha margaritifera), 6 g
- Ling zhi (ganoderma lucidum), 6 g
- Gan cao (radix glycyrrhizae), 6 g
- Da zao (fructus ziziphi jujubae), 5 pieces
- Sheng jiang (rhizome zingiberis officinalis), 6 g

Resource: You can find a certified practitioner of Chinese herbology near you by visiting the Web site of the National Certification Commission for Acupuncture and Oriental Medicine (NCCAOM), at *www.nccaom.org*, and clicking on "Find a Practitioner" on the home page. At "Certification Registry" you can enter your state and zip code to find all the practitioners certified by the NCCAOM in "Chinese Herbology."

Jake Paul Fratkin, OMD, LAc, TCM practitioner, Boulder, Colorado, author of *Chinese Herbal Patent Medicines* (Shya Publications).

Xiu-Min Li, MD, director of the Center for Chinese Herbal Therapy for Allergy and Asthma at Mount Sinai School of Medicine, New York City.

The Best Houseplants For Healthier Air

When you think of air pollution, you probably think of clouds of contaminants rising out of smokestacks and smog from car exhaust.

But if you're a typical twenty-first-century human being, you spend about nine out of every 10 hours indoors—and research shows that indoor air in cities is up to 100 times more polluted than outdoor air, says Stanley Kays, PhD, a professor in the Department of Horticulture at the University of Georgia.

The source of most pollutants are volatile organic compounds (VOCs) that "gas out" from indoor paints, varnishes, adhesives, furniture, furniture wax—even clothing (particularly if it's been dry cleaned). VOCs also are released by household products such as cleansers, detergents, disinfectants, spot removers and air fresheners.

VOCs aren't all bad. The fragrance of a rose and the aroma of an apple pie are VOCs. But many are bad. Very bad.

They can cause asthma and other respiratory problems—along with headaches, fatigue, eye irritation, skin rashes and long-term damage to the liver, kidney and central nervous system, says the Environmental Protection Agency. Some, such as benzene, are known carcinogens. In fact, experts estimate that indoor air pollution from VOCs is responsible for 65,000 to 150,000 deaths in the US every year!

"Unfortunately, there is currently little public awareness of the problem or health risks," says Dr. Kays.

Good news: Houseplants can remove VOCs from indoor air. The pollutants are absorbed through microscopic openings in leaves called *stomata*...detoxified in the plant...transported to the roots...and biodegraded by microbes, which turn the chemicals into substances both the plant and the microbes can use, explains B.C. Wolverton, PhD, author of *How to Grow Fresh Air* (Penguin), and founder of Wolverton Environmental Services, Inc.

Now: A new study from Dr. Kays and his colleagues at the University of Georgia show which houseplants do the best job at cleaning indoor air.

Pollutants and Purifiers

Dr. Kays and his colleagues tested more than two dozen "ornamental species commonly used for interior plantscapes" (in other words, houseplants) for their ability to rid indoor air of these five health-damaging VOCs:

- **Benzene and toluene** (two chemically related VOCs from petroleum-based indoor coatings, cleaning solutions, plastics, tobacco smoke and exhaust fumes that end up inside)

• **Octane** (from paint, adhesives and building materials)

• **Trichloroethylene, or TCE** (from tap water, cleansers and plastics)

• **Alpha-pinene** (from synthetic paints and air fresheners)

The five plants with the ability to remove the most VOCs (defined as "superior removal efficiencies") were…

• **Purple waffle (Hemigraphis alternata).** This standout plant had the highest removal efficiency for four out of the five VOCs.

• **English ivy (Hedera helix)**

• **Wax plant (Hoya carnosa)**

• **Asparagus fern (Asparagus densiflorus)**

• **Purple heart plant (Tradescantia pallida)**

The six plants with "intermediate removal efficiencies" were…

• **Weeping fig (Ficus benjamina)**

• **Ming aralia (Polyscias fruticosa)**

• **Silver net-leaf (Fittonia argyroneura)**

• **Snake plant (Sansevieria trifasciata)**

• **Guzmania bromeliad (Guzmania)**

• **False aralia (Schefflera elegantissima)**

Houseplants that didn't get the job done—those with "poor removal efficiency"—included (forgoing the Latin nomenclature): arrowhead vine, cast-iron plant, corn plant, croton, dumb cane, heart-leaf philodendron, peace lily, peacock plant, pothos, prayer plant, red rubber tree, rose geranium, sentry palm, spider plant, variegated red-edged peperomia and the variegated schefflera.

Use More Than One Type of Plant

"For maximum improvement of indoor air quality, multiple species are needed," says Dr. Kays. He also points out that it's difficult to determine the exact number and species of plants you'd need to clean your air.

You can grow the five VOC-eating lowering plants specified by Dr. Kays, or expand your list to the top 11.

And here are a few more plants, found by Dr. Wolverton in his research to be among the most effective at removing VOCs:

• **Boston fern** (*Nephrolepis exaltata 'Bostoniensis'*). "It's the best for removing air pollutants and adding humidity to the environment," he says. "It must have frequent misting and watering, or the leaves will quickly turn brown and begin to drop."

• **Bamboo plant** (*Chamaedorea seifrizii*). "They add a peaceful, tropical feeling wherever they are placed," says Dr. Wolverton.

• **Rubber plant** (*Ficus robusta*). "Bred for toughness, it will tolerate dim light and cool temperatures."

• **Gerbera daisy** (*Gerbera jamesonii*). "In early studies conducted by NASA, this plant proved to be extremely effective in removing chemical vapors from the air," he says.

• **Golden pothos** (*Epipremnum aureum*). "It is one of the easiest plants to grow under low-light conditions, and you can grow it on a trellis as a vine. That's especially important in a small space where room for an ornamental plant is limited."

Smart idea: Plants grown in *hydroculture* (without dirt, usually in water and pebbles or other open aggregate) are 30 to 50% more effective in removing VOCs than those grown in potting soil, says Dr. Wolverton. "This is mostly due to greater airflow through pebbles rather than soil to the plant root zone, where microbes break down the VOCs."

You can find information about growing indoor plants using hydroculture in Dr. Wolverton's book, *Plants: Why You Can't Live Without Them* (Roli).

Stanley Kays, PhD, professor, Department of Horticulture, University of Georgia, Athens

B.C. Wolverton, PhD, author of *How to Grow Fresh Air* (Penguin) and founder of Wolverton Environmental Services, *www.wolvertonenvironmental.com*.

Keep Your Nose Happy—Take Care of Your Cilia

If you suffer from hay fever (allergic rhinitis), you may dread the arrival of spring. As billions of pollen spores are released into the air, it's likely that your nose will start running or become stuffy, your eyes will itch, you won't be able to stop coughing and your head will ache.

At least 30% of people who suffer from hay fever go on to develop a related condition known as *sinusitis* (inflammation of the sinus cavities, usually due to a bacterial or viral infection). But airborne allergens aren't the only culprit.

If you're exposed to air pollution, smoke or dry or cold air, or even if you have a common cold, you also are at increased risk for sinusitis. In all of these instances, the mucous glands secrete more mucus to dilute the offending material. Unless the *cilia* (tiny hairs on the cells of the mucous membrane) move the mucus out, this creates an ideal breeding ground for infection.

When you have coldlike symptoms that last for at least 12 consecutive weeks, you are likely to have chronic sinusitis, the most commonly diagnosed chronic illness in the US. Most of the 37 million Americans who suffer from sinusitis each year turn to decongestants, antihistamines and antibiotics.

What most sinusitis sufferers don't know: You will have the best chance of preventing sinus problems in the first place if you take care of the cilia. *My secrets to improving the health of your cilia...*

Cilia: The Missing Link

The cilia play a crucial—though underrecognized—role in keeping the respiratory tract healthy. These tiny hairs wave rhythmically to carry tiny airborne particles and bacteria out of the nasal passages. When allergy symptoms persist for many days or even weeks, however, the cilia become overworked and quit moving.

Cilia also can be damaged if you regularly take antihistamines or breathe dry air—both of which decrease the liquid component of mucus that traps bacteria and is needed for good cilia movement. When the cilia no longer do their job, bacteria multiply, setting the stage for infection.

To test the health of your cilia: Many ear, nose and throat specialists (otolaryngologists) use the so-called saccharin test. With this test, the doctor places a particle of saccharin in your nose and times how long it takes you to taste it.

Normally, the patient tastes the saccharin in five to eight minutes. If the cilia are damaged, however, it may take 25 minutes or longer for the patient to taste it. If the damage is severe, special treatment, such as breathing exercises, may be required.

Keep Your Cilia Healthy

When allergy or cold symptoms persist or when nasal discharge becomes colored (usually yellow or green)—a symptom of sinusitis—there are some surprisingly simple steps you can take to ensure the health of your cilia. *Favorite methods...*

●**Drink hot tea with lemon and honey.** Compounds found in black and green tea help block the body's allergic response to pollen by inhibiting the production of *histamine*, the substance that causes nasal stuffiness and dripping due to a cold or hay fever.

Drinking five cups of hot tea a day helps the body mount its natural defenses against infection, scientific studies have shown. The moist heat stimulates the cilia, while lemon and honey thin mucus, allowing for better cilia movement.

●**Sing "oooommmmm" in a low tone.** You might feel a little silly at first, but singing the "oooommmmm" sound, which was used by the ancient yogis as a form of meditation, causes a vibration of air that stimulates the cilia. Make this sound often throughout the day. As an alternative, buy a toy kazoo and hum into it for 10 minutes daily.

●**Use pulsatile irrigation.** This highly effective strategy involves rapidly but gently rinsing your nose with a stream of saltwater (saline solution) that pulses at a rate matching the normal pulse rate of healthy cilia—hence the name pulsatile irrigation.

Clinical trials involving thousands of patients have shown that *pulsatile irrigation* increases blood flow to the nasal passages and helps restore function to damaged cilia.

Several pulsatile irrigation devices are available from Web sites specializing in allergy or medical products, such as National Allergy (*www.natlallergy.com*, 800-522-1448) or Health Solutions Medical Products (*www. pharmacy-solutions.com*, 800-305-4095). The typical cost is around $100 to $140. For best results, use this form of irrigation twice daily, as needed.

Murray Grossan, MD, otolaryngologist and head and neck surgeon with the Tower Ear, Nose and Throat Clinic at Cedars-Sinai Medical Center in Los Angeles. He is author of *Free Yourself From Sinus and Allergy Problems—Permanently* (Hydro Med).

Boost Your Ability to Fight the Flu

With the outbreak of the H1N1 virus (commonly known as the swine flu), most people relied solely on public health authorities for advice on the best ways to avoid infection.

While such recommendations can be helpful, there almost always are additional steps you can take to stay healthy when a highly contagious disease threatens large numbers of people.

Overlooked infection-fighting strategy: By enhancing your body's natural infection-fighting mechanisms (*immunity*), you often can avoid illness—even if you are exposed to infectious organisms that are making other people sick.

How Infections Begin

Bacteria and viruses are the main causes of potentially deadly infections. Whether bacterial or viral, these infections pass from person to person in much the same way—from people touching contaminated surfaces, through hand-to-hand contact or via coughs and/or sneezes. Hand-washing is the most widely recommended infection-control measure.

With the flu, antiviral medications can help prevent infection or at least lessen the severity of the infection, depending on the strain that has caused the illness. The *antivirals oseltamivir* (Tamiflu) and *zanamivir* (Relenza) have been shown in laboratory tests to shorten the duration of H1N1 symptoms by one to two days (when taken within 48 hours of the onset of symptoms).

As we all know, antibiotics are prescribed for bacterial infections—and should not be taken unnecessarily.

Reason: Antibiotics kill not only dangerous bacteria, but also "friendly" immune-boosting bacteria that help ward off dangerous bugs. Antibiotics are not effective against viral infections.

Simple Lifestyle Strategies

Our lifestyles play a critical role in whether our immune systems are able to fight off illness. *Recommendations for reducing your infection risk...*

● **Eat immune-boosting foods.** Blueberries and other berries (the darker, the better), purple grape juice and pomegranate juice are rich sources of plant-based compounds (*phytochemicals*) that boost the immune system.

Cruciferous vegetables contain *sulforaphane*, a compound with immunity-enhancing properties that help fight off infection.

Good sources of sulforaphane: Broccoli (especially BroccoSprouts, high-potency broccoli sprouts available at supermarkets and health-food stores)...cabbage...cauliflower... and brussels sprouts. Aim to eat at least one serving of immune-boosting foods with every meal.

● **Get eight hours of sleep a night.** Lack of sleep has been shown to weaken the immune system—especially the activity of natural killer cells, a type of white blood cell that's key to preventing infection.

Be Clean—But Not Too Clean

Keeping your environment too sterile will stifle your immune system's interactions with microorganisms, which is what primes it for action. According to Robert Rountree, MD, the regular use of antimicrobial soaps and other antimicrobial personal-care products can be counterproductive.

The best defense against common sources of infection is to wash your hands often with plain soap and water for at least 15 to 20 seconds.

Supplements to Consider

Most health-conscious adults take a multivitamin to ensure that they are getting enough key nutrients. In addition, certain individual supplements (which can be taken indefinitely with your doctor's approval) have important infection-fighting properties. *For example...*

●**Vitamin D.** Scientists have found that vitamin D helps protect against viral infections and stimulates the body to produce natural antibiotics.

Important: Studies now suggest that at least half of the people in northern latitudes (in the US, generally north of Atlanta) are vitamin D–deficient in the fall and winter, when the sun's angle is too low to stimulate the body's natural production of vitamin D.

Advice: Take a daily supplement of 2,000 international units (IU) of vitamin D-3 (the most readily absorbed form). It's best to take this vitamin with food high in fat, such as milk or cheese, which helps absorption.

After two to four months, ask your doctor to order a 25-hydroxy vitamin D blood test to see if the supplement is doing its job (a healthy blood level is 40 ng/mL to 50 ng/mL). If not, you may want to increase your daily dose of vitamin D-3.

●**Probiotics.** These "good" bacteria work in the gut to prime the immune system.

Advice: Look for a product that contains lactobacillus, acidophilus or bifidus and provides a total daily dose of 10 billion to 30 billion organisms (sometimes expressed as CFUs, or *colony-forming units*). Refrigerated probiotic supplements, which are sold in the supplement section of most health-food stores, are best—refrigeration helps preserve potency of the probiotics.

Also helpful: Products such as the yogurt Activia and the drinks DanActive and Yakult contain high amounts of probiotics.

●**Sulforaphane.** This antimicrobial compound found in cruciferous vegetables is believed to boost the immune system by replenishing nutrients in the dendritic cells in the membranes of the mouth, nose, bladder and gut. These cells bolster the body's defense against invading microorganisms.

Animal studies also have shown that sulforaphane is very effective at ridding the body of toxins in our environment that dampen the immune response. Such toxins could include arsenic, polychlorinated biphenyls (PCBs) and bisphenol A (BPA), the chemical used in certain plastic water and beverage bottles and the lining of many food cans.

In addition to BroccoSprouts (described earlier), scientists at Johns Hopkins have now developed a tea called Brassica Tea—both products provide concentrated doses of sulforaphane. To learn more, visit the product Web site, *www.brassica.com* or call 877-747-1277.

Robert Rountree, MD, physician in private practice and owner of Boulder Wellcare in Boulder, Colorado. He is co-author of *Immunotics: A Revolutionary Way to Fight Infection, Beat Chronic Illness and Stay Well* (Perigee).

Are You Showering Yourself with Germs?

You assume that when you're taking a shower, you're getting clean, not sick.

Surprising: A new study shows that your showerhead might be blasting bad-for-you bacteria into the air—bacteria that can give you a respiratory infection every bit as serious as tuberculosis.

The Bacterial Biofilm

Researchers at the University of Colorado analyzed 45 showerheads from homes, hotels and health clubs in nine cities around the US, including New York, Chicago and Denver.

They found that three out of every 10 showerheads were coated inside with slimy, hard-to-remove "biofilms" of *Mycobacterium avium*, a bacteria similar to the type that causes tuberculosis (*Mycobacterium tuberculosis*).

When the shower is turned on, those bacteria are "aerosolized" in tiny droplets that are suspended in air and inhaled into the deepest part of the lungs, explains Norman Pace, PhD, a study researcher.

"If you are getting a face full of water when you first turn your shower on, that means you are probably getting a particularly high load of Mycobacterium avium, which may not be too healthy," he says.

Warning: Scientists theorize that the recent rise in serious and even fatal lung infections caused by these *nontuberculous mycobacteria* (NTM) is because people are taking more showers and fewer baths, say the researchers, in the *Proceedings of the National Academy of Sciences*. In fact, cases of infection from NTM now outnumber cases of tuberculosis in many areas of the US.

What to Do

NTM can infect anybody, but the most likely victims are people with a compromised immune system or people with chronic lung disease. *If any item on this list describes you, infection with NTM from your showerhead is a concern…*

- Age 65 or older, with the thin, weak "frail" elderly at greatest risk

- Pregnant

- Chronic obstructive pulmonary disease (COPD)

- Undergoing chemotherapy or radiation for cancer

- Active leukemia, lymphoma or multiple myeloma

- HIV/AIDS

- Genetic immune-deficiency disease, such as cystic fibrosis

- Taking an immune-suppressing drug after a transplant

- Taking an immune-modifying drug for rheumatoid arthritis or another disease

- Excessive alcohol use

- Using illegal drugs such as heroin, cocaine or methylamphetamine

Symptoms of lung disease caused by NTM can include fatigue; a persistent, dry cough; shortness of breath; weakness and "generally feeling bad," says Dr. Pace.

- **See your doctor.** If you have the above symptoms, see your doctor immediately—and specifically mention NTM as a possible cause. "This type of infection is not on the radar of most doctors," says Laura Baumgartner, PhD, a study researcher.

Important: Infection from NTM is not transmissible, like a cold.

For a person with a weak immune system, any one of the following precautions may be effective in preventing infection from NTM, say both Dr. Pace and Dr. Baumgartner.

- **Take a bath.** "Shower usage possibly is contraindicated for individuals with compromised immune or pulmonary systems," write the researchers. "Taking a bath is the simplest way to avoid the problem," adds Dr. Baumgartner.

- **Change your showerhead every six months.** "We haven't seen strong biofilms on any showerhead newer than six months," says Dr. Baumgartner.

Buy a showerhead with an effective filter. The Pall Corporation manufactures filtered showerheads for the immunocompromised—the Pall-Aquasafe or Pall Kleenpak Shower

Filters. They are available at most medical supply stores and online.

● **Use a metal rather than a plastic showerhead.** Since plastic showerheads appear to "load up" with more bacteria-rich biofilms, all-metal showerheads may be a good alternative, says Dr. Pace.

● **Don't clean your showerhead with bleach.** The researchers tried that on one showerhead and re-installed it. Seven months later, they checked the showerhead again—and levels of NTM had tripled, covering 75% rather than 25% of the inside of the showerhead. "Chlorine might kill everything else and encourage the one bacteria you want to eliminate," says Dr. Baumgartner.

Norman Pace, PhD, distinguished professor, Department of Molecular, Cellular and Developmental Biology, University of Colorado, Boulder.

Laura Baumgartner, PhD, researcher, applied molecular microbiology, University of Colorado, Boulder.

Natural Ways to Prevent Pneumonia

Even though many people think of pneumonia as a wintertime illness, it can strike during any season of the year. It can be caused by one of many different types of bacteria, viruses, fungi—or even an injury, such as exposure to chemical fumes (from a chlorine spill, for example). People who are at greatest risk for pneumonia are older adults and newborns, smokers, heavy drinkers, people with pre-existing lung disease or compromised immune systems, or anyone who is bedridden or has limited mobility (which increases risk for buildup of mucus in the lungs). Fortunately, you can take steps to protect yourself. *My secrets to avoiding pneumonia...*

● **Consider getting a pneumonia vaccination.** Discuss the vaccine with your doctor if you are age 65 or older—or at any age if you have congestive heart failure, a compromised immune system, liver or lung disease or diabetes, or if you are a smoker or heavy drinker. The vaccine can help prevent a common type of pneumonia caused by the Streptococcus pneumoniae bacterium.

● **Take vitamin A daily.** Vitamin A deficiency can cause drying of the respiratory-tract lining and a reduction in cilia, the hairlike tissues that move mucus and debris out of the lungs. Both changes make the lungs vulnerable to infection and inflammation. A total daily dose of 10,000 international units (IU) of vitamin A can help keep your lungs healthy.

Caution: Vitamin A is toxic when consumed in high doses over long periods of time. Consult your doctor before taking more than 10,000 IU of vitamin A daily. If you have liver disease or are pregnant, do not take supplemental vitamin A. In addition, some research suggests that smokers should not take vitamin A supplements.

● **Get more vitamin C daily.** The results of studies on the immune-enhancing effects of vitamin C have been mixed. However, I'm convinced—based on my clinical experience—that a daily dose of vitamin C does, in fact, help the immune system resist disease and is essential to combating the immune-draining effects of stress, a chief cause of illness.

Recommended: A daily total of 1,000 mg of vitamin C.

● **Treat upper respiratory infections (URIs) promptly and effectively.** Quite often, pneumonia develops from the spread of inflammation caused by a viral infection, such as bronchitis.

Advice: Rest (forgo your usual activities, including going to work)...and hydrate (drink 68 ounces of water daily). For a cold or bronchitis, I recommend drinking a tincture made from extracts of the powerful antiviral botanical medicines elder, echinacea, eyebright and licorice—15 drops of each in one ounce of water, 15 minutes before or after meals, every four waking hours for several days.

Caution: Omit licorice if you have high blood pressure or heart disease—the herb may affect blood pressure or cause heart problems.

• **Don't delay a doctor visit if you suspect pneumonia.** Typical symptoms include a cough, fever, shortness of breath and fatigue. An early diagnosis increases your chance of a good outcome.

Jamison Starbuck, ND, naturopathic physician in family practice in Missoula, Montana.

Do-Re-Mi for COPD

Twenty-four million Americans have chronic obstructive lung disease (COPD), usually after a lifetime of smoking. In the earliest stage, you develop a chronic cough, constantly clearing sputum. Next, you find yourself short of breath while carrying groceries, climbing stairs or going for a brisk walk. As the disease advances, you wheeze, can't take a deep breath and sometimes feel like you can't breathe at all. Eventually, you may need oxygen therapy to keep going.

Surprising: If you have COPD and find breathing difficult, it may be time to start singing.

Less Breathlessness

A team of researchers from the School of Arts and Communication and the Medical School at Sao Paulo University in Brazil studied 30 people with moderate to severe COPD. (They were all former smokers, and none used oxygen therapy.)

They divided them into two groups. One group took weekly, one-hour singing classes; the other group took weekly, one-hour handicraft classes in drawing, origami (paper folding) and collage.

The singing classes consisted of relaxation exercises for neck and arm muscles for five minutes; breathing exercises for 10 minutes; vocalization exercises for 15 minutes (loudly pronouncing the vowels *le*, *la*, *mi* and *mu*, and then using those vowels rather than lyrics to sing the melody of a familiar song); and singing Brazilian folk songs for 30 minutes.

Results: After one singing class, those with COPD had less breathlessness (dyspnea), more ability to inhale (inspiratory capacity) and more ability to exhale (expiratory reserve volume). There was no change in those taking handicrafts.

After six months of singing classes, there was a small but significant improvement in average maximal expiratory pressure—a standard measurement of the strength and volume of exhalation, and an indicator of the severity of COPD.

Meanwhile, after six months of handicraft classes, there was a significant deterioration in maximal expiratory pressure.

Both groups had a similar improvement in quality of life, as determined by a questionnaire about the impact of COPD on everyday activities, such as talking a shower, getting dressed, household chores and walking.

"Regular practice of singing may improve quality of life and preserve the maximal expiratory pressure," conclude the researchers, in the *International Journal of Chronic Obstructive Pulmonary Disease*.

Why it works: "People who sing are practicing a particular type of respiratory exercise" that strengthens the muscles involved in inhaling and exhaling, say the researchers. The "better breathing coordination" of singing can also reduce the anxiety and fear that accompanying breathlessness. And singing can boost mood and alleviate depression—a common problem for people with COPD.

Important: No one in the singing classes complained of severe breathlessness, chest pain or dizziness—though there was "a high prevalence of coughing and sputum expectoration" after the 15-minute vocalization exercises and again after the 30 minutes of singing. That was a good sign, explain the researchers—singing was promoting "bronchial hygiene," helping people with COPD mobilize clogging secretions up and out of their lungs.

Anyone Can Learn to Sing

"Singing classes," say the researchers, "could be a practical and pleasant way of training expiratory [exhalation] muscles"—and, they point out, other research on COPD expiratory training shows that it leads to more endurance, strength, improvement in exercise performance, reduction of symptoms and better quality of life.

"Singing classes are an amusing, nonrisky and well-tolerated activity" for COPD, they conclude.

But what if your singing voice sounds like those rejected contestants that tunelessly embarrass themselves in the auditions for American Idol? What if you just can't sing?

"Anyone can learn to sing," says Timothy Kelly, author of *Teach Yourself Singing: If You Can Talk, You Can Sing* (CreateSpace). "That's because the human voice was designed to sing.

"You probably don't talk in a monotone—you use pitch, rhythm and melody. In fact, you go about your day using a wider voice range in talking than you would use in singing most songs.

"When you realize that you already know how to sing—when you look at talking as being a type of singing, and that you've been 'practicing' for years—then it's easy to take the next step and learn how to sing."

Kelly provides online singing lessons using his unique approach at *www.teachyour selfsinging.com*, where you can also order his book and/or CDs to teach yourself to sing. Or write, Timothy Kelly, Teach Yourself Singing, 2211 Lady Leslie Lane, Pearland, TX 77581.

Other resources for singing lessons include:

● **www.takelessons.com,** a Web site that connects you to singing teachers in any one of 2,800 cites across the US, or call 877-231-8505.

● **www.singingvoicelessons.com,** which offers the Singing Voice Lessons Series on CD, from voice coach Shelley Kristen.

● **www.easysinginglessons.com,** providing downloadable "Singing Is Easy" lessons.

● *Singing for the Stars: A Complete Program for Training Your Voice* (Alfred Publishing) by Seth Riggs, a book and 2-CD set.

● *Singing for Dummies* (For Dummies) by Pamelia S. Phillips.

Timothy Kelly, author of *Teach Yourself Singing: If You Can Talk, You Can Sing* (CreateSpace), *www.teachyourself singing.com*.

Natural Prescriptions For Laryngitis

There's no mistaking the husky, whispered voice that accompanies laryngitis. Often due to a viral infection, laryngitis also can cause your voice to sound hoarse or crackle into a variety of unexpected pitches. Typically occurring with a sore or dry throat, a cough and, in some cases, fever and fatigue, laryngitis frequently is related to a cold, bronchitis or sinusitis. It also can be due to overuse of the voice or irritation from smoke or air pollution. Because there are so many potential causes of laryngitis, it's a good idea to see your doctor for an exam to rule out a bacterial infection, such as from strep. Fortunately, there are a number of natural strategies that are safe and effective at limiting the length and severity of laryngitis.

Since laryngitis indicates inflammation of the vocal cords, it's crucial to rest your voice as much as possible for several days.

To accelerate healing of laryngitis—or a sore throat (without laryngitis)...

● **Use slippery elm.** This *demulcent* (soothing) herb relieves inflamed mucous membranes including those of the throat. Lozenges, which are available at health-food stores, are probably the most convenient form of slippery elm. Use the lozenges according to the instructions on the label. Another option is slippery elm powder.

How to prepare: Add one teaspoon of slippery elm powder to one-quarter cup of applesauce. Eat this four times a day.

● **Soothe your throat with a botanical spray.** Typically made from demulcent and antiseptic herbs (such as those mentioned below), a throat spray can effectively relieve the symptoms of laryngitis. Look for a botanical throat spray at a health-food store or make your own by combining equal parts of the individual tinctures of echinacea, hyssop, osha and marshmallow.

How to prepare: To six ounces of warm water, add one-half ounce of each tincture. Add two teaspoons of honey and stir until the honey dissolves. Put this mixture in a small spray bottle and spray directly on the back of the throat every two waking hours. (You can store this mixture in a sealed jar.)

● **Try homeopathic remedies.**

Patients have reported very good results when using either of these homeopathic remedies: Causticum, used when hoarseness is accompanied by a raw sore throat and/or cough or a sore throat due to overuse of the voice…or Phosphorus, used when laryngitis is painless or accompanied by extreme thirst and anxiety.

What to do: Take two pellets of a 30C potency of either remedy (under the tongue), 20 minutes before or after eating, twice daily for no more than three days. (Taking the remedy longer may lead to irritation.) If your laryngitis lasts for more than two weeks or recurs every few weeks,

If your laryngitis lasts for more than two weeks or recurs every few weeks, there may be a more serious problem. Heavy smoking, gastroesophageal reflux disease (chronic heartburn) or benign or malignant growths on the vocal cords can lead to chronic laryngitis. See your doctor for an evaluation.

Jamison Starbuck, ND, naturopathic physician in family practice in Missoula, Montana.

Hidden Dangers of Snoring

S noring may not strike you as a serious health problem. But that belief could cause you to unwittingly increase your risk for a variety of medical conditions, including some that are life threatening.

It's been known for some time that the sleep disorder sleep apnea—commonly marked by snoring—is associated with an increased risk for cardiovascular disease, heart failure and stroke. Recent scientific evidence now links sleep apnea to erectile dysfunction and even eye disorders, such as glaucoma.

Latest news: New treatments are relieving sleep apnea symptoms at an unprecedented rate.

Are You at Risk?
Up to 20 million Americans—including one in every five adults over age 60—have sleep apnea, a condition in which breathing intermittently stops and starts during sleep. Most people who have sleep apnea snore—but not all snorers have sleep apnea.

And contrary to popular belief, sleep apnea also can affect women. About 9% of middle-aged women have the disorder and 24% of middle-aged men.

Even Mild Cases Are Dangerous
Doctors once thought that only severe forms of sleep apnea posed cardiovascular risks. Now, research shows that patients who stop breathing more than five times an hour have double or even triple the rate of hypertension as those who breathe normally. With sleep apnea, breathing may stop several dozen or even hundreds of times during the night compared with one to four times an hour during sleep in a healthy adult. The frequent interruptions in breathing that characterize sleep apnea can lead to a potentially harmful decrease in oxygen levels.

What Causes Sleep Apnea

It's not widely known, but there are two forms of sleep apnea...

• **Obstructive sleep apnea (OSA),** the most common form, occurs when the muscles of the throat relax and collapse during sleep, interrupting the flow of air.

• **Obesity is a main cause of OSA.** Fatty deposits surrounding the airways may interfere with breathing, and the weight of excess tissue makes it harder for muscles to retain their normal position during sleep. People with large neck sizes (17 inches or more for men, 16 inches or more for women) are at increased risk.

• **Central apnea,** in which the brain doesn't send the appropriate signals to the respiratory muscles, is relatively rare. It is not associated with obesity and sometimes occurs in the presence of a stroke, which affects brain function.

Sitting and Sleep Apnea

Sitting at a desk all day can cause sleep apnea. When you sit for long periods, blood and water pool in your legs. If you sit long enough and collect a great deal of fluid in your legs, when you lie down to go to sleep, gravity causes this fluid to flow to your neck. In some people, so much fluid moves to their necks that it puts pressure on the throat, causing it to collapse from the pressure, leading to obstructive sleep apnea and making it difficult to breathe and get a good night's sleep.

Self-defense: Take a walk every hour while you're at work to prevent fluid retention in your legs.

T. Douglas Bradley, PhD, professor of medicine and director, Centre for Sleep Medicine and Circadian Biology, University of Toronto, Canada, and leader of a study published in *American Journal of Respiratory and Critical Care Medicine.*

Best Treatment Options

Patients who are slightly overweight and suffer from mild OSA (defined as five to 15 interruptions in breathing per hour) may improve if they lose just a few pounds. Most patients, however, need medical help. *Best approaches for both types of apnea...*

• **Change sleep position.** Up to 50% of patients with mild OSA and 20% of those with a moderate form of the disease (16 to 30 interruptions in breathing per hour) stop breathing only when they sleep on their backs. This form of OSA, positional sleep apnea, can be completely eliminated if the sufferer sleeps on his/her side or stomach.

New development: A product called Zzoma, which is worn around the chest like a belt, has a padded back that prevents people from sleeping on their backs. Developed by researchers at Temple University School of Medicine, Zzoma has been approved by the FDA for patients diagnosed with "positional snoring." It is available at *www.zzomasleep.com.*

Cost: $69.95.

Other treatments (all are available at medical-supply stores)...*

• **Continuous positive airway pressure (CPAP).** This is the standard treatment for OSA and central apnea.

How it works: CPAP delivers room air under pressure through a mask to a patient's nose and/or mouth. The slightly pressurized flow of air helps keep the airways open and helps prevent snoring as well as apnea.

CPAP can be uncomfortable because patients must wear a mask all night. For this reason, the device is used as prescribed—for example, worn all night, every night—only about half of the time.

Helpful: Before choosing a CPAP device, try on different masks until you find one that's comfortable enough to wear all night.

*You should undergo a sleep evaluation at a sleep disorders clinic before buying one of these devices. Insurance won't pay for the device unless you've been diagnosed with sleep apnea by a doctor. To find a sleep disorders clinic near you, consult the American Academy of Sleep Medicine (708-492-0930, *www.aasmnet.org*).

Typical cost: Starting at about $200.

Alternative: Some people with mild OSA prefer to wear a nighttime oral device, such as the Thornton Adjustable Positioner (TAP), which moves the lower jaw forward so that the tongue and throat tissue don't block the airway. The TAP is available online for about $1,800.

• **Bi-level positive airway pressure (Bi-PAP)** is similar to CPAP, except the machine delivers more air pressure when patients inhale and less when they exhale. This is helpful for OSA patients who find it uncomfortable to exhale "against" air pressure—and for obese patients who tend to breathe too shallowly.

Cost: Starting at about $800.

• **Adaptive servo-ventilation (ASV)** is an air-flow approach that also involves wearing a mask. An ASV unit, which is used for central apnea, analyzes normal breathing patterns and stores the data in a computer. If a patient stops breathing, the machine automatically delivers pressurized air—and then stops when the patient's normal breathing resumes.

Cost: About $7,000.

If You Still Need Help

For most sleep apnea patients, surgery is a last resort. It makes a significant difference in only 20% to 30% of cases.

Common procedures...

• **Uvulopalatopharyngoplasty (UPPP)** involves removing tissue from the back of the mouth and the top of the throat. This procedure often stops snoring, but is less effective at eliminating frequent interruptions in breathing during sleep.

• **The Pillar,** a relatively new procedure, involves the placement of small synthetic rods in the soft palate in the mouth. The rods stiffen the tissue and reduce sagging during sleep. Like UPPP, it's effective primarily for snoring.

Samuel Krachman, DO, professor of medicine and director of the Sleep Disorders Center in the division of pulmonary and critical care medicine at Temple University School of Medicine in Philadelphia.

Chapter 15

SKIN CONDITIONS

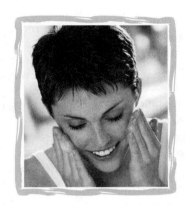

A Dream Come True—Erase Wrinkles While You Sleep

It's Dermatological Utopia. You go to sleep and wake up in the morning with fewer wrinkles—having done nothing more than spent the night with your face resting on your pillowcase.

Well, that's exactly what a new study in the *International Journal of Cosmetic Science* says can happen—if the pillowcase you're sleeping on has fibers that have been treated with *copper oxide*, a mineral that can regenerate skin.

The Power of Copper

The study, led by Gadi Borkow, PhD, was conducted at a medical center affiliated with the prestigious Hebrew University of Jerusalem Medical School.

Fifty-seven people (55 women and 2 men, aged 40 to 60) were divided into two groups.

For one month, one group slept on a pillowcase treated with 0.4% copper oxide. The other group slept on a look-alike "placebo" pillowcase that hadn't been treated with copper.

At the beginning of the study, two weeks later, and at the end of the month, each person had three photographs of their face taken—from the right, left and front. Each time photos were taken, a dermatologist and cosmetologist looked at the photographs and graded each person from 1 (none) to 5 (severe) based on:

- Wrinkles
- Crow's feet and fine lines
- Blemishes
- Skin glow
- Texture
- Overall appearance

Result: After two weeks, those sleeping on the copper pillowcases had a significant decrease in wrinkles, in crow's feet and fine lines and an improvement in general appearance, compared with the non-copper group.

By the end of the four weeks, the copper group had continued improvement in wrinkle reduction…fewer crow's feet and fine lines…new improvements in skin texture… and overall better general appearance.

A Safe Stabilizer of Protein

How it works: Copper helps synthesize and stabilize collagen, the protein that maintains firm, youthful-looking skin, explains Dr. Borkow. It also stabilizes *fibronectin,* a protein that strengthens cell-to-cell connections.

"Triggered by the humidity of the face, the copper oxide ions are released slowly from the pillowcase into the skin, affecting collagen and fibronectin, which leads to a fresher, younger appearance," he says.

Important: Copper—an essential trace mineral found in foods and nutritional supplements, and in many medical devices—is very safe, says Dr. Borkow.

There are a few, rare reports of copper allergy in the medical literature, but the allergy was usually due to an impurity in copper rather than the copper itself.

The Pillowcase

You can purchase the pillowcase—the Cupron Anti-Aging Appearance-Enhancing Satin Pillowcase—at the Cupron Web site (*www. cupronsales.com*), and other online stores, or at retail stores such as Bed, Bath & Beyond. (Also called the SkinGlow Cupron Copper Technology Pillow Protector.)

"Using this pillowcase along with moisturizers and other anti-aging skin care products will produce the best results in controlling and reversing skin aging," says Dr. Borkow.

Red flag: A silicon-containing, laundry "softener" deactivates the copper ions in the pillowcase.

Gadi Borkow, PhD, virologist and professor, Hebrew University of Jerusalem Medical School.

Antioxidant Creams That Smooth Aging Skin

Anti-aging creams are big business in both the cosmetic and natural-health industries. Everyone wants healthy, youthful-looking skin.

Antioxidants for Damage Control

When it comes to anti-aging products, some of the most popular natural creams contain *antioxidants*, nutrients that neutralize harmful molecules called free radicals. We associate antioxidants with foods, particularly fruits and vegetables, that can reduce *oxidative stress* (an increase in cell-damaging free radicals caused by stress, eating fried and processed foods, and breathing pollutants) and subsequent inflammation.

The same idea applies when these nutrients are in topical form—what is good inside the body also is good outside. Our skin incurs oxidative damage from excessive sun exposure and through *glycation,* a process in which dietary sugar alters the molecular structure of collagen and other skin components. Eventually, in the course of normal aging, these factors overwhelm the skin's natural antioxidant capability.

Contrary to moisturizers that provide on-the-surface fixes (such as mineral oil, which slows evaporation of water from the skin), antioxidant creams work at the cellular level, making lasting changes to the skin and reducing wrinkles and blemishes. As with many products on the market, the potency of antioxidant creams varies.

For best results, try products that contain one or two of the antioxidants noted on page 292. (Or try the products recommended.) Give the product a chance to work. Don't expect any changes in a week. Instead, use it for six to 10 weeks. Then check to see whether there is a noticeable improvement in the quality of your skin. Look to see if blemishes have diminished and if your skin is softer, clearer or more radiant. If there is no improvement, try a different anti-aging cream formulation.

Big News on Natural Wrinkle Reversers

"Many natural compounds can reduce inflammation and oxidation, which drive the aging process in the skin and throughout the body," says Alan Logan, ND, a naturopathic physician in Connecticut and coauthor of *Your Skin, Younger: New Science Secrets to Reverse the Effects of Age* (Cumberland House). "Taken orally or applied topically, these compounds also help protect the skin against 'photoaging' and 'photodamage' from the UVB and UVA radiation of sunlight."

Here are highlights from recent research on natural compounds that help control skin aging.

●**Korean ginseng (red ginseng).** Korean researchers gave an herbal product containing Korean ginseng to 82 women over 40, for six months. By the end of the study, "facial wrinkles were significantly improved," say the researchers.

Dr. Logan recommends 200 milligrams (mg) a day of a standardized extract.

●*Glycosaminoglycans* **(GAGs from fish cartilage).** "GAGs are small peptides, or protein complexes, that make their way to the deeper, or *dermal* layer of the skin, where they are used as raw material for building collagen," says Dr. Logan.

In a study on GAGs, researchers in Thailand divided 60 women, age 35 to 60, into two groups. One group took a supplement with GAGs (which also contained several antioxidants, such as Coenzyme Q10). The other took a placebo.

After three months, those taking the supplement had a 21% improvement in fine wrinkles and depth of skin roughness, compared with a 1.7% improvement in the placebo group.

Product: Radiance, from Blackmores, which you can purchase online at *www.blackmores.com.au/products*.

●**Dead sea minerals.** Researchers in Israel tested a product containing Dead Sea mud and water—"known for their unique composition of minerals, and their therapeutic properties on psoriasis and other inflammatory skin diseases"—on human skin cells exposed to UVB radiation.

They found the Dead Sea combo preserved cell-protecting antioxidants, limited the production of inflammatory compounds called cytokines by 70%, and, in general, kept the skin cells more "viable."

"The minerals magnesium, calcium and zinc are probably the key antioxidant and anti-inflammatory players in this mud pack," says Dr. Logan.

Product: Dermud, from Ahava, which is widely available in retail specialty stores and online.

●**Multi-ingredient anti-aging cream.** Noting that "very few over-the-counter cosmetic anti-aging products have been subjected to a rigorous trial of efficacy," researchers in England decided to test one of them—No7 Protect & Perfect Intense Beauty Serum, from Alliance Boots Ltd, a UK company. (The product contains a range of nutrients, herbs and other natural compounds, including vitamin E, vitamin A, ginseng, white mulberry and white lupin.)

They studied 60 photoaged (skin damaged by prolonged exposure to the sun) people, dividing them into two groups—one used the anti-aging cream every day for six months, and one used a fake, lookalike placebo cream.

After the first six months, 43% of those using the product had an improvement in their facial wrinkles, compared with 22% of those using the placebo.

No7 Protect & Perfect Intense Beauty Serum is widely available in retail and online stores.

Bonus: These natural skin ingredients are all considered very safe. If any product causes skin irritation or redness, stop using it and try another.

To Enhance Moisture Content

• **Vitamin C.** This well-known antioxidant was one of the first to be used in anti-aging creams. A Brazilian study showed that vitamin C (*ascorbic acid*) and several of its derivatives enhanced skin moisture content when it was applied daily for four weeks. A review of studies conducted by a US researcher concluded that vitamin C is effective for treating photoaging (sun damage) and that combining it with other vitamins (A, B-3 and E) is more effective than using individual compounds.

Good brands: Avalon Organics Vitamin C Renewal Facial Cream (877-263-9456, *www.avalonorganics.com*, $20.95 for two ounces)...or MyChelle Dermaceuticals, The Perfect C Serum, All Skin Types (800-447-2076, *www.mychelle.com*, $41.79 for 0.5 ounce). These products may seem expensive, but they last for a long time because you apply just a pea-size dab at a time.

Best for: Dry, sun-damaged skin.

To Restore Elasticity

• **Green tea.** When ingested, green tea protects us against illness, including cardiovascular disease, diabetes and even some cancers. So it isn't surprising to find out that it also can help the skin.

A study conducted at Emory University found that an eight-week regimen of a topical cream containing 10% green-tea extract and a 300-mg twice-daily green-tea oral supplement resulted in tissue improvements that could be seen under a microscope, although the improvements were not visible to the naked eye. Researchers noted that it may take longer than eight weeks to see visible improvements.

Good brands: Green Tea Skin Natural Anti-Aging Cream (781-326-1700, *www.greenteaskin.com*, $19.95 for 1.7 ounces)...or OriginBioMed Green Tea Skin Cream (888-234-7256, *www.originbiomed.com*, $34.95 for 0.7 ounce).

Plus: Take 600 mg daily of an oral green-tea supplement.

Best for: Wrinkles, age-related loss of skin elasticity.

To Smooth Wrinkles and Improve Skin Health

• **Coenzyme Q10 (CoQ10).** This natural substance exists in every cell of the body and is a popular ingredient in anti-aging creams. Several studies indicate that it may be able to enhance the skin's ability to combat signs of aging at the cellular level—for example, making skin cells look younger. At an American Academy of Dermatology meeting, researchers reported that CoQ10 cream seemed to reduce fine wrinkles around the eyes without harmful side effects, such as itching.

Good brands: Avalon Organics CoQ10 Wrinkle Defense Night Creme (877-263-9456, *www.avalonorganics.com*, $24.95 for 1.75 ounces)...or Botanic Spa CoQ-10 Wrinkle Cream (800-644-8327, *www.botanicchoice.com*, $14.99 for two ounces).

Mark A. Stengler, NMD, naturopathic medical doctor in private practice, La Jolla, California, and author of the *Bottom Line/Natural Healing* newsletter. *www.drstengler.com*.

Skin Infections That Are Often Overlooked

MRSA (*methicillin-resistant Staphylococcus aureus*), once a threat primarily in hospitals, long-term-care facilities and other health-care settings, is now appearing in a slightly mutated form in gyms, schools, military barracks and other settings where people may have skin-to-skin contact and/or share towels, linens or other items that can become contaminated. MRSA may turn life-threatening if the bacteria penetrate the skin, become blood-borne and reach other areas of the body, such as the heart or lungs.

What most people don't realize: The skin can harbor dozens of infectious organisms.

Example: The average handprint on a dinner plate might contain up to 35 species of bacteria, viruses or fungi.

Most of these organisms are harmless—and even those that are capable of causing disease are usually blocked from entering the body by the skin's protective barrier and/or destroyed by immune cells just beneath the skin's surface.

Danger: The skin typically has thousands of microscopic nicks or other openings that provide entry points for harmful germs—even if you don't have an obvious cut. To help prevent harmful bacteria from entering these tiny openings, wash your hands often with mild soap and warm water, and shave carefully. *Infections to avoid…**

Cellulitis

This skin infection, which can be mistaken for a scrape, bruise or spider bite, is caused by bacteria that enter the body through dry, flaky and/or cracked skin or other skin openings such as those caused by a cut, splinter or surgical wound.

Cellulitis typically occurs on the legs but can occur anywhere on the body—even on your hand. The infection usually originates in the upper layers (the *dermis* and *epidermis*) of the skin but can also occur in deeper (*subcutaneous*) tissues, including the muscles and muscle linings. Infections in deeper tissues are more likely to cause serious symptoms and extensive tissue damage, such as severe swelling and pain, and formation of abscesses. Everyone is at risk for cellulitis, but those with weakened immunity (such as diabetes and dialysis patients) are at greatest risk.

What to look for: The affected area will be red, hot and tender. The redness spreads very quickly, and you may develop a fever (101°F or higher) and body aches. If the infection is severe, confusion or fecal inconti-

---

*To see examples of the many ways these infections can appear on the body, go to www.images.google.com and type in the name of each infection. Beware: Many of the images are graphic.

nence also may occur. People with any of the severe symptoms described earlier should seek immediate medical care at a hospital emergency department.

Treatment: Oral antibiotics, such as *dicloxacillin* (Dycill) or *cephalexin* (Keflex). These are effective against *Streptococcus* and about half of the *Staphylococcus* organisms—common causes of cellulitis—and usually start to relieve symptoms within two days. Patients with more severe infections may require hospitalization and intravenous antibiotics.

To reduce your risk of developing cellulitis: Take a daily shower or bath. People who wash often and use plenty of mild soap are less likely to develop cellulitis or other skin infections.

Necrotizing Infections

The media often refer to these infections as "flesh-eating." This isn't entirely accurate. Several bacterial species can cause the *necrosis* (death) of infected tissue, but the bacteria don't eat the flesh, per se. Rather, they secrete toxins that break it down.

Necrotizing infections are rare—fewer than 1,000 cases occur each year in the US—but the fatality rate is quite high at 25 to 30%. These infections spread very rapidly—if you marked the edge of an infection with a pen, you might see the redness creep past the mark in as little as one hour.

What to look for: Skin redness and/or swelling that's warm to the touch. The initial infection, which can follow even a minor cut or puncture wound, resembles cellulitis. But a necrotizing infection is far more painful. As the infection progresses, you may develop very large, fluid-filled purple blisters (*bullae*), a high fever (104°F or higher), disorientation and a rapid heartbeat. If you develop any of these symptoms, seek immediate medical attention at a hospital emergency department.

Treatment: Intravenous antibiotics and surgery, sometimes requiring amputation, to remove infected tissue.

To reduce your risk of developing a necrotizing infection: Thoroughly clean even minor cuts and scrapes. Apply an over-the-counter antibiotic ointment, such as Neosporin or bacitracin, and keep the area covered with a clean dressing until the area is completely healed.

Folliculitis

This skin infection occurs at the root of a hair (follicle) and may produce a small pimple—or, less often, a larger, more painful pimple called a boil. Folliculitis tends to be more common in people with diabetes (which reduces resistance to infection) and those who live in hot, humid climates (excessive perspiration promotes growth of the bacterium that causes folliculitis).

What to look for: A small, white pimple at the base of a hair. Boils, also called abscesses, are larger than pimples (sometimes an inch or more in diameter), with a greater volume of pus. They tend to be warmer than the surrounding skin and can be intensely painful.

Treatment: The small pimples caused by folliculitis often disappear on their own within several days. Applying a topical antibiotic several times a day can prevent the infection from spreading. Apply a warm, moist compress (for 15 minutes four times daily for one to two days) to tender pimples or boils to help them drain.

Painful or unusually large boils should be lanced, drained and cleaned by a doctor. Do not "pop" them yourself. The risk for infection is high—and boils can be caused by MRSA. Antibiotics usually aren't necessary when boils are professionally drained and cleaned.

To reduce your risk of developing folliculitis: Wash your hands several times daily with soap...and take a daily shower or bath. If you have chronic, recurrent boils, use antibacterial soap.

Lawrence Eron, MD, associate professor of medicine at the John A. Burns School of Medicine at the University of Hawaii in Honolulu and infectious disease consultant at Kaiser Foundation Hospital, also in Honolulu.

Itchy Skin? Play a Computer Game

Our first natural response to any itch is a scratch. But that's not the best way to go...especially if the itch is incessant. There are three common skin conditions that can cause a lot of itching:

• **Eczema,** or what doctors call atopic dermatitis, a genetic disorder that afflicts 20 million Americans with dry skin that becomes severely itchy, itchy, itchy...

• **Psoriasis,** an autoimmune disorder that produces patches of red, flaky, scaly lesions that can crack, bleed, hurt and itch, itch, itch...

• **Hives,** a reaction to stress or an allergen (such as a food, medication or dye), triggering the cellular release of *histamine*, which produces red bumps on the skin that itch, itch, itch...

Or you could have a chronic illness such as diabetes, liver disease or kidney disease that has among its bothersome symptoms itching, itching, itching...

You find yourself scratching, scratching, scratching...

And before long, you also may find yourself caught up in what medical experts call the itch-scratch cycle.

What happens: Although scratching temporarily relieves the itch, it also irritates already irritated skin, causing more itching, more scratching and more itching—in a cycle that produces redder, sorer, infected skin that never stabilizes or heals.

Is There a Way Out?

"The first step in treating any itch should be a good medical evaluation," says Ted Grossbart, PhD, a clinical psychologist in Boston, assistant professor of psychology at Harvard Medical School and author of *Skin Deep: A Mind/Body Program for Healthy Skin* (Health Press).

"Your dermatologist or allergist may discover 'trigger factors' in your diet and environment, and encourage you to minimize or eliminate them. He may suggest wearing different clothes or washing them in a different detergent and avoiding certain foods and chemicals. If there is an underlying disease, such as diabetes, he will refer you to a specialist for treatment."

Beyond that, medical care simply aims to reduce the itch itself, he explains. Anti-itch baths and tar ointments suppress inflammation and lubricate the skin. Antihistamines such as *hydroxyzine* (Atarax) relieve some itching. The most frequently used drugs are the *corticosteroids,* such as *cortisone,* which reduce the inflammation that intensifies itching.

However: "For many people, these conventional approaches are not enough," says Dr. Grossbart.

Best: "Psychological techniques can relieve itching, regardless of its medical cause," he says.

And one of those techniques is distraction. "Imagine what would happen to your itching if a tiger walked into your room—your itching would instantly go to the 'back burner,'" says Dr. Grossbart. "That's because itching has no ultimate physical reality. Like pain, it's an experience, not a disease—so substituting another, distracting experience can temporarily relieve it."

And in a recent study, Israeli scientists tried to find out what kind of distracting experience might work best.

Distraction Techniques

Noting that "pharmacological means of therapy have not yet provided satisfactory results for the cure of itching and its link to the desire to scratch," researchers in the Department of Dermatology at Hadassah University Hospital in Jerusalem used a nondrug method to treat 24 people with eczema and psoriasis and help "break the vicious itch/scratch cycle."

They divided them into two groups. One group practiced a distraction technique using "virtual reality immersion"—playing a computer game while wearing a special visor and headphones (earbuds) that blocked out all distractions. The other group played the same game without the visor and earbuds.

Result: Both distraction techniques reduced the feeling of itching—the virtual reality technique by 78%, and the computer game without the extra equipment by 50%.

"Both methods of distraction captured the attention of patients as they focused their concentration on playing the interactive computer game, which resulted in a significant reduction of reported intensity of itch, and scratching that was mostly absent or mild," say the researchers, in *Pain Research & Management.*

But, add the researchers, a computer game without virtual reality equipment is "easier to use, cheaper to obtain," and perhaps already available in your home.

Helpful: "Itching is most severe during the evenings and nights, when people are free to concentrate on their symptoms," say the researchers. "Some patients who complain of nighttime itching make use of extremely harmful measures, such as very hot showers and applications of lemon juice to get relief. The audiovisual distraction method may serve to shorten itching episodes at night."

Redirect Your Spotlight

"Distraction works because attention is like a spotlight," explains Dr. Grossbart. "If your attention is on the itching, you feel it. If the spotlight swings to something else, the itching recedes into the shadows.

"For example, if you get a mosquito bite at a fascinating garden party, you barely notice it. If you get a mosquito bite during the middle of the night, that itch might be all you think about, and it gets worse and worse."

● **Mindfulness works.** Along with distraction techniques, Dr. Grossbart also recommends mindfulness techniques—rather than not paying attention to the itch, you pay attention to it in a different way.

"Often, if you can focus on the itch, and sit on your hands for a couple of seconds—if you observe it with detachment and compassion, rather than do anything about it—you can take some of the sharpness out of it," he says.

One way to observe the itch is by rating its severity from 1 to 10. "Just doing that—just that degree of objectivity—can provide quite a bit of relief."

Dr. Grossbart describes another psychological method that he created and uses with his patients:

●**Scratching hand to soothing hand.** You've been trying to stop scratching with willpower? It simply doesn't work. Your itch keeps building, keeps calling out for help. Your hand finally reaches to relieve it, almost of its own accord. The hand is quicker than the will.

Rather than struggling to restrain your scratching hand, you can convert it, turning it into a powerful ally. You can use this technique as you would use steroid cream to gain control over your itch. Once you break the cycle, you may find that your skin heals itself.

First, enter into a state of relaxation, or what Dr. Grossbart calls the "healing state."

●**Close your eyes.** Let all your muscles loosen and relax. Breathe evenly. As you breathe out, say the word "one" to yourself. As distracting thoughts enter your head, ignore them, without struggling to push them away. Keep repeating "one" to yourself every time you breathe out. Do the exercise for a few minutes.

Now, imagine your hand as a deep reservoir of whatever sensations are most healing and soothing for your skin. When your hand is full almost to the bursting point, move it to each of the areas that sometimes itch. Just rest the soothing hand lightly on your skin. You needn't rub or press. Feel the soothing sensations flow out your fingers, taking over so totally that there is no room at all for an itch. Give each area as much help as it needs. If your hand needs replenishing, just take it away from your skin and let it fill up again.

Focus on the idea that your scratching hand will be automatically transformed into a soothing hand.

Go through this procedure at least daily, preferably twice a day.

Be prepared for a discouraging period before you master this challenging but ultimately effortless mental magic. When it works—when your hand reaches for an itch and automatically soothes with a touch— you'll feel more like an amazed spectator than someone who's "broken a habit" by heroic willpower.

Important: There are many different psychological methods that can help overcome the itch-scratch cycle, says Dr. Grossbart.

"Try a number of them and find out what works for you."

You'll find those methods in Dr. Grossbart's free e-book available on his Web site. The book also teaches the relaxation and self-hypnosis techniques.

(For more information on self hypnosis, see page 19 in "Aches and Pains.")

Ted Grossbart, PhD, clinical psychologist in Boston, assistant professor of psychology at Harvard Medical School and author of *Skin Deep: A Mind/Body Program for Healthy Skin* (Health Press). *www.grossbart.com.*

The Whole-Body Cure For Chronic Hives

I f you're one of the millions of Americans with repeated outbreaks of hives—histamine-sparked eruptions of raised, red and very itchy bumps—you've probably been to doctor after doctor, trying to find relief.

You've received prescriptions for antihistamines to short-circuit the outbreaks, and for topical medications such as steroid creams to ease the itching.

You've had allergy tests to detect the allergen—the food, food additive, medication or other factor that is supposedly triggering the outbreaks. But if you're like 95% of people with hives, the allergen was never found.

Maybe you even have to carry an EpiPen with injectable epinephrine (*adrenaline*), just in case an outbreak of hives cascades out of control into anaphylactic shock, with your tongue and throat swelling up so much you can't breathe.

And in spite of all that, your hives still aren't under control. In fact, you feel really bad. And not just when you're having another one of those maddeningly itchy outbreaks.

"I've never seen a case of chronic hives where the person isn't also generally ill—with allergies, digestive problems and constant fatigue," says Kamila Kingston, a certified practitioner of Traditional Chinese Medicine (TCM) at the White Lotus Cosmetic Acupuncture and Longevity Center in Brisbane, Australia. "Most of these people have been in the medical mill for 10 to 15 years, seeing doctor after doctor, trying everything that's medically recommended, while their problem gets worse and worse."

But a recent scientific study shows that an alternative treatment for chronic hives may be more effective than the conventional treatments of modern medicine.

That treatment is *acupuncture*—small, pain-free needles are placed strategically along invisible channels of energy called *meridians*, unblocking and balancing the flow of energy, which restores ease and harmony to the body, alleviating symptoms.

70% Reduction

Doctors in the Department of Acupuncture and Moxibustion at the Chinese Academy of Chinese Medical Sciences in Beijing treated 31 people with chronic hives. Their patients were four to 82 years old, and hives had bothered them anywhere from one month to 30 years.

The doctors explain that acupuncture treats both the hives—"the incidental"—and the imbalances underlying the hives—"the fundamental." And the treatment works.

Of the 31 people treated, eight were cured—they had no more outbreaks.

Another 17 were improved—they had at least a 70% reduction in number of hives, longer time between outbreaks and their symptoms (such as itching) were alleviated.

Overall, 25 of the 31 people treated—81%—experienced significant relief.

How it works: In their study, the doctors point out that the main cause of hives is a body weakened by deficiencies of *qi* (pronounced CHEE) and blood.

"Qi is the fundamental energy in the body and in the universe," explains Kingston. "When there isn't enough qi, the body isn't able to make sufficient blood. A deficiency of qi and blood causes fundamental weakness in the internal organs, which produces symptoms such as hives."

Better Than Western Medicine

"In my experience, Chinese medicine is better than Western medicine at treating long-standing problems such as chronic hives," says Kingston.

●**Find a practitioner.** She recommends finding a practitioner of Traditional Chinese Medicine (TCM) who specializes in skin disorders, and who uses both acupuncture and Chinese herbal medicine, which she says go hand-in-hand in treating qi and blood deficiency.

Resource: To find a practitioner of TCM near you, go to the Web site of the National Certification Commission for Acupuncture and Oriental Medicine (*www.nccaom.org*) and click the link "Find a Practioner." You can then search by country, state and zip code.

(Please see page 23, in the chapter "Aches and Pains," for more information about ways to find a good acupuncturist. See appendix page 354 for more general information on acupuncture.)

●**Understand the treatment isn't short-term.** In the study, the doctors followed up on the patients six months later, and found that those experiencing a recurrence of hives had stopped their acupuncture treatments after about one month, as soon as the outbreaks cleared up. "This suggests that continuous treatment after alleviation of the symptoms is effective for decreasing recurrences of hives," they say.

"Treatment for a chronic problem is not short-term," agrees Kingston. "Within the first month, you should start to notice an improvement in the frequency and intensity of your outbreaks. But for long-term relief—to address the underlying qi and blood deficiency, so that the problem doesn't come back—

you probably need a minimum of three to six months of acupuncture, with a treatment every three to four weeks.

"Your health and energy levels are going to improve so much, that you'll probably be happy to continue the treatments!"

● **Don't stop conventional treatment on your own.** "As symptoms decrease, it will be natural to use less medication, with your dermatologist's approval and supervision," says Kingston.

"Since most conventional doctors have tried everything for their patients without avail, they're usually very happy to cooperate with the TCM practitioner in this way. And once the medications are lessened, the practitioner can begin to introduce Chinese herbal medicines.

"Acupuncture and Chinese herbal medicine—by addressing the symptoms and the imbalances causing the symptoms—can give hope to hopeless, suffering people with chronic hives, who've probably concluded nothing will ever solve their problem."

Kamila Kingston, certified practitioner of Traditional Chinese Medicine (TCM) at the White Lotus Cosmetic Acupuncture and Longevity Center in Brisbane, Australia. *www.whitelotus.com.au*.

Rescue Your Winter Skin

By the time February rolls around, your skin has been contending with months of dry indoor heating and bitter outdoor air. (Even in temperate climates, temperature dips take a toll.) Dryness, flaking and cracking may have set in—and more extreme problems can arise, such as eczema and other types of inflammation. *Natural solutions to help you well past the cold weather...*

● **Skip long showers and baths.** Lengthy exposure to hot water strips away the skin's natural moisture. Limit showers and baths to no more than five minutes.

● **Use mild soaps.** Commercial products may contain harsh, drying chemicals. Try mild soaps with *Calendula officinalis* (marigold), a botanical that promotes healing. One good product is made by Weleda (800-241-1030, *www.usa.weleda.com*). Scented soaps can irritate sensitive skin. Until spring, consider switching to an unscented soap, such as Dove Sensitive Skin Unscented Beauty Bar.

● **Apply a moisturizer with a humectant.** Moisturizing is a must. Look for lotions that contain humectants, such as glycerine, sorbitol and alpha-hydroxy acids that attract moisture to the skin.

Good choice: Aveeno Skin Relief Moisturizing Cream (available in drugstores and at *www.drugstore.com*).

● **Relieve the driest patches.** For especially distressed areas, such as fingertips, that are cracked, painful, even bleeding, apply topical creams. Try salves or repair creams made by Burt's Bees (866-422-8787, *www.burtsbees.com*).

● **Take oral supplements for severely dry skin.** For excessive discomfort, including itchiness or cracking, try fish oil—1,500 mg of combined *eicosapentaenoic acid* (EPA) and *docosahexaenoic acid* (DHA)—plus 1,000 mg of *gamma linoleic acid* (GLA). Together, they help the skin retain moisture.

Mark A. Stengler, NMD, naturopathic medical doctor in private practice, La Jolla, California, and author of the *Bottom Line/Natural Healing* newsletter. *www.drstengler.com*.

Clothes That Can Save Your Skin

Here comes the sun, and it's all right, sang the Beatles.

But if the band members had been four dermatologists, they would have been singing, *Here comes the sun, and it's not all right for you to be outside without adequate protection...*

Warning: A lifetime of exposure to the ultraviolet-B (UVB) rays of the sun can scramble the DNA in skin cells, triggering a *squamous cell* or *basal cell carcinoma*, the two skin cancers that account for 95% of all cases. (The link between sun exposure and *melanoma*—the deadliest skin cancer—is still a matter of debate among scientists, though most believe that excessive sun exposure raises the risk for some types of this cancer.)

And even if you don't get cancer, you get older faster. Those DNA-damaging rays gradually shred protein fibers in the skin called *elastin*. Eventually, once-firm skin stretches and sags, creasing your body with wrinkles. (Sun damage can also cause age spots, dilated blood vessels and sallow coloring.)

Maybe you're sun-savvy and slather on sunscreen every day, particularly during the summer, when UVB rays are at their most direct and damaging.

But can the color of the clothes you wear provide maximum protection from UVB?

A new study from scientists in sunny Spain provides the answer.

Blue and Red Are Best

The team researchers tested different colored cotton clothing to find out which were the best at blocking UVB rays.

The winners: blue and red.

The loser: yellow.

"The color of cotton woven fabrics is a factor that has a remarkable influence on their protection against ultraviolet rays," say the scientists, in *Industrial & Engineering Chemistry Research.*

What happens: Darker colors absorb more UVB rays, explains Ascension Riva, PhD, the study leader. (Even though it wasn't tested in this study, black is the most protective color, she says.)

"People think that any piece of clothing will sufficiently protect them from the UV radiation of the sun, and that's not true," she adds. "The lighter and more porous the fabric, the less it will protect."

Sun-Protection Laundry Secrets

"Yes, the sun's UV rays can go right through your clothes," says Cynthia Bailey, MD, a dermatologist in private practice in Sebastopol, California.

Problem: One-third of what you wear during the summer does not protect you, she adds.

That includes clothes with these types of fabrics…

- Light colors
- Lightweight and thin
- Cotton
- Linen
- Rayon
- Wet and stretched (*example:* wet cotton T-shirt)

However: "Fuzzy, new, unbleached cotton sometimes provides good sun protection when it's dry," she says.

Wear protective fabrics as much as possible. To provide maximum protection, consider wearing fabrics that are more protective, she says. *They include…*

- Dark colors
- Thick and tightly woven threads
- Polyester
- Nylon
- Wool

Unfortunately, points out Dr. Bailey, these are just the type of clothes you're least likely to wear during the summer.

But don't give up. You can wash some extra sun protection into your light-colored, lightweight summer clothes.

- **Wash your laundry in Sun Guard.** "This product contains *Tinosorb*, which binds to fabric and absorbs UV rays," says Dr. Bailey. "I've used it many times—in the washing machine, and in a hotel sink to wash a new cotton knit shirt while on vacation—and it's never damaged or changed the look of a fabric."

The protection lasts for 19 launderings, she says.

- **Use a laundry detergent with an "optical brightener."** The optical brightener absorbs UV rays, releasing the energy as "fluorescence"—which is why your clothes look brighter, she explains.

●**Don't bleach.** It decreases sun protection, so try to avoid it, especially for cotton and rayon, she says.

●**Buy sun-protective clothing.** For sun-intensive activities—like hiking, gardening and cycling—consider buying special sun protective clothing from companies such as REI, Sun Precautions or Coolibar, says Dr. Bailey. "Sun protective garments often contain hidden vents and zippers that open for ventilation, plus other clever tricks to keep you cool in sunny, hot places."

Resources: The Web site of REI is *www. rei.com*, and includes a store locator. The Web site of online retailer Sun Precautions is *www.sunprecautions.com*. The Web site of online retailer Coolibar is *www.coolibar. com.*

Follow these other sun-guarding precautions. Dr. Bailey counsels her patients—many of whom have precancerous lesions, or who have already had skin cancer—to make use of the following strategies to minimize sun exposure...

●**Use multiple forms of sun protection, rather than just one.** "Wear sunscreen, a hat, sun-protecting clothes and stand in the shade," says Dr. Bailey. "It's these multiple forms of sun protection that allow you to avoid having to reapply sunscreen every two hours, which is the standard recommendation, but which few people ever do." (However, she adds, multiple applications are important if you're out in the sun for extended periods of time, or after you've gotten wet.)

●**Be prepared in advance.** Put your sunscreen on first thing in the morning, and keep an extra hat and sun umbrella in the car, she says.

●**Use the best sunscreen ingredient.** It's 5% micronized zinc oxide. It provides excellent protection, she says, has almost no risk of side effects (unlike chemical sunscreens) and blends into the skin completely, without

leaving a white residue. And it provides protection from ultraviolet-A (UVA), which also damages skin, and is a year-round threat.

Bottom line: "Learn the practical strategies that work for you in everyday life to minimize sun exposure, and put them into place," says Dr. Bailey.

Ascension Riva, PhD, professor, Universitat Politècnica de Catalunya, Terrassa, Spain.

Cynthia Bailey, MD, dermatologist in private practice in Sebastopol, California. *www.otbskincare.com*.

Beta-Carotene for Better Sun Protection

In a new meta-analysis of seven studies, researchers at Münster University Hospital in Germany found that oral beta-carotene supplements help protect against sunburn. How long you take these is key, however—protective benefits kicked in at 10 weeks, and the longer a person had been taking supplements, the more protective benefit they received. Scientists also stressed that beta-carotene alone is not the answer to sunburn prevention. With an equivalent SPF (sun protection factor) of four, at most, it should be used in addition to—not instead of—regular sunscreen.

Andrew L. Rubman, ND, explains that as an antioxidant, beta-carotene helps your body better withstand a variety of free radical challenges, including those posed by exposure to the sun's ultraviolet (UV) rays. UV radiation consists of particles of energy called *photons*—when these strike and penetrate your skin, they set off oxidative changes that can damage tissue. Beta-carotene makes your skin more resistant to these harmful effects.

Practice Sun Smarts

Sun exposure is a must for good health. Your body needs a daily dose of at least 15 minutes to produce the vitamin D you need for bone growth, immune resistance and other physiological and mental processes. It's nonetheless important to avoid painful and potentially dangerous sunburn—apply water-resistant sunscreen with an SPF of at least 15 every two hours...wear protective clothing such as wide-brimmed hats and long-sleeved cover-ups...and seek shade as appropriate, especially when the sun's rays are at their most intense between 10 a.m. and 4 p.m.

If you want to add beta-carotene to your sun protection plan, a daily dose shouldn't exceed six to 15 milligrams. Better than supplements, however, is to get your beta-carotene from dietary sources—consume five servings of fruits and vegetables daily, which naturally provide six to eight milligrams of beta-carotene. Carrots, green leafy vegetables, sweet potatoes, winter squash, cantaloupe and broccoli are all rich dietary sources.

Andrew L. Rubman, ND, medical director, Southbury Clinic for Traditional Medicines, Southbury, Connecticut. www.southburyclinic.com.

Three Alternative Remedies for Bruises

After you've been bumped and know a bruise is on the way, reduce swelling by applying an ice pack to the area—about 30 seconds on and 30 seconds off three times—twice daily. Rub one teaspoon of arnica lotion or oil into the area three times daily for five days to alleviate swelling and stimulate the healing action of white blood cells. Also, take 500 mg of the herb gotu kola three times daily for two days to help skin cells knit together. (Products are sold in health-food stores.)

To minimize future bruising, strengthen the blood vessel walls by taking 1,000 mg of vitamin C daily, continuing indefinitely. Several times a week, eat blueberries or other berries—these are rich in flavonoids, which improve circulation.

Laurie Steelsmith, ND, a naturopathic doctor and acupuncturist in private practice in Honolulu and author of Natural Choices for Women's Health (Three Rivers), www. naturalchoicesforwomen.com.

Natural Treatments For Psoriasis

Remember those 1960s advertisements about the "heartbreak of psoriasis"? The ugly patches and tremendous discomfort that characterize psoriasis have been shown to lead to low self-esteem and even depression and anxiety in some patients. Research has also shown that people with the disease may be at risk for cardiovascular problems and arthritis. Psoriasis can, indeed, be a heartbreak.

It's unfortunate that, decades later, mainstream medicine doesn't have much to offer in terms of a cure. Pharmaceutical drugs can help but, as always, carry significant side effects—in fact, the FDA issued a public health advisory on one, called Raptiva, which can cause severe brain infection (the manufacturer has voluntarily withdrawn the product from the US market). Side effects of other psoriasis drugs include an increased risk of kidney problems and blood disorders.

There are natural remedies for psoriasis, including sunlight and dietary adjustments—according to naturopathic physician Eric Yarnell, ND. These are not as quick to work but do bring a measure of relief, sometimes significantly so.

Testing Indigo Naturalis Treatment

A study from Taiwan recently demonstrated the efficacy of a Chinese botanical ointment called *indigo naturalis*. The research involved 42 patients with severe psoriasis who had tried but not found relief from at least two conventional medical approaches, including pharmaceutical drugs. All patients had psoriasis on both sides of the body. On one side, participants were instructed to spread a soothing ointment made of petroleum jelly, yellow wax and olive oil—on the other side, to rub on an ointment made with those ingredients plus indigo naturalis, a traditional Chinese medicine derived from the plant *Strobilanthes formosanus*. It turned out that both versions of the ointment were at least somewhat soothing—however, for three

301

quarters of the patients (31 of the 42) the one containing indigo naturalis brought complete or nearly complete clearing of the plaques in 12 weeks. There is one problem, however—the dark blue indigo left temporary unattractive stains on the skin, which researchers say wash away with soap and water.

Other Natural Treatments For Psoriasis

Dr. Yarnell carefully tailors psoriasis treatments to meet each individual's unique set of needs. Along with the indigo naturalis, he recommends some combination of the following strategies to reduce stressors and strengthen the body's immune system...

- **Identify and avoid triggers.** Psoriasis often flares up in response to triggers such as physical illness or trauma, poor diet, smoking, stress, changes in the weather or the seasons and/or menstrual irregularities.

- **Examine and adjust your diet.** Diet is the core of a naturopathic program for people with psoriasis, emphasizes Dr. Yarnell. *He advises...*

- **Consume whole-foods.** Increase your intake of omega-3-fatty-acid-rich cold-water fish such as salmon and sardines, as well as fresh fruits and vegetables (especially carotenoid-rich leafy greens, sweet potatoes, carrots, mangos, etc.).

- **Liven up your cooking with anti-inflammatory turmeric (in curry powder), ginger, onions and garlic.** At the same time, keep your body's inflammatory response under control by avoiding excess sugars, saturated fats, hydrogenated oils, processed and deep-fried foods, and fast foods, all of which promote inflammation.

- **Try to identify your individual trigger foods and/or food allergies by following an elimination/challenge diet.** This is a process your doctor should supervise over several weeks. It involves removing from your diet specific foods and ingredients that you suspect cause food allergies or sensitivities that contribute to psoriasis. Common allergens are milk, eggs, nuts, wheat and soy.

- **Get tested for celiac disease.** A subset of people with psoriasis simultaneously have this other autoimmune disease, in which they experience difficulty digesting the protein gluten in wheat, rye and barley. (Learn more about celiac disease at the Celiac Disease Foundation Web site, *www.celiac.org*.)

Consider Fish Oil and Other Treatments

- **Fish oil.** This anti-inflammatory supplement is slow-acting, but critically important in reducing psoriasis symptoms, says Dr. Yarnell. He adds that fish oil is especially effective when coupled with lowering your omega-6-fatty acid intake—he advises eating fewer grains overall, limiting consumption of hydrogenated vegetable oils, if not eliminating them altogether...and when possible opt for grass-fed instead of grain-fed animal products.

- **Immune-strengthening botanical medicines.** To balance underlying immune disturbances, Dr. Yarnell often prescribes some combination of Asian ginseng (*Panax ginseng*), devil's club (*Oplopanax horridus*), Siberian ginseng (*Eleutherococcus senticosus*), ashwagandha (*Withania somnifera*), Schisandra (*Schisandra chinensis*) or licorice (*Glycyrrhiza glabra*).

- **Vitamin D-3 supplements.** In his practice, Dr. Yarnell uses natural and inexpensive vitamin D-3 supplements, noting that like fish oil it works slowly but effectively.

- **Folic acid.** Psoriasis sufferers are often deficient in folic acid, which is necessary for DNA synthesis, cell formation and growth and more. For optimal absorption, take folic acid together with a multi-B vitamin or get it from dietary sources such as broccoli, leafy vegetables, orange juice, dried beans and peas.

Other Natural Remedies

You can get immediate relief with creams and ointments. To relieve itching and inflammation and keep skin moisturized, Dr. Yarnell recommends topical treatments such as *capsaicin*, which helps itching, and topical vitamin D-3. (Note: Capsaicin may cause an initial burning sensation, which won't last.) To a lesser degree, aloe can also be helpful, he says.

Light therapy, whether in the form of natural or artificial ultraviolet (UV) light, slows skin cell turnover and helps reduce scaling and inflammation. Short, daily exposure of the affected areas to natural sunlight is best, says Dr. Yarnell, although too much sun can backfire and worsen symptoms. Work with your doctor to determine the level that is best for you.

●**Apple cider vinegar.** This is an old folk remedy that many psoriasis patients swear by. Dr. Yarnell agrees it is beneficial for people with *hypochlorhydria* (low stomach acid), which often accompanies psoriasis.

Practice Stress Management

If stress and anxiety act as triggers of your psoriasis, take active measures to get them under control. Since different stress relievers work for different people, explore what works best for you. For instance, try a yoga or tai chi class, keep a journal or practice meditation, breathing exercises or visualization. You may find it helpful to connect with others facing the same challenges by visiting psoriasis blogs such as *www.mypsoriasis treatment.com/blog.*

Psoriasis is a stubborn disease that requires considerable time, patience and expertise to successfully treat. While naturopathic treatments may not work quickly, you'll get the best and most lasting results by working with a naturopathic practitioner who resorts to only minimal use of strong conventional medicines on an as needed basis. In the long run, addressing the underlying causes of your symptoms this way will give you a greater likelihood of bringing psoriasis under control.

Eric Yarnell, ND, founding member and current president of the Botanical Medicine Academy, assistant professor of botanical medicine at Bastyr University and author of numerous textbooks and articles.

Chapter 16

STRESS, INSOMNIA & FATIGUE

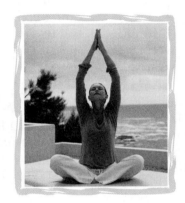

Mellow Out with Melon Extract

You're weary, irritable and can't concentrate. Your body is peppered with vague aches and pains. Hanging out with your family or friends seems more burdensome than fun. You're having trouble sleeping. And you're tired all the time.

What's wrong?

Maybe you've OD'd—on stress.

You're not alone. Most of us are overdosing on stress these days, as we try (and sometimes fail) to creatively cope with our 24/7 lives.

Well, if you've OD'd, maybe it's time for SOD—*superoxide dismutase*, a super-powerful antioxidant that a recent study shows can ease the symptoms of stress.

Less Stress, More Energy

When cells are barraged by hyperactive molecules called *reactive oxygen species* (ROS)—the same molecules that spark the inflammation that fuels chronic disease and aging—scientists say your body is under oxidative stress.

New thinking: Scientists have begun to link oxidative stress with perceived stress—the physical, mental and emotional toll from the relentless demands of modern life.

That's why French scientists decided to see if they could lessen perceived stress with a nutritional supplement containing the antioxidant *superoxide dismutase* (SOD). This enzyme is found in every cell of the body, where it helps prevents the formation of ROS. Scientists discovered it in 1968, dubbing it the "enzyme of life."

The researchers studied 70 healthy people who (like all of us) were doing their best to deal with everyday demands, and divided them into two groups.

At the beginning of the study, the researchers evaluated both groups for the typical symptoms of perceived stress:

- Negative feelings about life
- Pain

- Anxiety
- Disinterest in socializing
- Irritability
- Depression
- Poor concentration
- Fatigue and weariness
- Doubt and indecision

Then one group started taking a daily supplement of 140 international units (IU) of SOD. The other group took a placebo.

One month later, the researchers compared the stress symptoms of both groups. The SOD group had:

- 50% more energy
- 38% less insomnia
- 30% less pain
- 26% less weariness/fatigue
- 22% more concentration
- 22% less irritability
- 18% more interest in socializing

"Oral supplementation with SOD, which is known to have antioxidant activity on the cellular level, fighting against oxidative stress, could have a positive effect on several signs and symptoms of perceived stress," conclude the researchers, in *Nutrition Journal*.

The Melon Connection

"SOD is a unique antioxidant that is a natural part of the body's defense system against ROS," says Claire Notin, a nutritionist and study researcher. "I participate in sports—running and volleyball. After starting to take SOD, I find that even after a long, stressful day at work, I still have energy in the evening for training or competition."

Product: The supplement used in the study was Extramel, a freeze-dried concentrate of juice from a hybridized cantaloupe rich in SOD.

"Although there are no contraindications for taking a product that contains Extramel, if you have a medical condition you should talk to your doctor before taking it or any nutritional supplement," says Notin.

Extramel is an ingredient in several nutritional supplements sold in the US.

They include:

- Melonx, by O-Life
- Longevity Antioxidants, by MDR
- Defenze, by Enzymedica
- Body Boost, by Nature's Code
- Genesis, by Symmetry
- Xyngular Super Fruit Global Blend, by Xyngular
- Oriyen E3 Fruit and Vegetable Diet Mix, by E3
- Power Repair Spa Vitamins, by ClariPlex
- RAW Cleanse, by Garden of Life

Good news: In a recent animal study, Extramel blocked the formation of artery-clogging plaque by up to 85% in hamsters fed a high-fat diet. In another recent animal study on weight loss, researchers concluded that taking Extramel regularly "may represent a new alternative to reduce obesity induced by a high-fat diet."

"The widespread applications of this unique antioxidant are just beginning to be discovered," says Notin.

Claire Notin, nutritionist and study researcher, *Nutrition Journal*.

The Four Best Anti-Stress Foods

Recommendations to reduce stress are pretty standard.

Breathe deeply. Be assertive—say no to requests and demands you can't handle. Practice a technique that triggers the "relaxation response," such as meditation.

What you may not know: What you eat can also reduce stress.

That's because stress involves challenge—from avoiding a hazard in the road to meeting a deadline at work. To respond to that challenge, your body pumps out cortisol and several other "stress hormones." If you have balanced body chemistry, you pump out just enough cortisol to handle the challenge. If you have imbalanced body chemistry, you're flooded with cortisol—which can debilitate digestion, clog your bloodstream with extra fat, see-saw normal blood-sugar levels and weaken your immune system. In other words, you feel even more stressed!

To keep your body chemistry balanced and your cortisol under control, you need to eat right.

"Good eating habits play an enormous role in your capacity for adaptation—your ability to healthfully deal with stress—by keeping your body chemistry better balanced and preventing excessive production of cortisol and other stress hormones," says Charles Moss, MD, a physician in La Jolla, California, and author of *The Adaptation Diet: The Complete Prescription for Reducing Stress, Feeling Great and Protecting Yourself Against Obesity, Diabetes and Heart Disease* (iUniverse).

Now: Recent research shows that several superfoods are particularly effective at keeping body chemistry balanced and stress under control.

Today's De-Stress Specials

• **Dark chocolate.** A team of researchers from Germany and Switzerland found that eating dark chocolate (not milk chocolate) every day for two weeks lowered the production of stress hormones in people who rated themselves as "highly stressed."

"Eating dark chocolate significantly impacts the metabolism of people with high levels of stress, and chocolate can be a part of a healthy, balanced diet," says Sunil Kochhar, PhD, a study researcher.

Recommended: Dr. Kochhar recommends one ounce of dark chocolate a day, with a minimum of 60% cocoa solids (also called cocoa and cacao), the nonfat portion of chocolate that researchers think may deliver the most stress-lowering compounds.

• **Green tea.** Researchers in Japan analyzed diet and health data from more than 42,000 people and found that those who drank five or more cups of green tea a day had a 20% lower risk of developing "psychological distress." The findings were in the *American Journal of Clinical Nutrition*.

"The compound in tea that accounts for its stress-reducing effect is *theanine*, which increases neurotransmitters in the brain that help modulate cortisol production," says Dr. Moss.

Recommended: Dr. Moss suggests drinking two to three cups of green tea a day. "Choose it over black tea or coffee as a hot beverage."

• **Fish.** Researchers in Canada studied more than 800 people and found that those with the lowest intake of omega-3 fatty acids (found primarily in fatty fish) were 44% more likely to have psychological distress.

"Omega-3s are incorporated into brain cells, and have a significant effect on reducing cortisol production," says Dr. Moss.

Recommended: He recommends eating a serving of fatty fish (wild salmon, anchovies, herring, mackerel, sardines, sturgeon, low-mercury tuna) at least three days a week, and taking a supplement of 1,000 milligrams (mg) (1 gram) of omega-3 fish oil on days you don't eat fish.

If you consider yourself "significantly stressed," he recommends 2,000 mg a day (2 grams) of an omega-3 supplement.

Also helpful: "A study shows that flax seed powder, rich in a plant form of omega-3, is particularly effective in lowering cortisol, and I've recommended it to patients for many years," says Dr. Moss. He advises using two tablespoons a day in salads, smoothies and other foods. For maximum freshness and potency, grind the flax seeds in a coffee grinder immediately before use.

• **Vegetables and fruits.** Researchers from the Mayo Clinic analyzed diet and health data from 2,000 people and found that those who ate two to four servings of fruits and vegetables a day had a 41% lower risk of "frequent mental distress," compared with people who ate one or no servings.

"Eating a diet low in animal protein and high in complex carbohydrates raises levels of feel-better brain chemicals such as serotonin and also inhibits cortisol production," says Dr. Moss.

"The flavonoids in fruits and vegetables also reduce inflammation, which in turn cuts the body's production of cortisol."

Recommended: "The largest portion of every meal should be vegetables," he says.

Here are some of the guidelines he offers for putting more vegetables and fruits in your diet:

• **Eat one cup of cruciferous vegetables per day** (broccoli, Brussels sprouts, kale, cauliflower and cabbage), and liberally use onions, shallots and garlic.

• **Have at least one vegetarian dinner every week.**

• **Drink juice with organic green vegetables,** including kale, Swiss chard and spinach mixed with carrots at least three days a week.

• **Incorporate colorful vegetables and fruits** (carrots, squash, cabbage, tomatoes, blueberries, pomegranate, cherries, etc.) in every meal, with at least seven portions a day.

Sunil Kochhar, PhD, head of BioAnalytical Department, the Nestlé Research Center, Lausanne, Switzerland.

Charles Moss, MD, physician in La Jolla, California, and author of *The Adaptation Diet: The Complete Prescription for Reducing Stress, Feeling Great and Protecting Yourself Against Obesity, Diabetes and Heart Disease* (iUniverse). *www.integrativemedicinelajolla.com.*

How to Reduce Stress in Tough Times

It is no surprise that a new study by the American Psychological Association reports that 80% of Americans are stressed by the economy, with 60% feeling angry and irritable and 52% having trouble sleeping at night.

In tough economic times, it's understandable that many people feel financially vulnerable and emotionally stressed. But even in a national crisis, we're never as helpless as we think. Those who develop mental fitness are in a much better position to weather this and other stressful times.

To achieve mental fitness, we need to open our "locks," behaviors or habits that prevent us from finding solutions to problems and keep us from reaching our full potential.

Example: One of my clients coped with his high-stress job by eating too much and drinking heavily after work. These negative strategies (his locks) eased his stress momentarily but did nothing to increase his overall resilience and, in fact, undermined his mental fitness.

People who handle stress well use a series of skills, or "keys," to overcome obstacles and unlock their full potential. *The main ones…*

Direct Your Attention

Your brain can focus on one issue at a time (the *laser mode*), or it can expand its attention to everything around you (*glow mode*). Both skills are useful. An air-traffic controller, for example, has to keep track of fast-moving and constantly changing situations. He/she needs to be comfortable with the glow mode. But when you're dealing with a specific problem, the laser mode is more efficient.

Many of us have a hard time meeting deadlines not because we have too much to do, but because too many things compete for our attention. We jump around from thought to thought and task to task. We're mentally scattered, which means we excel at nothing—and stress builds. *What to do…*

• **Decide what has to be done first.** The process of prioritizing requires that we rank tasks along two dimensions—what is most important and what is most urgent. Maybe there's a project that you have to finish by the end of the day or a meeting later in the week to prepare for. Establish these as your one or two priorities, nothing more. Then selectively ignore everything else. Keep communication flowing when others are involved, and let them know where they are on the waiting list.

●**Create reminders.** Jot down your immediate goal on an index card. Keep the card somewhere in your field of vision. If your attention begins to wander, seeing the card will remind you to stay on target. Some people also find it helpful to set an alarm or cell phone to ring every 15 or 30 minutes as a reminder to focus on the goal.

Stay Alert

We all get distracted when life is stressful. We forget to pay attention to what's going on around us. That's when we do stupid things, such as forget where we put our car keys or bounce a check because we forgot our account balance.

People who handle stress well almost always are observant. They watch what's going on around them in order to acquire information and choose the best course of action.

What to do: Practice observing every day. When you put down your car keys at home, for example, notice the whole environment, not just the spot where you put them. Notice the table you put them on, the lighting in the room and so on. Not only will you find your keys more quickly, you'll sharpen your ability to acquire new information.

Know the Objective You

We all have two visions of ourselves. There's our subjective self-image, which often is colored by self-doubt and insecurity. Then there's the objective self, which usually is closer to reality.

Many experienced people with impressive résumés fall apart when they lose their jobs and have to find new ones. They're paralyzed with self-doubt because all they see is their subjective (inferior) self. It's the equivalent of stage fright. Even though they have done the same type of work a thousand times, an inner voice tells them that they're not good enough.

What to do: Do a reality check. Suppose that you have spent three months looking for work without success. Before doubting yourself, get objective verification. Show your résumé to different people in the field in which you're applying. Ask them what they think about your qualifications.

Maybe you're not qualified for the jobs you're applying for. More likely, you've just had a run of very bad luck. Trust your objective history of accomplishment.

Boost Willpower

This is one of the most vital skills during difficult times. Someone with strong willpower, for example, will find it relatively easy to cut back on spending. Most people think that willpower just means resisting temptations. It's much more than that. It's a set of skills that you can use to achieve specific goals.

Example: Suppose that you're in debt and know you need to create a budget and stick to it, but you've never been very good at that. Willpower means knowing your weakness... identifying ways to correct it...and then taking the necessary steps to improve it. These might include taking a personal finance class at a community college or getting a book on that topic from the library.

What to do: Some people naturally have more willpower than others, but everyone can develop more. The trick is to start small. Maybe your goal is to save 10% of your paycheck each month, but the first step is to reduce your credit card debt by paying off 10% more than the minimum payment each month.

Replace Negative Patterns

We're creatures of habit. Any behavior that's repeated a few times can become an automatic pattern. These patterns can be positive (such as arriving at work on time) or negative (thinking you're going to fail).

Negative patterns are particularly hard to manage because they're often internalized—we don't always know that we have them. People often have an inner voice that says things such as, I can't succeed...I'm not smart enough...It's not worth my trouble.

Negative self-talk has real-world effects. It guides our behavior and prevents us from coping effectively with difficult situations.

What to do: Pay attention to the thoughts that go through your mind. Are they helpful and affirming? Or do they inspire fear and anxiety?

When your thoughts are negative, create opposite mental patterns. When you think, I'll never get this project done, consciously come up with a positive alternative and say it aloud if you can or to yourself if the situation warrants. Be specific. Rather than something general, such as *I can do it*, say something such as, *I'm glad to be completing this project with pride, on time*. Say it three times.

This might sound like a gimmick, but our brains like routines. Focusing your mind on positive outcomes—even if it seems artificial at first—causes the automatic part of the brain to build more positive thought patterns that enable us to achieve more. The key is to constantly monitor yourself. Are you aiming at the center of the target? If not, refocus on the bull's-eye.

John Ryder, PhD, psychologist in private practice in New York City. He is author of *Positive Directions: Shifting Polarities to Escape Stress and Increase Happiness* (Morgan James). *www.takepositivedirections.com.*

Log On and Nod Off

Maybe instead of Rx, your doctor's prescription pad should read Rzzz—because people who don't get enough sleep are more likely to get sick.

Newest research: Chronic insomnia has been linked to a higher risk for...

- Anxiety
- Depression
- Diabetes
- High blood pressure
- Heart attack
- Stroke
- Substance abuse
- Suicide

(And that's not to mention the fatigue and brain fog that often follow a poor night's sleep, hobbling daily performance.)

The official definition of chronic insomnia is having trouble falling asleep or staying asleep, or waking up too early, at least three times a week, for more than a month.

An estimated 30 to 45 million Americans fit that definition. Another 50 to 60 million have the symptoms of insomnia, but less frequently.

Yet out of those 100 million poor sleepers, only an estimated 7% receive treatment for insomnia, according to a survey from the National Sleep Foundation.

And most of them are treated with sleeping pills—which are only a short-term solution, don't treat the causes of insomnia and can have dangerous side effects, says Gregg Jacobs, PhD, an insomnia specialist at the Sleep Disorders Center at the University of Massachusetts Medical School, and author of *Say Good Night to Insomnia* (Holt).

What most people don't realize: There's a drug-free treatment for chronic insomnia that studies show is every bit as effective as sleeping pills—*cognitive-behavioral therapy* (CBT).

This psychological approach teaches you how to change two sleep-robbing factors: the everyday behaviors that can cause or complicate insomnia (*example:* an irregular sleep schedule) and the negative thoughts about sleep that are a setup for more sleeplessness (*example:* "This is going to be another night of insomnia").

"CBT treats the underlying issues that cause insomnia, while medication only treats the symptoms," says Lee Ritterband, PhD, associate professor in the Department of Psychiatry and Neurobehavioral Sciences at the University of Virginia Health System, in Charlottesville, Virginia. "And the beneficial effects of CBT—in contrast to those produced by sleeping pills—last long after the treatment ends."

Researchers in the US and Canada have figured out how to deliver CBT for insomnia via the Internet. And not just information about CBT. What they're offering is a self-help "Internet intervention" very similar to CBT, but without face-to-face contact with a therapist.

And after logging on, a lot of chronic insomniacs are sawing logs.

WWW.ZZZ

In the US, Dr. Ritterband and his colleagues studied 43 people who had chronic insomnia for ten years or longer, enrolling half of them in an Internet program and putting half on a waiting list.

Like face-to-face CBT for insomnia, the online program—Sleep Healthy Using the Internet, or SHUTi—offered weekly instruction in the behavioral and mental changes that can help a person overcome the problem.

The study participants learned and adopted a new set of skills and behaviors. For example, they…

- Went to bed only when sleepy;

- Got out of bed when unable to sleep;

- Limited "sleep-incompatible" activities in the bedroom, such as watching TV and reading;

- Avoided daytime napping;

- Got up at the same hour every day;

- Increased exercise;

- Avoided nicotine, caffeine and alcohol before bedtime;

- Learned "cognitive restructuring" for unhelpful beliefs, thoughts and worries about sleep and

- Learned strategies to prevent relapse.

Result: After nine weeks, those receiving therapy online had a 59% decrease in their "Insomnia Severity Index," a standard measurement for insomnia.

They also had improvements in two other measurements—a 55% decrease in the time spent awake during the night, and a 16% increase in "sleep efficiency" (the time spent sleeping while in bed).

Meanwhile, those on the waiting list didn't have significant changes in any of the measurements.

In all, 16 of the 22 participants in SHUTi, or 73%, were considered "in remission"—not insomniacs—after completing the program.

Six months later, 61% were still in remission.

That level of improvement, says Dr. Ritterband, is "almost identical" to typical improvements from face-to-face CBT and sleeping medications.

In Canada, researchers in the Department of Clinical Health Psychology at the University of Manitoba also designed an online treatment for insomnia using CBT. To test the program, they studied 79 people with chronic insomnia, assigning half to the program and half to a waiting list.

After five weeks, those enrolled in the program experienced "significant improvements in insomnia severity, daytime fatigue and sleep quality," compared with the waiting list group, says Norah Vincent, PhD, a clinical psychologist and the study leader, in the journal *Sleep*. Overall, four out of five participants said their sleep was improved.

"Our participants found the online program much more convenient than having to come into the therapist's office for treatment," she adds.

Online Resources for a Good Night's Rest

The SHUTi program from Dr. Ritterband is not yet available to the general public, although you can apply for enrollment in a large, national study of the program, at *www.shuti.net*. E-mail study@SHUTi.net or call 434-243-2704 or 800-251-3627, ext 3-2704.

An updated and commercial version of Dr. Vincent's program is available online, at *www.insomniasleepsolutions.com*.

There are several other online CBT programs for insomnia. They are available at *www.myselfhelp.com* (click "Sleep Better" on the home page) and *www.cbtforinsomnia.com*, which uses techniques developed by Dr. Jacobs at Harvard Medical School.

There are also self-help books for insomnia using CBT methods, including *Relief from Insomnia* (Main Street) by Charles Morin, PhD (the techniques in this book were used by Dr. Ritterband to develop the Internet intervention for his study) and Dr. Ritterband's *Say Good Night to Insomnia*.

Gregg Jacobs, PhD, insomnia specialist at the Sleep Disorders Center, University of Massachusetts Medical School and author of *Say Good Night to Insomnia* (Holt).

Lee Ritterband, PhD, associate professor, Department of Psychiatry and Neurobehavioral Sciences at the University of Virginia Health System, in Charlottesville, Virginia. *www.shuti.net*.

Norah Vincent, PhD, clinical psychologist, Department of Clinical Health Psychology, University of Manitoba. *www.insomniasleepsolutions.com*.

Bedroom Makeover for More Restful Sleep

If a busy schedule prevents you from getting the full seven-and-a-half to eight hours of sleep per night that the vast majority of adults require, it's no wonder that you often feel drowsy during the day.

But what if you spend plenty of time in bed yet still never feel fully rested? Something in your sleep environment may be keeping you up or creating disturbances that, even without waking you fully, interfere with the normal progression of sleep stages that you need to feel truly rested.

Concern: Chronic sleep deprivation negatively affects virtually every aspect of life—energy, alertness, work performance, mood, sex drive.

New finding: Sleep deprivation also contributes to weight problems. Studies show that losing sleep for just a few nights raises levels of hormones linked with overeating and weight gain and makes a person more likely to reach for fattening comfort foods instead of nutritious fare.

Even worse: Sleep deprivation increases the risk for diabetes and heart disease as well as car crashes and other accidents.

What to do: Speak to your doctor—sleep problems sometimes signal a potentially serious condition, such as *sleep apnea* (repeated cessations in breathing during sleep) or depression. If you still have trouble sleeping well even after underlying medical problems are ruled out or treated, chances are that your bedroom is not offering an optimal sleep environment.

Recommended: Follow the eight simple guidelines below to create a space conducive to restful, restorative slumber...

1. Clear out clutter. Ideally, a bedroom should be simply furnished and decorated so that there isn't a lot to distract you from the primary purpose of sleep. Keeping the bedroom neat and well organized helps minimize anxiety.

Reason: A messy room often is an oppressive reminder of other things that need to be done, making it harder to fall asleep.

2. Don't work—or play—in the bedroom. Keep your computer, checkbook, to-do list, briefcase and other paraphernalia related to your chores, job or responsibilities in your home office, where they are less likely to intrude on your thoughts during the night. If you must have a phone in the bedroom, use that extension only for emergencies, not for potentially exciting or disturbing conversations.

Recreational activities (other than sex, of course) also should be done elsewhere—so remove the TV, DVD player, stereo and anything else that shifts the bedroom's focus to entertainment. If you play music in your room every night before bed, for instance, and then wake up in the middle of the night, you may be unable to fall back to sleep unless you turn on the music again.

3. Banish dust bunnies. Dust mites are microscopic creatures that provoke nasal congestion and/or asthma attacks in allergy-prone people. Because airways naturally constrict at night, allergy flare-ups are likely to interfere with sleep.

Best: Regularly wash bedding in hot water, vacuum under furniture, and dust all surfaces.

4. Block the light. Light sends a strong message to the brain to wake up. Of all the external cues that keep the body clock operating on a 24-hour cycle, light striking the eyes—even when they are closed—is the most influential. Though you may not become fully conscious, light can move you out of deep-stage sleep and into lighter, less restful stages.

Solution: Hang shades, blinds or curtains made from "blackout" material over windows. Remove or cover any electronics that light up, including your alarm clock. If you cannot block ambient light, wear a sleep mask.

For safety's sake: It is fine to use a low-level night-light—for instance, to see your way to the bathroom.

5. Hide the clock. When you have insomnia, repeatedly checking the clock only makes the problem worse by providing an unwelcome reminder of just how much rest you are missing. Turn the face of the clock away so it won't taunt you as you toss and turn.

6. Muffle or mask sounds. Noise is extremely disruptive.

Recent findings: People whose partners suffer from sleep apnea (which causes loud snoring and gasping) lose about the same amount of sleep each night as the apnea patients themselves do. Also, people who live near airports often experience blood pressure elevations and disturbances in the heart's normal resting rhythm when planes fly by.

Self-defense: Use heavy draperies, double-paned windows and rugs to muffle outside sounds. Earplugs are very effective—try an inexpensive foam or silicone drugstore product. If you find earplugs uncomfortable, turn on a fan or white-noise machine (sold at household-goods stores) to create a low, steady background sound that masks more disruptive noises.

7. Make the bed comfortable. The older the mattress, the less support it generally provides (and the more dust mites it may harbor), so if you have had yours for more than 10 years, consider getting a new one. Take your time testing mattresses to see which brand and level of firmness feel best to you, and lie on your favorite one for as long as you need to before you buy to make sure it is comfortable.

Helpful: Replace pillows when they no longer feel comfortable. Avoid products filled with natural down if you are prone to allergies. Keep extra blankets at the foot of the bed—body temperature drops a few degrees during sleep, so you may wake up chilled during the night.

8. Keep a pen and paper on your bedside table. If you are fretting over impending tasks or feeling excited about a new idea as you're trying to fall asleep, jot down some notes about the situation. This way you won't worry about not remembering your thoughts in the morning—clearing your mind for a good night's sleep.

Lawrence J. Epstein, MD, instructor in medicine at Harvard Medical School in Boston, medical director of Sleep HealthCenters, based in Brighton, Massachusetts, and author of *The Harvard Medical School Guide to a Good Night's Sleep* (McGraw-Hill).

Boost Your Energy in Eight Minutes or Less

When you feel drowsy or droop with fatigue, every task you undertake seems monumental—and even fun activities you normally enjoy feel like work.

Helpful: Take a double-pronged approach to invigoration—including on-the-spot techniques for an immediate energy burst...plus simple strategies that take just minutes to do, yet give you long-lasting stamina day after day.

For an Instant Energy Surge...

• **Wake up your nose—and the rest of you will follow.** Aromatherapy stimulates the brain's olfactory center and heightens awareness of your surroundings. Dab a drop of therapeutic-grade rosemary essential oil (sold at health-food stores) on the pulse points behind both ears, as you would perfume...or dampen a cloth with cool water, sprinkle it with four drops of therapeutic-grade lemon essential oil, then place it on your forehead or the back of your neck for five minutes. Do not dab full-strength essential oil directly under your nose—it could be too strong.

• **Belt out a few bars.** As you sing, you inhale deeply, bringing more energizing oxygen into your lungs and increasing circulation throughout your body...and exhale through your mouth, efficiently expelling the waste product carbon dioxide.

Bonus: Choosing a favorite cheerful song lifts your mood.

• **Give yourself a good stretch.** Stretching opens the chest, straightens the spine, expands the lungs and relieves energy-sapping tension in neck and shoulder muscles. *Try...*

• **Seated stretch.** Sit in a sturdy chair, feet flat on the floor, hands clasped in front of 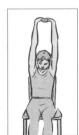 you. As you inhale, straighten arms and slowly raise them over your head, turning your wrists so palms face the ceiling. Gently press arms as far back as possible, holding for a count of five. Slowly exhale, lowering arms to the starting position. Repeat three times.

• **Doorway stretch.** Stand 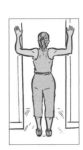 in a doorway, a few inches behind the threshold, with feet about six inches apart. Raise arms out to your sides and bend elbows to a 90-degree angle, placing hands and forearms on either side of the doorjamb. Keeping your back

Illustrations by Shawn Banner

straight, lean forward slightly to feel a stretch across your chest. Hold for 15 seconds. Repeat three times.

• **Take 800 steps.** A moderately brisk walk—at a pace of about 100 steps per minute—is an excellent way to get blood flowing to your heart and brain. Exercise also triggers the release of *endorphins*, brain chemicals that make you feel alert and energetic. If possible, walk outdoors—the sun's rays activate the synthesis of mood-enhancing vitamin D.

• **Just breathe.** The beauty of this is that you can do it anytime, anywhere, and instantly feel more alert.

Good deep-breathing technique: Inhale deeply through your nose, filling your lungs for a count of four...hold your breath for a count of seven...slowly and deliberately exhale through pursed lips (to regulate the release of air) to a count of eight. Take three normal breaths, then repeat the deep-breathing exercise twice more.

Rationale: This technique pulls the diaphragm downward and creates a negative pressure that draws more blood into your heart. As the heart pumps this blood around your body, all your tissues receive extra energizing oxygen.

To Refuel Energy Reserves...

• **Eat a stamina-boosting breakfast— one cup of fortified, whole-grain cereal.** Whole grains are complex carbohydrates that enter the bloodstream slowly, providing sustained energy by keeping blood sugar levels stable. Avoid starting your day with simple carbohydrates, such as white toast or a doughnut, which cause blood sugar and energy levels to spike and then plummet by mid-morning.

Also: With your cereal, have one-half cup of low-fat milk or fortified soy milk. Its calcium and vitamin D nourish your bones...its protein is used to build and repair muscle and other tissues.

• **For snacks, go nuts.** A handful of almonds, cashews, walnuts or other type of nut provides a sustained energy boost, thanks to blood sugar–stabilizing complex carbohydrates and tissue-building protein.

More benefits: Though relatively high in calories at about 160 per ounce, nuts tend not to cause energy-depleting weight gain because they promote long-lasting satiety and stave off hunger. Nuts also are rich in unsaturated fats that promote cardiovascular health.

• **Take a green tea break three or four times a day.** Green tea contains *catechins*, antioxidant plant chemicals that support the immune system by neutralizing cell-damaging free radicals, fighting bacteria and easing inflammation. When your immune system is operating at its peak, you have more pep. Green tea also boosts metabolism, stabilizing blood sugar and helping to ward off weight gain…and protects against many debilitating chronic conditions, including heart disease and diabetes.

Convenient: If you are going to be out and about during the day, before you leave the house, brew up enough tea to fill a thermos and take it with you.

While green tea does contain some caffeine—enough to provide a slight energy lift—its caffeine content generally is low enough not to interfere with sleep, provided that you avoid drinking it within four hours of bedtime. If you want to minimize caffeine, let the green tea bag steep for just 30 seconds, then discard that water and replace it with fresh hot water, allowing it to steep for several minutes.

If you prefer coffee: Be aware that, with its higher caffeine content, coffee may leave you feeling even more sluggish once the caffeine buzz wears off. Limit caffeinated coffee to no more than 16 ounces per day, and consume it prior to midafternoon so it doesn't interfere with your sleep.

• **Try energizing supplements.** Various herbal and dietary supplements help support immune function and/or reduce energy-sapping stress. Each has its own benefits as well as risks (such as possible side effects or interactions with medications or other supplements), so it is important to discuss their appropriateness and dosage guidelines with your doctor before taking them.

Options to consider: Astragalus…calcium plus magnesium…coenzyme Q10…ginseng… rhodiola…vitamin B complex.

• **Express yourself to lower stress.** Play the piano, pen a poem, paint a picture or just doodle.

The purpose: Creative self-expression is stimulating—it alleviates energy-draining stress by helping you reconnect with your deep inner well of emotional well-being.

Evangeline Lausier, MD, director of clinical services at Duke Integrative Medicine and assistant clinical professor of medicine at Duke University School of Medicine, both in Durham, North Carolina.

Natural Ways to Boost Energy

Exhaustion is an underrecognized epidemic in the US. Up to 75 million Americans report feeling "extreme" fatigue at work. Fatigue is among the top five complaints that people discuss with their doctors—even though it's estimated that two-thirds of people with chronic exhaustion never mention it to their doctors.

Every physical activity, from the beating of the heart to running to catch a train, depends on *adenosine triphosphate* (ATP), chemical energy produced inside cells. Nearly everyone can significantly increase daily energy by increasing the cellular production of ATP and reducing unnecessary consumption of ATP. *Most people know that exercise boosts energy—but you also can boost your ATP in other ways…*

Stress Reduction

Stress activates the sympathetic nervous system, which triggers thousands of chemical reactions that consume tremendous amounts of energy—energy that is then unavailable to the body. People who experience chronic stress may have insufficient energy even for normal body repairs. It is estimated that up to 80% of all illnesses are due in part to stress. *What to do...*

●**Keep a stress log.** Every day, write down the events or situations that put you over the edge. These might include rush-hour traffic or dealing with a difficult boss. Once you recognize your flash points, try to eliminate them—by taking a different route to work, for example, or avoiding unnecessary encounters with difficult people.

●**Create the perception of control.** People who feel helpless experience more stress than those who take a proactive approach—even when they're exposed to similar stressful events.

Example: Maybe your job involves daily, high-pressure meetings. The source of stress won't go away, but you can blunt the impact by deciding to do something about it—by taking a brisk walk before each meeting, perhaps, or simply telling yourself to stay calm.

●**Take frequent breath breaks.** Harvard mind-body researcher Herbert Benson, MD, found that the body's energy expenditure dropped by as much as 17% during meditation. A less formal approach, when you notice signs of stress, is to take a "breath break."

How to do it: Inhale slowly to the count of four, pause for one second, then exhale slowly and completely to the count of six. Pause for one second, then repeat four more times.

People who take a breath break every one to two hours usually notice that they have more energy throughout the day. They also have a slower pulse, lower blood pressure and lower levels of cortisol (the primary stress hormone).

High-Energy Foods

A Harvard study found that the majority of American adults are deficient in vitamins and minerals. These deficiencies usually aren't severe enough to cause diseases, but they can impair the body's ability to manufacture usable forms of energy. *Helpful...*

●**Choose a "rainbow diet"**—including blueberries, broccoli, carrots, spinach, toma-

toes and even dark chocolate. A variety of colors is important because different plant pigments, such as *carotenes* and *flavonoids*, help prevent metabolic by-products from damaging the *mitochondria* (energy-producing machinery) within cells.

●**Eat fish two to three times a week.** The omega-3 fatty acids in cold-water fish reduce inflammation—saving the energy that is normally needed to fight it. To avoid the risk of excessive mercury, eat small fish, such as sardines, anchovies or trout. Large, predatory fish, such as tuna and sea bass, tend to have the most mercury.

●**Avoid refined carbs.** White bread, sweets and other refined carbohydrates are rapidly converted to blood sugar. This causes an energy surge that is followed by a longer-lasting energy decline. Spikes in blood sugar also cause *glycation*, a process that prevents cells from working efficiently.

Better: Whole grains, lentils, beans and other foods high in complex carbohydrates. These are digested more slowly and provide the materials for longer-lasting energy.

●**Drink water—at least six glasses a day.** The majority of my patients are dehydrated. Water supports the body's ability to eliminate *free radicals* (cell-damaging molecules) and other toxins that impair energy production.

The Juice Cleanse

Juice fasts allow the digestive tract to rest while promoting detoxification, reducing inflammation and dramatically increasing energy. One study even found that people who fasted once a month were 39% more likely to have healthy hearts than nonfasters.

Once a month, consume nothing but juice for an entire day. Use a juicer to combine a variety of organic vegetables, such as spinach, carrots and broccoli. Add a small amount of apples, cherries or other fruits as a natural sweetener.

It's normal to feel a little worse during the day of the fast. That's when the body is shedding the most toxins. Most people feel much more energized and clear-headed on the day after the fast.

Caution: If you have a severe chronic disease, diabetes or are pregnant, consult your physician before fasting.

Supplements Can Help

Woodson C. Merrell, MD, coauthor of *The Source* (Free Press), recommends supplements only to patients who don't notice significant energy improvements within a few weeks of eating a healthier diet or making other lifestyle changes. *If this is the case for you, try...*

●**Ashwagandha.** It's an "energy-balancing" herb that improves the body's ability to metabolize sugars as well as cortisol.

Standard dose: 250 milligrams (mg) twice daily.

●**Probiotics that include acidophilus and bifidophilus.** People who take probiotic supplements have improvements in immunity and digestive function.

Standard dose: One to two daily supplements containing at least 10 billion organisms per dose.

●**Multivitamin that includes at least 400 international units (IU) of vitamin D.** People who have been diagnosed with low vitamin D need 1,000 IU to 2,000 IU daily. Vitamin D is very important for immune strength and cardiovascular health—and is crucial for maintaining healthy circulation and energy.

Woodson C. Merrell, MD, chairman, Department of Integrative Medicine at Beth Israel Medical Center, New York City, and author, with Kathleen Merrell, of *The Source: Unleash Your Natural Energy, Power Up Your Health, and Feel 10 Years Younger* (Free Press). *www.woodsonmerrell.com.*

Stop Worrying About Chronic Fatigue—Take Probiotics

No one knows the cause of *chronic fatigue syndrome* (CFS), a condition that affects an estimated three to six million Americans. But if you have CFS, you definitely know the main symptom—severe and constant fatigue.

And nearly everyone with CFS also experiences a "variety of symptoms in the emotional realm," says Alan Logan, ND, a naturopathic physician in Connecticut, and coauthor of *Hope and Help for Chronic Fatigue Syndrome and Fibromyalgia* (Cumberland House). "Of these emotion-related symptoms, anxiety and depression are the most prevalent, with approximately 50% of those with CFS meeting the medical criteria for an 'anxiety disorder' or 'major depressive disorder.'"

Good news: In a recent study, Dr. Logan and researchers from the University of Toronto found a new, simple, natural (and surprising) treatment for the anxiety that often accompanies CFS—a probiotic supplement.

Likeable Bacteria

Probiotics (also called *microfloras*) are the friendly bacteria that populate our intestines in the trillions, digesting food, disarming toxins and keeping unfriendly bacteria and fungi in check. What do microfloras have to do with CFS and anxiety?

Along with emotional upset, people with CFS are prone to gastrointestinal upset, particularly the bloating, gas and abdominal cramping of *irritable bowel syndrome* (IBS), says Dr. Logan. "Over 50% of people with CFS meet the diagnostic criteria of IBS. And anxiety itself is often a hallmark symptom in those with IBS."

The reasons for this common overlap of IBS and CFS aren't understood, says Dr. Logan. But recent research shows that people with CFS often have imbalances in microfloras, with low levels of friendly bacteria and high levels of unfriendly.

New thinking: Recent animal and human research shows that gut health and brain health are linked, says Dr. Logan. Researchers gave experimental animals a dose of toxic bacteria so small it didn't even spark an immune response—but the animals had a marked increase in anxiety-like behavior. Intestinal microorganisms cause a "direct activation" of pathways in the central nervous system, concluded the researchers.

Animal research also showed that probiotics boost the levels of *serotonin* and *dopamine*, brain chemicals that play a key role in emotions and mood.

When researchers in Wales gave 132 people a probiotic drink, it boosted the mood of those who were depressed.

"Based on these and other studies, my colleagues and I decided to see if probiotics might make a difference in the symptoms of anxiety and depression in people with CFS," says Dr. Logan.

To find out, they studied 39 people with CFS, dividing them into two groups—one group received daily supplements of probiotics and one group didn't.

After two months, those taking the probiotic had a "significant rise in both *lactobacilli* and *bifidobacteria*" (friendly intestinal bacteria) and a "significant decrease in anxiety symptoms." There was little change in either bacteria levels or anxiety levels in the group not taking probiotics. The study was reported in *Gut Pathogens*.

Boost Bacteria, Improve Your Mood

"It's becoming clear that there is ongoing communication between the microbes in the gut and the brain," says Dr. Logan. He encourages people with CFS to try a probiotic supplement to see if it improves their mood. In fact, a probiotic supplement might do a lot more than relieve anxiety.

Latest development: Commenting that "disturbances in intestinal microbial ecology…have been implicated" in the development of CFS, researchers at the world-famous Karolinska Institute in Sweden recently gave 15 people with CFS a daily probiotic supplement. After four weeks, six people said they had more energy, fewer symptoms and better physical and mental health. The findings were in *Nutrition Journal*.

Product: Dr. Logan recommends several different brands of probiotics, based on his clinical experience. "Choose a product and try it for about six weeks to see if it makes a difference. If it doesn't, try another." These products are available at the manufacturer's Web site and from many retail and online outlets where probiotics are sold.

●Align. "This is one of the most researched probiotic products, and you get the amount you need in a single, daily supplement," says Dr. Logan. *www.aligngi.com*, 800-208-0112.

●Culturelle. "This product also has been widely researched," he says. *www.culturelle.com*. 800-722-3476.

●Jarrow. The product he recommends is Ideal Bowel Support. *www.jarrow.com/probiotics*, 800-726-0886.

●Yakult. This probiotic drink, popular worldwide and being introduced into the US, was the probiotic supplement used in Dr. Logan's study on CFS and anxiety. *www.yakultusa.com*, 310-542-7065.

Alan Logan, ND, a naturopathic physician in Connecticut, and coauthor of *Hope and Help for Chronic Fatigue Syndrome and Fibromyalgia* (Cumberland House).

What to Do When Your Willpower Wears Out

Your body gets tired—that's why you go to sleep every night.

Your mind gets tired—that's one reason why you take breaks during the day at work, and go on vacations.

Even your emotions can get tired—one example of this phenomenon is what experts call "compassion fatigue."

But did you know that your willpower can get tired too?

Important: Knowing how to keep the power in willpower can make all the difference in whether or not you form and sustain stay-healthy habits, such as regular exercise.

Willpower Is Limited

Research by psychologist Roy Baumeister, PhD, at Florida State shows that using your willpower (which psychologists also call self-control and self-regulation) is just like using your muscles in a session of lifting weights.

Like muscles, when you use your willpower repeatedly in a set period, it weakens and then fatigues completely—and you have to wait for willpower to recover before you can use it again.

If your will is weakened from recent and intense use and you try to use it again—to will yourself out the door for your daily walk, or to stop yourself from eating that second helping of ice cream—you're likely to fail.

Psychologists call this the "limited strength model of self-regulation."

"The limited strength model theorizes that willpower is a finite, renewable resource that is drained when you try to control your behaviors, thoughts or emotions," says Kathleen Martin Ginis, PhD, a professor of health and exercise psychology at McMaster University in Canada.

Dr. Ginis is a psychologist and an exercise enthusiast. "Exercise is such a great way to reduce stress—not to mention reduce depression and anxiety, and improve mood," she says. "It's cheap, it's as effective as drugs or psychotherapy for mental and emotional health, it typically doesn't have any side effects—and it helps you stay physically healthy in the bargain."

Only 30% of us exercise regularly, she points out. And 50% of people who start an exercise program drop out within six months.

Could weakened willpower help explain people's inability to exercise regularly—to plan exercise...go out and exercise...and stick with regular exercise over time?

Dr. Ginis and her colleagues decided to conduct a study to answer that question.

Study Details

They asked 61 university students to show up at an exercise laboratory, and then divided them into two groups.

The complex study proceeded in several steps.

1. Both groups were asked to work out intensely on a stationary bicycle for 15 minutes.

2. Both groups were then given a form and asked to create a plan to use the 10 pieces of high-tech exercise equipment in the lab.

3. Group one then took the Stroop Test—a psychological test that requires (and depletes) willpower. During the test, the participant is shown words that designate a color, such as red, yellow or blue. However, each word is printed in another color—red is printed in yellow, yellow is printed in blue, etc. The participant is required to say the color (not the word) aloud—and it requires an intense output of willpower to ignore the color-indicating word and say the different color it's printed in. Group two took a test in which the word and its actual color were the same.

4. After the tests, both groups were asked to once again make an exercise plan for using the equipment in the lab.

5. Then they were asked to once again ride the stationary bicycle intensely for 15 minutes.

6. In the last part of the study, the researchers tracked group one for the next two months, to see how much they exercised day-to-day.

Result: Group one—the students who had their willpower depleted by the Stroop Test—didn't exercise as hard during the second round of bicycling. Their exercise intensity was 47% less than that of group two.

Group one put together a second exercise plan that was 89% less ambitious than that of group two.

And as the researchers tracked the day-to-day exercise habits of group one for the next two months, they found that those who had put together the least ambitious second exercise plan also exercised the fewest times.

In other words, depleting willpower...

- Decreased exercise intensity and

- Decreased exercise planning.

"When people's self-regulatory resources are depleted, they plan to do less exercise, and they exert less effort during exercise," says Dr. Ginis, summing up the results. "Furthermore, people who are more susceptible to the acute effects of self-regulatory depletion are more likely to skip workouts."

So, when you get home after a hard day at the office and you just can't bring yourself to exercise, you're not being "weak" or "bad." Your willpower has been depleted!

What can you do about it?

Replenishing Your Willpower

"There are strategies to help you conserve your willpower or rejuvenate it after it's been depleted," says Dr. Ginis.

She recommends:

• **Make a plan.** "This is a particularly important for people starting an exercise program," she says.

"You have to think through where you're going to exercise, what exercise you'll do when you get there, how you'll fit the exercise into your day, and what you'll do if and when the exercise starts to feel uncomfortable.

"Because there's so much thinking and planning around exercise—all of which deplete willpower—the best strategy is to plan your exercise in advance. For example, at the beginning of the month, or the beginning of the week, take out a calendar and figure out the days you'll be exercising, and the time of day you'll do it.

"This type of advance planning removes the need for a lot of daily self-control. When the planned time for exercise rolls around, you don't have to use your limited willpower making a decision whether or not to exercise—the decision is already made. Just get up out of your chair and go.

"Planning is an astoundingly effective strategy for not draining willpower—and for maintaining regular exercise," she says.

• **Exercise in the morning.** This is an effective strategy for those who are morning people. "You exercise before other activities drain self-regulation," says Dr. Ginis.

• **Take a break—and then exercise.** "Rest is always the best way to replenish self-con-

trol," she says. "Take 10 to 15 minutes, close your eyes, and meditate or catnap. Then go out and exercise."

• **Boost your mood.** "A good mood helps you muster up self-control," says Dr. Ginis. "Listen to music you like. Read a joke book."

• **Be sweet to yourself—literally.** "Self-control is a brain activity, and when the brain's glucose reserves are depleted it's more difficult to self-regulate," she says. "Drink something with a little bit of sugar in it."

• **Strengthen your willpower by using it.** "If you consistently use your willpower—resisting a second piece of chocolate cake, stopping yourself from checking your e-mail every 15 minutes, resisting the urge to hit the snooze button when your alarm goes off in the morning—you'll gradually increase the strength of your willpower, so that it more readily responds when you need it for any activity," says Dr. Ginis.

"Willpower is like a muscle," she emphasizes. "Using it is temporarily draining, but builds greater strength for the next time you want to 'exercise' self-control."

Roy Baumeister, PhD, Francis Eppes Professor of Psychology, Florida State University, Tallahassee, Florida, and author of numerous books, including *Is There Anything Good About Men?* (Oxford University).

Kathleen Martin Ginis, PhD, professor of health and exercise psychology at McMaster University in Canada.

Reiki-Inspired Relaxation Exercises

Reiki (pronounced ray-kee) is a system of natural healing that can be used for stress reduction and relaxation. It's an old laying-on of hands technique that claims to use life force energy to heal and balance the body's subtle energies that affect each of us physically, mentally and spiritually. Receiving Reiki can be a richly relaxing and balancing experience, but not everyone has time or money to get the treatments regularly.

Reiki practitioner Phylameana Iila Désy, author of *The Everything Reiki Book*, (Adams

Media) has adapted exercises for people to do themselves that may help them experience some of the calming, centering benefits of Reiki. This is unlikely to deliver the same level of energetic balance a trained Reiki master can, but doing this self-treatment ritual regularly may help you maintain equanimity on a day-to-day basis. Désy describes it as a way of loving yourself each day.

Reiki Basics

There are 12 basic Reiki hand placements, but Désy says it is fine to use your hands in whatever placements you find most relaxing and comfortable. It's recommended that each hand placement be held for five minutes, especially in the beginning. Désy recommends one-hour daily sessions for 30 consecutive days in order to get your energy flowing, after which you may find that once or twice weekly is enough. However, if you don't have an entire hour, remember that some time is better than none. You can also use one or two particular positions if you feel tension in one part of your body. "There's no right or wrong way to invite Reiki energies into your life," says Désy. "Just do it."

Sit comfortably. You may place your hands directly on your body or an inch or two above—it's a matter of individual preference. You may or may not feel a tingling or heat sensation in your hands as you go through the Reiki-derived hand positions. If you do, then this is an indication of the Reiki energy flow. Not everyone feels the sensation but everyone should feel some degree of relaxation, stress reduction and greater mental clarity.

First Position: Hands over Eyes

This position is good for reducing stress and for increasing clarity of thought and concentration. Hold arms parallel to the floor, bending your elbows so that your palms go toward your face, covering your eyes. Direct the energy toward your eyes. This position assists in activating the "third eye," which can help you see the divine in everything.

Second Position: Temples

This position can be restorative to the brain and helpful for relieving worry and depression. It's also good for headaches. Place your hands, palms facing inward, on the sides of your head (temples) and focus the energy in this same direction. This position is helpful in integrating the left (analytical) and right (creative) sides of the brain.

Third Position: Base of the Skull

This position enhances relaxation, calms thoughts and relieves pain. Slide or place your hands behind your head at the base of the skull, elbows out. The third finger of each hand may be slightly touching the other. You may feel heat in your hands in this position.

Fourth Position: Throat and Jaw

This position improves self-confidence and relieves anger and hostility. Slide (or place) your hands over the sides of your face, fingers pointing up, from about the ear down to the throat, covering the jaw as though you are supporting it. Practitioners believe we hold many intense emotions in the jaw, including anger and helplessness. As you focus your healing energy in this area, you may find it easier to "speak your truth," saying what you mean and meaning what you say.

Fifth Position: The Heart

This position improves the capacity both to love and be loved. Slide (or place) hands over the chest, palms facing the body, third fingers touching, elbows relaxed. Focus the energy on your heart. Some people report a sensation that is like breaking down a protective wall, which can lead to an increased willingness to be vulnerable.

Sixth Position: Solar Plexus

This position helps to center yourself and also to release fears. Slide (or place) hands over the solar plexus, underneath the chest and on the rib cage. This is the power center of the body. Focus your energy there and you may experience a feeling of increased confidence, security and strength.

Seventh Position: Abdomen

This position helps you to release the past, including negative feelings of frustration and bitterness. Slide (or place) your hands at your waistline. The hands can point slightly downward. Bringing energy to this area can help release negative thoughts, since such feelings are so often "stuffed" down inside of us. This position is very calming and may also assist in digestion.

Eight Position: Pelvis

This position enhances feelings of well-being. Slide (or place) your hands over the pelvis and hip area, slightly angled down. The area is the center from which we express ecstasy and creativity, as well as resentments toward the opposite sex. Sending positive Reiki energy to this area may also sooth some digestive problems.

Ninth Position: Shoulder Blades

This position facilitates the release of burdens. Slide (or place) your hands on your shoulders, right hand to left shoulder and vice versa, as if you are patting yourself on the back, fingers aimed down. Most of us experience tension in this area—we "carry the weight of the world on our shoulders." At stressful times, placing your hands in this position while you focus on sending energy to the area may help release the burdensome feeling and make it easier to relax.

It may be difficult to achieve the hand placements for the 10th, 11th and 12th positions without the help of a Reiki practitioner. However, you can modify them by placing your hands along your sides, elbows out, then reaching behind your back in the following three positions at rib level, lower back and tailbone.

Tenth Position: Upper Back

This position helps increase the capacity to give and receive love. Slide (or place) the right hand comfortably over the heart, fingers pointing slightly up, then place your left hand at your waist, on the right side, fingers pointing slightly down. After 2½ minutes, reverse positions so that the left hand moves up toward the heart area and the right hand goes to the left side of your waist. Since many of us feel tension in our backs, focusing the energy in this area helps bring a soothing sense of peace to the body.

Eleventh Position: Lower Back

This position helps to release self-criticism. Slide (or place) your hands in the small of your back. The palms can be facing either forward or backward, whichever is more comfortable for you. The lower back is another area where many people feel tension—focusing positive energy here helps to release negative feelings, particularly self-blame. You may feel lighter and clearer after doing this position.

Twelfth Position: Coccyx

The *coccyx* is the "seat of power" and the center of creativity. Slide (or place) your hands down to cover your tailbone. When focusing your energy here, envision all that you want to experience in your life and imagine reaching your full potential.

Reiki Resources

Though many advanced Reiki practitioners speak about how each position relates to specific organs and/or physical symptoms, the truth is that Reiki energy is systemic—positive energy flow throughout the body, no matter where the hands are placed. You can use any of these positions to focus positive energy that can help melt away the physical tensions and negative emotions you are holding throughout your body. It's not magical or mysterious—these positions are merely tools to help in focusing energy to flow freely through every part of our bodies. Try it. There's nothing to lose and a great deal to gain.

Those wishing to learn how to practice Reiki on others and on themselves should take Level One training. You can find out more at The International Center for Reiki Training (*www.reiki.org*). If you wish to experience a Reiki session, you can locate a certified practitioner through the International Association of Reiki Professionals (*www.iarp.org*). There are some excellent short videos on YouTube showing exactly what a Reiki session looks like (put Reiki into the search engine at *www.youtube.com*). Désy's book, *The Everything Reiki Book*, serves as a wonderful introduction as well.

(For more information on energy healing, see appendix page 343.)

Phylameana Iila Désy, Master Reiki Practitioner and author of *The Everything Reiki Book* (Adams Media).

Chapter 17

WOMEN'S HEALTH

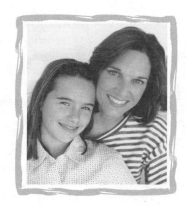

Prevent UTIs at Any Age With Cranberries

"One out of three women will experience a urinary tract infection (UTI) sometime in her life," says Elizabeth Kavaler, MD, a urologist in private practice in New York and author of *A Seat on the Aisle, Please!: The Essential Guide to Urinary Tract Problems in Women* (Springer). Up to 30% of those women will have a second UTI—and two-thirds of those will have several a year. Men, on the other hand, rarely have UTIs. Why the discrepancy?

Reason: On average, women have a two-inch urethra, the tube between the genital opening and the bladder. In men, the average urethra is eight inches long. Which means that, in women, the E. coli bacteria that harmlessly hang around the rectum and vagina have an easy scoot upstream to the bladder, where they morph from harmless passengers into infection-causing pests.

If you think you have a UTI—with symptoms such as urgent, frequent, and burning urination; cloudy (and maybe bloody) urine; and, in severe cases, back and groin pain—visit your doctor, who will determine if you have the infection. If you do, you'll probably receive a prescription for bacteria-killing antibiotics. In four out of five cases, that's that—infection defeated, once and for all.

But for the millions of women who have recurrent UTIs, there's a proven, effective and natural strategy for preventing the problem—cranberry juice and cranberry supplements.

Why it works: Scientists at the Worcester Polytechnic Institute in Massachusetts found that cranberry juice cripples *fimbriae*—the sticky, hairlike projections that E. coli use to attach themselves to bladder walls.

Newest Research

Several recent studies show cranberry is effective in preventing UTIs in children, girls, young women, pregnant women, and middle-aged and older women.

●**Preventing recurrent UTIs in older women.** Researchers at the University of Dundee in Scotland studied 137 women aged 45 and older who had two or more UTIs in the past year, dividing them into two groups. For six months, one group took 500 milligrams (mg) of a cranberry supplement daily, while the other group took a daily dose of 100 mg of the antibiotic *trimethoprim* (Trimpex, Proloprim, Primsol), which is used to prevent recurrent UTIs.

Both treatments performed about the same, in terms of preventing UTIs, but the cranberry supplement caused fewer side effects. "Older women with recurrent UTIs should weigh the options with their doctors, says Marion E.T. McMurdo, MD, the study leader. "Do they want to use a cheap, natural product like a cranberry extract or a drug that poses the risk of antibiotic resistance, fungal infections and super-infection with *Clostridium difficile bacteria*—all possible side effects of antibiotic treatment." The findings were in the *Journal of Antimicrobial Chemotherapy*.

●**Reducing recurrence in young women.** Researchers at the University of Minnesota reviewed the research on cranberry and UTIs and reported that an analysis of several studies on cranberries and UTI prevention showed the remedy lowers the risk of recurrence by 35% in young women.

●**Preventing UTI (and premature births) in pregnancy.** UTIs in pregnant women (even without symptoms, a condition called *asymptomatic bacteriuria* or ASB) are more than a discomfort for the mother-to-be— they're linked to premature birth. Doctors in the Department of Obstetrics and Gynecology at the University of California–Irvine studied 188 pregnant women, dividing them into three groups—a group drinking two glasses of cranberry juice a day, a group drinking one glass a day and a group not drinking the juice.

Those who drank the juice twice a day had 57% fewer cases of ASB than those not drinking juice. Those drinking juice once a day had 41% fewer cases.

Our study "provides support for a unique approach toward the reduction of ASB in pregnancy," say the researchers, in the *Journal of Urology*.

●**Preventing UTIs in girls.** Researchers in the Department of Pediatrics at Catholic University in Rome studied 84 girls, ages three to 14, with recurrent UTIs. For six months, some of the girls drank one glass of cranberry juice daily and some didn't. Those not drinking the juice had more than twice as many UTIs.

Increase Cranberry Intake

"Regularly taking a low-dose antibiotic to prevent recurrent UTIs may not be the best strategy, because antibiotic resistance can develop," says Amy Howell, PhD, an associate research scientist at the Marucci Center for Blueberry and Cranberry Research at Rutgers University in New Jersey. (Dr. Howell and her colleagues discovered the compound in cranberries—*proanthocyanidins*—that prevent E. coli from sticking to bladder walls, publishing their landmark research in the *New England Journal of Medicine* in 1998.)

Red flag: "Overuse of antibiotics is a major contributor to the rise of antibiotic resistance around the world," she continues. "In West Africa, Spain and China there is already massive resistance to the first- and second-line antibiotics routinely used to treat UTIs." (Her research shows that cranberry juice can even stop antibiotic-resistant strains of E. coli from adhering to bladder cells.)

Her recommendations: One glass a day. Drink an eight-ounce glass of cranberry juice every day to prevent recurrent UTIs, says Dr. Howell. And any kind of cranberry juice works—cranberry cocktails…"lite" cranberry juice with artificial sweeteners, if sugar is a concern…and 100% cranberry juice, which you'll need to dilute for palatability (otherwise it's too tart).

"There is no 'resistance' to cranberry juice, because it's not killing the bacteria," she adds. "You can have a glass a day until you're 80, and you won't see much change in efficacy. You couldn't find a better mechanism for dealing with this problem. If you're getting fewer infections, you know it's working." ("But if you do get a UTI, be sure to see the doctor for antibiotics to stop the infection," she adds. "Cranberry is preventive, not curative.")

And, she points out, proanthocyanidins are also powerful antioxidant and anti-inflammatory compounds—and may help prevent heart disease and cancer.

● **Eat dried cranberries.** "Our research shows that Craisins—dried cranberries—create the same anti-adhesion effect as cranberry juice," says Dr. Howell. A single serving —about 1½ ounces, or a handful of Craisins—can do the trick.

Smart idea: "Girls going through puberty have a spike in hormones that leads to UTIs, and having them eat a handful of Craisins a day is a good way to get them through that time of increased risk," says Dr. Howell.

● **Use cranberry sauce.** About ½ cup produces the desired effect, she says.

● **Take a cranberry supplement.** Dr. Howell's research and that of other scientists around the world shows that there are two supplements that have the amount of proanthocyanidins, with the necessary bioactivity (it prevents E. coli from adhering) to protect you from recurrent UTIs.

"Seventy-five percent of the cranberry supplements on the market are just junk," she says. "Many companies don't know the right dosage of proanthocyanidins or whether the proanthocyanidins they're using actually have biological activity."

Among the well-formulated products she recommends are…

● CraLief, from Nutramax

● TheraCran, from Theralogix

Both products are available online and in some retail stores that sell supplements. "Take the supplement daily to maintain urinary tract health," she says, following the dosage recommendations on the label, says Dr. Howell.

Smart idea: "I do a lot of traveling, including to countries where there is a high level of antibiotic-resistant bacteria, and I always travel with and take a daily cranberry supplement."

● **Don't take a D-mannose supplement to prevent UTIs.** This solution is widely promoted on the Internet, but no definitive scientific studies prove that it works, and it could do more harm than good, says Dr. Howell.

"I've done studies on D-mannose, which is a simple sugar," she says. "You have to take so much of the product—a tablespoon to two tablespoons a day—that you could put yourself in a prediabetic state. And although the compound can prevent the adherence of certain strains of E. coli in laboratory studies, it is only proven to work in horses, where it is injected directly into the uterus of mares."

Elizabeth Kavaler, MD, a urologist in private practice in New York and author of *A Seat on the Aisle, Please! The Essential Guide to Urinary Tract Problems in Women* (Springer). *www.nyurological.com.*

Marion E.T. McMurdo, MD, professor and director of aging and health, University of Dundee, Scotland.

Amy Howell, PhD, associate research scientist, Marucci Center for Blueberry and Cranberry Research, Rutgers University, New Jersey.

The Baffling Bladder Condition Antibiotics Can't Cure

Perplexing, painful and inconvenient, the chronic condition *interstitial cystitis/painful bladder syndrome* (IC/PBS) affects women more than nine times as often as men. Its symptoms, including bladder pain and frequent urination, often are mistaken for those of a bladder infection—yet tests reveal no bacteria, and antibiotics bring no relief.

Though IC/PBS affects up to 6% of American women, its cause is a mystery.

What is known: The bladder wall becomes inflamed and supersensitive…pinpoints of bleeding and ulcers often appear…stiffness and scarring may develop.

Many women suffer for years without a proper diagnosis, taking antibiotics for infections that they do not actually have. This delay causes needless pain…raises the odds of becoming resistant to antibiotics…and increases the risk that an IC/PBS–triggered inflammatory reaction will spread to other organs. In severe cases, surgery may be needed to remove part or all of the bladder. IC/PBS cannot be cured—but treatment can relieve symptoms and reduce complications.

Getting Diagnosed

If you have symptoms that suggest IC/PBS, visit your doctor. If no infection is found or symptoms persist despite treatment, consult a urologist or urogynecologist.

IC/PBS symptoms…

- Bladder pain or pressure
- Frequent urination (more than eight times in 24 hours)
- Urgent need to urinate
- Discomfort, pain or pressure in the lower pelvis or vulva
- Pain during or after sex
- Flare-ups during menstruation

There is no definitive test for IC/PBS. Diagnosis involves excluding other conditions, such as a bladder infection, overactive bladder or bladder cancer. Testing may include blood and urine tests, bladder biopsy and *cystoscopy* (exam of the bladder using a viewing instrument).

Good news: For about 70% of patients, natural remedies ease symptoms with few or no side effects.

Soothing Dietary Strategies

Your diet affects how your bladder feels. *Helpful…*

- **Identify foods that spark symptoms.** A chief culprit is cranberry juice. Yes, this juice combats bladder infections—but with IC/PBS, you aren't fighting an infection. And cranberry juice is acidic, so it irritates a sensitive bladder.

Other top troublemakers: Alcohol…artificial sweeteners…caffeine (coffee, soda, tea)…carbonated drinks…citrus fruits, citrus juices…spicy foods…and tomato products. For a comprehensive list of problematic foods, visit the Web site of the Interstitial Cystitis Association (*www.ichelp.org*, click on "Patient Resources" and then "Tools for Living with IC"). To identify your personal triggers, for one month do not eat anything on the ICA list. Then, reintroduce one food from the list every three to five days. If symptoms flare up, swear off that food.

- **Drink more, not less.** You may think that limiting fluids reduces your need to urinate—but skimping on water makes urine more concentrated and thus more irritating. Drink six to eight cups of water daily—and sip, don't gulp.

- **Take supplements.** *With your doctor's okay, try the following…*

- Prelief (sold at drugstores) contains calcium glycerophosphate, which makes food less acidic.

- CystoProtek (sold at *www.cysto-protek.com*) has antioxidants and anti-inflammatories (*glucosamine, quercetin, rutin*) that help repair the bladder lining.

Note: If you take a multivitamin or other supplement that contains vitamin C, choose one with ascorbate, not ascorbic acid.

Mind Over Bladder

Try any or all of the following mind-body therapies…

- **Bladder retraining.** Urinating temporarily relieves pain, so patients use the toilet often—in some cases, up to 60 times a day—but this habit further reduces the bladder's capacity to comfortably hold urine.

Best: Try to increase your typical time between bathroom trips by 15 minutes. After two weeks, increase by another 15 minutes. Continue until you can wait at least two hours.

•**Stress reduction.** Practice relaxation techniques daily, such as deep breathing, meditation and yoga. Also consider cranio-sacral therapy (gentle head and spine massage).

Practitioner referrals: Upledger Institute, 800-233-5880, *www.upledger.com.*

•**Acupuncture.** This reduces IC/PBS pain for some patients.

Referrals: American Association of Acupuncture and Oriental Medicine, 866-455-7999, *www.aaaomonline.org.*

Medical Treatment Options

Persistent bladder pain eventually can cause pelvic muscles to spasm, worsening IC/PBS. *Helpful...*

•**Intravaginal Thiele massage.** To relieve spasms, a physical therapist massages muscles inside the vagina and/or rectum... and patients learn to do the procedure themselves at home. In one study, this reduced symptoms for 90% of patients.

•**Electrical nerve stimulation.** Stimulating the sacral nerves in the back with a mild current helps pelvic floor muscles function normally. If symptoms are severe, a urologist or urogynecologist can implant a nerve stimulator under the skin near the tailbone for continuous stimulation.

•**Medication.** About 5 to 10% of IC/PBS patients must resort to narcotic prescription painkillers—but these can have adverse effects, including a risk for dependence.

Better: First consider one or more of the following non-narcotic prescription drugs, discussing the pros and cons with your doctor...

•**Dimethyl sulfoxide (DMSO).** This pain-relieving anti-inflammatory and antispasmodic is infused into the bladder through a catheter and kept in place for about 20 minutes. The procedure typically is done once a week for six weeks. Relief lasts three to 12 months...treatment is repeated as needed. Side effects may include garlic taste in the mouth, headache and dry nasal passages. DMSO is the only drug approved for this treatment, but for some patients, other anesthetics (such as *lidocaine*) work as well with fewer side effects.

•**Pentosan (Elmiron).** This oral drug helps heal the bladder lining. It can thin the blood, however, so it may be inappropriate if you use a blood thinner, such as *warfarin* (Coumadin).

•**Potassium citrate (Urocit-K).** Taken orally, this makes urine more alkaline. Possible side effects include nausea, muscle weakness and irregular heartbeat.

•**Urelle.** This brand-name oral medication is a five-drug formulation that reduces pain and spasms. Side effects may include nausea, dizziness and blurred vision.

Lifestyle Changes

To make day-to-day life with IC/PBS more comfortable, try...

•**Modified exercise routines.** When symptoms flare up, reduce the intensity and duration of workouts—for instance, by walking instead of running. Rinse off after swimming to remove irritating chlorine.

•**Bathing.** Soak in bathwater mixed with colloidal oatmeal (sold at drugstores). Avoid bubble baths and bath oils—these can be irritating.

•**A personal lubricant for sex.** This makes intercourse more comfortable.

Try: The organic Good Clean Love line (541-344-4483, *www.goodcleanlove.com*).

Kristene E. Whitmore, MD, professor and chair of urology and female pelvic medicine and reconstructive surgery at Drexel University College of Medicine, and medical director of the Pelvic and Sexual Health Institute, both in Philadelphia. She is coauthor of *Overcoming Bladder Disorders* (Harper Perennial). *www.pelvicandsexualhealthinstitute.org.*

Prevent BV with Probiotics

Vaginitis is a group of conditions—*bacterial vaginosis* (BV), yeast infections and trichomoniasis—that prompt 10 million doctor visits a year.

BV is the most common vaginitis, accounting for 40 to 45% of cases.

What most people don't realize: BV is not an infection. It is an overgrowth—of *anaerobic bacteria*, a type that doesn't need oxygen to live and that normally co-exists in the vagina alongside oxygen-requiring aerobic bacteria, explains Cherie A. LeFevre, MD, founder and director of the Vulvar and Vaginal Disorders Specialty Center at the Saint Louis University School of Medicine.

The typical symptoms of BV include a thin, grayish discharge, slight irritation, burning during urination and a fishlike odor.

BV is triggered by a change in the vagina's pH, from a healthy "acidic" level of 3.8 to 4.2, to an unhealthy "basic" level of 4.5 or more. Basic pH allows anaerobic bacteria to thrive.

Many factors can undermine the natural acidity of the vagina, says Dr. LeFevre. *The most common include...*

• The menstrual period, because of hormonal factors and the basic pH of menstrual blood;

• Intercourse, because ejaculate has a basic pH;

• Douching and

• Heavily scented soaps, laundry detergents and fabric softeners.

If you've never had the symptoms before, you need to see a doctor and receive an accurate diagnosis, says Dr. LeFevre. If your doctor diagnoses BV, the standard treatment is an antibiotic such as *metronidazole* (Flagyl), taken twice a day for seven days. You can also use a topical antibiotic gel.

If you're having recurrences (more than twice a year)—you need to confirm the problem is BV and find a way to stop it from recurring.

Now: Several new studies shows that one of the best ways to prevent the recurrence of BV (or to stop it from ever occurring in the first place) is with probiotics—a nutritional supplement or topical application of the "friendly" bacteria that live throughout the body, keeping disease-causing bacteria in check.

Probiotics Are Anti-BV

Probiotics work to beat BV because they lower the pH, replenish the normal vaginal *microflora* (the microbial environment of the vagina), and force out unfriendly BV-causing bacteria, explains Gregor Reid, PhD, chair in human microbiology and probiotics at the Lawson Health Research Institute in Ontario, and professor of microbiology and immunology at the University of Western Ontario.

Recent research demonstrates their effectiveness...

• **Probiotics boost the power of antibiotics.** Brazilian researchers studied 64 women with BV, dividing them into two groups. One group received an antibiotic, while the second group received an antibiotic and a probiotic supplement containing two different strains of the probiotic *lactobacillus* (*Lactobacillus rhamnosus GR-1* and *Lactobacillus reuteri RC-14*). After four weeks, 87% of those taking the antibiotic and the probiotic were cured, compared with 50% of those taking just the antibiotic.

The doctors also found that 75% of the women taking the antibiotic/probiotic combination had normal vaginal bacteria, compared with 35% in the antibiotic-only group.

"Probiotic lactobacilli can provide benefits to women being treated with antibiotics" for BV, say the researchers, in the *Canadian Journal of Microbiology.*

• **Probiotics work alone.** Researchers in Italy studied 39 women with BV, dividing them into two groups. One used a lactobacillus-containing vaginal suppository for seven days and one didn't. "After completion of the therapy, all the patients in the lactobacillus-treated group were free of BV," say the researchers, with tests showing that 83% had normal vaginal microflora. Only two patients in the non-probiotic group were free of BV, and none of them had normal flora.

• **Many studies, many successes.** Researchers at the University of Wisconsin Medical School analyzed 25 studies on probiotics and BV.

Their conclusion: "Lactobacilli were beneficial for the treatment of patients with BV." The findings were in the *Journal of Chemotherapy.*

Proven Probiotic

"The best probiotic for preventing and treating BV is RepHresh Pro-B—it's the only one consistently proven in scientific studies to work," says Dr. Reid. (One of the studies reported above used RepHresh Pro-B.)

Studies show this probiotic works better than an antibiotic when applied topically (the vaginal gel)…improves cure rate when combined with antibiotics…and helps prevent recurrence of BV, he says.

The product is widely available in superstores, supermarkets and pharmacies.

The Best Detergents for BV Prevention

Avoiding factors that undermine the natural acidity of the vagina is one of the best ways to lower your risk for recurrent BV, says Dr. LeFevre.

● **Use a detergent free of dyes and perfumes** on any clothes and linens that come in contact with your vulva (the external genitalia, including the outer and inner lips, or labia majora and minora). That list includes underwear, exercise clothes, pajama bottoms and towels (*example:* All–Free and Clear).

● **Don't use a fabric softener in the washer or dryer on those same articles.**

● **If you use a stain-removing product on your underwear or towels,** soak and rinse them in clear water and then wash in a regular washing cycle.

● **Wear all-white, all-cotton underwear,** not nylon with a cotton crotch.

● **Avoid pantyhose.**
Better: Thigh-high nylons.

● **Avoid bath soaps, lotions, gels, etc.** that contain perfume. That includes baby products and feminine hygiene products labeled "gentle" or "mild."

Best: Dove Hypoallergenic, Neutrogena, Basis, Pears.

● **Avoid all bubble baths, bath salts and scented oils.**

● **Use white, unscented toilet paper.**

Avoid all feminine hygiene sprays, perfumes, adult or baby wipes. If urination causes burning, pour lukewarm water over the vulva after urinating.

● **Avoid deodorized pads and tampons.** Tampons are safe for most women, but wearing them too long or when blood flow is light can cause BV.

Best: use when blood flow is heavy enough to soak one tampon in four hours or less.

● **Do not douche.** A five- to 10-minute soak in lukewarm water with 4-5 tablespoons of baking soda can soothe itching and burning. Soak one to three times a day for 10 to 15 minutes to rinse away extra discharge and decrease odor.

● **Keep dry.** Do not wear pads daily… choose cotton fabrics…and keep an extra pair of underwear with you and change if you become damp during the day.

Smart idea: Apply Gold Bond Powder or Zeasorb Powder to the vulva and groin area one or two times a day to help absorb moisture.

Gregor Reid, PhD, chair in human microbiology and probiotics, Lawson Health Research Institute, and professor of microbiology and immunology, University of Western Ontario.

Cherie A. LeFevre, MD, founder and director of the Vulvar and Vaginal Disorders Specialty Center at the Saint Louis University School of Medicine.

Stop Menstrual Pain with Electromagnetism

"Cramping and pain are common problems for many women during the menstrual period," says Barry Eppley, MD, DMD, a plastic surgeon in Indianapolis, Indiana, whose 225 scientific papers include several on relieving pain after plastic sur-gery—and two on relieving menstrual pain.

"Usually, sharp pains in the lower abdo-men begin at the start of menstruation, and continue for three or four days," he says. "The pain can range from mild to severe, and for many women it interferes with everyday activities."

The most commonly used self-care treat-ment for menstrual pain is an over-the-coun-ter *non-steroidal anti-inflammatory drug* (NSAID), such as *ibuprofen* (Advil, Motrin, Nuprin) or *naproxen* (Aleve).

However: "These drugs don't work for ev-erybody, and some women experience stom-ach upset," says Dr. Eppley. "Doctors and their women patients are always searching for a nondrug approach to ease menstrual pain."

Good news: Dr. Eppley's two studies on menstrual pain show that there is an effec-tive nondrug pain-relief method—pulsed electromagnetic field therapy (PEMF).

Five Days of Relief

PEMF therapy—using a device that topically applies a gentle and imperceptible high-fre-quency electrical current—has been exten-sively researched for 40 years, with hundreds of scientific studies showing it can help re-lieve pain, reduce swelling and speed up the healing process.

"The number of people who have received substantial benefit from electromagnetic field therapy is certainly in the millions worldwide and increasing rapidly as new uses emerge," says Arthur A. Pilla, PhD, a professor in the Department of Biomedical Engineering, at Columbia University, in New York. "Electro-magnetic therapies are an alternative to many pharmacologic treatments, with virtually no toxicity or side effects."

"Exactly how PEMF works isn't known," says Dr. Eppley. "It's theorized that it reduces pain levels by enhancing the release of nitric oxide, an anti-inflammatory molecule. It's also theorized that it stabilizes the cell mem-brane, or outer covering, so swelling resolves more quickly."

"I have used a small, convenient, inexpen-sive, over-the-counter PEMF device called an Acti-Patch in my plastic surgery and spa practices for the past few years," he contin-ues. "I've found it effective for postoperative pain relief and to reduce swelling after breast augmentation, liposuction, and certain types of facial surgeries. I've also personally used it for muscle and joint pain, as have members of my family, and I recommend it to all my patients for those problems.

"This positive experience with the device started me wondering. Could PEMF help with menstrual pain, which is such a common problem among my women patients?"

To answer that question, Dr. Eppley con-ducted a study on 23 women, aged 19 to 27, who regularly experienced menstrual pain.

The women rated their pain on a 1-to-10 scale during a menstrual period when they didn't use the PEMF device.

Then they used the device during their next period, again rating their pain.

Result: During the first period, the aver-age pain rating was 7.8—with pain on days 1 to 5 averaging 8.3, 7.9, 7.4, 6.5, and 5.7.

During the next period, when PEMF was used, the average pain rating was 5.4—with pain on days 1 to 5 averaging 5.7, 4.8, 4.3, 3.4, and 2.1.

"These impressive findings weren't sur-prising to me, because they're consistent with what I've observed using PEMF for pain relief after numerous plastic surgery proce-dures," he says.

"The fact that the device is easy to use, inexpensive and can be combined with other pain-relieving approaches—such as NSAIDS and heating pads—makes it an ideal thera-peutic option for many women."

A Second Success

After this first study, Dr. Eppley and a col-league, Sheena Kong, MD, a physician in San Francisco, conducted a second study on PEMF for menstrual pain.

They studied 91 women, age 18 to 35, with moderate to severe menstrual pain, dividing them into two groups—half used the PEMF device during a period, and half didn't.

Of those who used the PEMF device, 77% reported either complete elimination or significant reduction in their typical menstrual pain symptoms. Of those using a fake, look-alike device, 20% reported a reduction in pain (typical for a "placebo response").

"Devastatingly painful periods have been such an issue in my life," said one user of the device. "I hate taking medicine, but each month, like clockwork, I am forced to take it to have any relief whatsoever from the pain. I've tried all the natural remedies that work for some women, such as heating pads and yoga, but those options didn't work for me. The PEMF device worked really well—when I tried it, the sharp pains I was feeling dissolved almost immediately."

Resource: As of this writing, the company that manufactures the Acti-Patch device used by Dr. Eppley in his two studies is in the process of gaining FDA approval to sell their menstrual pain PEMF device (Allay Period Relief Patch) over-the-counter. The patch may soon be available in stores.

If it's not, you can call the office of Dr. Kong, who sells her patients and other interested individuals the Allay Period Relief Patch. Contact her office at 415-673-7600.

"Wear the patch continuously on your skin, over your lower abdomen, during your menstrual period," says Dr. Kong. "If you have pain relief, you can take it off for awhile every eight hours or so. If the pain returns, put it back on."

Barry Eppley, MD, DMD, plastic surgeon in Indianapolis who has written scientific papers on relieving menstrual pain.

Sheena Kong, MD, physician, Internal Medicine Associates, San Francisco.

Arthur A. Pilla, PhD, professor, Department of Biomedical Engineering, Columbia University, New York.

Hot Flashes— Alternative Therapies to Cool the Heat

Menopause is a natural biological process—not an illness. Still, about 75% of women going through this "life change" experience considerable discomfort in the form of hot flashes.

While the exact cause of hot flashes is not known, it appears to involve the overreaction of the heat-regulating system in the brain caused by the natural decrease in hormones, in particular estrogen and progesterone. Simply put, the brain sends out chemicals signaling the body to release heat in, literally, a flash—causing warmth to spread across a woman's chest and up the neck and face. When the flash occurs during sleep, it's called night sweats. While taking hormone medication can help keep the heat-regulating system from misbehaving, many women now are wary of the heightened health risks associated with hormone replacement therapy (HRT), including increased risk for heart attack, stroke, blood clots in the lungs and legs, breast cancer and uterine cancer (associated with estrogen-only HRT).

The Often-Missed First Step

Many physicians, both traditional and holistic, prescribe estrogen therapy without taking a critical first step—testing hormone levels to determine if estrogen is the problem. In reality, low progesterone or testosterone also can cause hot flashes, in which case estrogen replacement is completely unnecessary and unhelpful. Some women are helped by small amounts of hormones. For example, for patients with low levels of progesterone or testosterone, natural hormone treatments, including transdermal creams or oral supplements can help. When women have severe, debilitating hot flashes, doctors might prescribe low doses of bioidentical hormones, which have the same structure as hormones produced by the body. (Synthetic hormones are not identical in structure and function to those produced by the endocrine system.) These women are carefully monitored and stay on hormone replacement for only as long as necessary to keep them comfortable. More conclusive research is needed on bioidenticals.

Alternative Therapies

With the effectiveness of natural substances, there is no reason for women to accept the risks of traditional pharmaceutical treatments and to continue to suffer from hot flashes. (Before using any of these supplements, check with your doctor.) *Here are recommendations by Mark Stengler, NMD...*

● **Black cohosh.** This herb, often used in Europe and America for hot flashes, has been the subject of controversy concerning its effectiveness and relationship to breast cancer. That black cohosh is effective for hot flashes is nothing new. At least eight studies have shown that it can relieve menopausal symptoms, including hot flashes.

The controversy focuses on whether women who have breast cancer should take black cohosh. A recent study in *Cancer Research* found that black cohosh did not increase breast cancer risk in mice, but it did prompt its spread in mice that already had cancer. However, several studies—in humans—show otherwise.

Example: A study, published in *Maturitas: The European Menopause Journal*, found that black cohosh extract not only had no hormonal effect but also decreased estrogen formation in normal breast tissue. In addition, a very interesting population-based National Institutes of Health–sponsored study, published in *International Journal of Cancer*, looked at possible factors for getting or not getting breast cancer.

Result: Women who took black cohosh had, on average, a 61% lower risk for breast cancer! Check with your doctor first before taking black cohosh if you have a history of breast cancer. The dosage Dr. Stengler typically prescribes is 80 mg daily of an extract standardized to 2.5% triterpene glycosides.

One good brand is Enzymatic Therapy (800-783-2286, *www.enzymatictherapy.com*).

● **Topical progesterone cream.** Studies show that these over-the-counter creams are beneficial and safe.

Example: A study in *Obstetrics and Gynecology* showed that transdermal natural progesterone cream reduced hot flashes in 83% of women compared with 19% of those using a placebo.

Another benefit: The cream could have an anticancer effect among postmenopausal women taking synthetic estrogen because it prevents the buildup of the *endometrium* (the lining of the uterus) and the potential proliferation of abnormal cells.

Recommendation: Apply 20 mg twice daily. Try Emerita ProGest (800-648-8211, *www.emerita.com*).

● **Pycnogenol.** Studies show that Pycnogenol, a pine bark extract that has anti-inflammatory and antioxidant properties, is a safe and effective supplement for curbing hot flashes. In a study in *Acta Obstetricia et Gynecologica*, 155 women in perimenopause (the years of transition to menopause) took either 200 mg of Pycnogenol daily or a placebo. For six months, they kept track of the severity of their symptoms, including hot flashes, poor concentration, depression and menstrual abnormalities.

Result: Women taking Pycnogenol reported a rapid and significant improvement in all symptoms.

Recommendation: Take 100 mg twice daily of Pycnogenol. Check with your doctor first if you are taking a blood-thinning drug, including a daily aspirin or *warfarin* (Coumadin)...or medication for diabetes, because Pycnogenol can lower blood sugar.

The Unique Problem of Hysterectomy

Women whose hot flashes are triggered by a hysterectomy face a different problem. Estrogen on its own is the standard postsurgery therapy.

Reason: Progesterone minimizes the thickening of the uterus, which is unnecessary for these women. But Dr. Stengler believes that these women do need both estrogen and progesterone because the two hormones work together intricately. One role of progesterone is to "oppose" estrogen—while estrogen stimulates cell division, progesterone regulates it. Dr. Stengler recommends bioidentical progesterone.

Homeopathic Help

Several homeopathic preparations could work for hot flashes. They pose no risk, including for women who have had a hormone-related cancer (breast, uterus, ovarian or other). Select the preparation that might be best for you by matching your symptoms to the descriptions below. Take two pellets, 30C potency, twice daily for one week. If symptoms improve, stop taking the remedy and then use it only as needed. If you experience no change after one week, try one of the other homeopathic remedies.

• **Lachesis for women with hot flashes that they can feel on the top of the head.** Also for hormonal changes triggering anger and suspicion.

• **Pulsatilla for hot flashes in women who feel much worse in a warm room** (hot flashes are followed by chills)...those experiencing mood swings and weepiness.

• **Sepia for women with hot flashes who also are fatigued,** depressed, irritable and have low libido.

• **Sulphur for hot flashes that cause discomfort everywhere,** including the head, hands and feet, and that also cause extreme thirst.

"Solutions" to Avoid

Conventional Western medicine physicians now prescribe low doses of antidepressants, such as *fluoxetine* (Prozac), for hot flashes. While these drugs can be effective,

the potential side effects include weight gain, insomnia and reduced libido.

These side effects make antidepressant therapy for hot flashes extremely unappealing. Other pharmaceutical drugs that are sometimes prescribed include *neurontin* (Gabapentin), developed for epilepsy, and *catapres* (Clonidine), used to treat high blood pressure, drug withdrawal and hyperactivity in children. These drugs also have troubling side effects, including fatigue and dizziness—hardly a healthful trade-off for hot flashes.

Mark A. Stengler, NMD, naturopathic medical doctor in private practice, La Jolla, California, and author of the *Bottom Line/Natural Healing* newsletter. *www.drstengler.com.*

How Women Can Halt Hair Loss

Say the words "hair loss" and people think of balding men, yet the problem affects many women, too.

The causes and patterns of hair loss are quite different between the sexes. In men, the primary culprit is a sensitivity of certain hair follicles—typically at the top and front of the head—to hormones called *androgens*. This "male-pattern baldness" often is treated by chemically blocking the hormones and/or by surgically transplanting hair.

Women typically experience overall thinning of the hair rather than obvious bald spots. This "female-pattern hair loss" may especially affect the top of the head.

The causes of hair loss are more varied in women than in men, so the underlying problem is harder to diagnose...though once identified, it can be treated successfully.

Avoid Hair Abuse

The average person loses about 100 hairs per day. When the rate exceeds this, you may notice an increased number of hairs in your brush or shower drain...a hairstyle that feels skimpier than it used to...and/or an increasingly visible scalp. These are signs of *alopecia*, the medical term for hair loss.

If you have developed alopecia, first consider whether you are treating your hair too harshly with any of the following...

●**Too-tight hairstyles.** Ponytails, buns, braids and cornrows that pull hair taut can yank out strands. When such a hairstyle is worn regularly, many hairs at the stressed sites stop growing back, a condition called *traction alopecia*. Changing the hairstyle helps prevent further thinning, but hairs already lost generally do not grow back.

●**Hair-straightening chemicals.** These can damage hair follicles if you are particularly sensitive to them or if they are applied too close to the scalp. You may experience a burning sensation during the straightening process, then notice hair loss in the following weeks. Affected hair may or may not grow back depending on the extent of the damage.

Best: Get hair straightened only by a professional stylist. If you already have thinning hair, avoid straightening chemicals.

●**Styling techniques.** Strong detergent shampoos, styling products with a high alcohol content and high-heat styling tools (blow-dryers, curling irons, straightening irons) are unlikely to cause hair to come out at the roots—but they can cause hair breakage, which makes already thinning hair look worse.

What to do: Choose gentle, alcohol-free products...and lower the heat setting.

Medical Roots of Hair Loss

Once you realize that your hair is thinning, consult a dermatologist familiar with hair loss in women. The sooner the problem is identified and treated, the less severe alopecia is likely to become.

Helpful: American Academy of Dermatology, 888-462-3376, *www.aad.org*.

What to expect: The doctor may gently tug on a group of hairs and see how many come out to gauge the severity of your problem. Blood may be drawn and/or a tiny sample of scalp may be removed and examined under a microscope to check for underlying medical problems. Correcting such conditions often can minimize hair loss and may even allow lost hair to grow back. *Possible underlying causes include...*

●**Hormones.** A common cause of female-pattern hair loss is a genetic sensitivity to androgens, which can lead to alopecia even when hormone levels are normal. Less commonly, excessive production of androgens is the culprit—as with *polycystic ovary syndrome* (PCOS), a disorder characterized by thin scalp hair, excess facial and body hair and irregular periods. In either case, treatment often includes androgen-lowering drugs.

In addition, a woman with PCOS may need medication to control high blood sugar, blood pressure and/or cholesterol. Iron deficiency. Hair follicles need iron. If blood tests reveal low iron levels (for instance lowering drugs. In addition, a woman with PCOS may need medication to control high blood sugar, blood pressure and/or cholesterol.

●**Iron deficiency.** Hair follicles need iron. If blood tests reveal low iron levels (for instance, due to heavy periods), your doctor may prescribe iron supplements to help with hair loss and guard against anemia.

●**A highly stressful experience.** A major ordeal—childbirth, surgery, crash dieting, a severe emotional upset—can trigger *telegen effluvium*. This type of hair loss typically begins a few weeks after the event and continues for several months. Fortunately, hair usually begins to grow back after about six months.

●**Medications and supplements.** Hair loss can be a side effect of certain heart disease drugs or megadoses of some supplements, such as vitamin A. Tell your dermatologist about all medications, vitamins and herbal supplements you take, and consider alternatives if necessary.

●**Thyroid disease.** Thyroid hormone regulates metabolism, the interplay of chemical processes that release energy and replenish cells—so it affects the entire body. An overactive or underactive thyroid gland can produce many varied symptoms, including hair loss.

The fix: Thyroid-regulating medication.

•**Autoimmune disorders.** With alopecia areata, the immune system attacks hair follicles, causing patchy hair loss on the head and body. It usually clears up on its own within 12 months—but during that time, oral immune-suppressing drugs and/or injections

Natural Remedies for Hair Loss

To determine the underlying cause of your hair loss, see your primary care physician. By examining your pattern of hair loss, he/she will gain clues to the type of alopecia you may have.

For any type of hair loss, it's especially important to get adequate levels of B vitamins, zinc and fatty acids.

Recommended daily regimen until hair health improves: A B-complex vitamin that contains at least 75 mg each of vitamins B-1, B-2, B-3, B-5 and B-6, as well as 800 micrograms each of vitamin B-12 and folic acid…along with 2,000 mg of fish oil…and 45 mg of zinc.

The herb gotu kola also promotes normal hair growth and calms the nervous system. Take the herb in tincture form (one-quarter teaspoon in two ounces water) 15 minutes before or after eating, once daily. Gotu kola, taken until hair health is restored, is generally safe for adults (except for those with liver disease). Pregnant women should not take gotu kola. Check with your doctor if you want to take the herb for more than six weeks.

You can also try a shampoo that contains oil of rosemary to soothe the scalp and promote hair growth. Rosemary is an herb that has a long history of use for hair and scalp health. (Such shampoos can be found online and in health-food stores.)

Jamison Starbuck, ND, naturopathic physician in family practice in Missoula, Montana.

of corticosteroids into the scalp can help control hair loss. Another autoimmune disorder, *cicatricial alopecia*, leads to scarring of the follicles, requiring ongoing medication to minimize hair loss.

Hair-Saving Treatment Options

If no underlying health problem is found or if natural remedies or lifestyle changes do not bring sufficient improvement, consider these options. They often are most effective when used in combination.

•**Minoxidil (Rogaine).** This nonprescription topical medication is very effective at halting certain types of hair loss, but it may be less effective at regrowing hair already lost—so the sooner you start treatment, the better. Products marketed to women typically contain 2% minoxidil—but the extra-strength 5% products marketed to men are more potent and generally are safe for women.

Best: Use the 5% formula, switching to 2% if you develop side effects (scalp dryness or itchiness, increased facial or body hair). Hair loss resumes if treatment is stopped. Do not use minoxidil when pregnant or nursing.

Price: About $30 at drugstores for a one-month supply.

•**Low-level laser therapy (LLLT).** An LLLT device emits a special light that penetrates the scalp and stimulates hair follicle cell metabolism, encouraging hair growth. Hair restoration clinics typically use a hood-style device (like a hair dryer). For home use, a handheld, hairbrush-like device can be purchased online or through a hair restoration clinic ($200 to $600). While LLLT has not been as rigorously researched as hair-loss medication, evidence suggests that it can help.

•**Hair-replacement surgery.** This involves taking hair follicles from areas where hair grows well and transplanting them onto balding areas. It is not appropriate for diffuse thinning throughout the scalp, but it successfully treats various types of hair loss in women, including traction alopecia from tight hairstyles…scarred areas from cicatricial alopecia (once it is no longer active)…and female-pattern hair loss.

Consult a cosmetic surgeon who does hair-replacement procedures.

Helpful: International Society of Hair Restoration Surgery, 800-444-2737, *www.ishrs. org.*

Kenneth Washenik, MD, PhD, clinical assistant professor of dermatology at New York University Langone Medical Center in New York City. He is chief medical officer of Bosley Medical, Beverly Hills, California. *www.bosley.com.*

Acupuncture and Exercise for PCOS

One out of every 10 American women of reproductive age has *polycystic ovarian syndrome* (PCOS).

Doctors call a health problem a syndrome when they can describe a predictable pattern of symptoms and complications, but don't know their cause. *In PCOS, symptoms and complications can include…*

• Small cysts around the outer edge of the ovary;

• High levels of testosterone and other "male" hormones (androgens);

• Irregular or absent menstrual periods;

• Excess facial and body hair;

• Acne;

• Overweight;

• Infertility and

• Blood sugar (glucose) and blood fat (cholesterol, triglycerides) problems, which dramatically increase the risk for type 2 diabetes, heart attack and stroke.

The medical treatment for PCOS is usually a prescription for birth control pills, which cuts testosterone production, and for *metformin* (Glucophage), an anti-diabetes drug that helps balance blood sugar.

Problem: "These drugs can have terrible long-term side effects," says Katie Humphrey, a personal trainer in Palm Beach Garden,

Florida, and author of *Freedom from PCOS: 3 Proven Steps to Naturally Overcome Polycystic Ovarian Syndrome and Insulin Resistance.*

The drugs used to treat PCOS can have adverse effects, agrees Elisabet Stener-Victorin, PhD, at the University of Gothenburg in Sweden.

Solution: Studies show that acupuncture treatments can help balance hormones and regulate periods in PCOS—"with no negative side effects," says Dr. Stener-Victorin. (In acupuncture, small, painless needles are inserted into points along meridians, invisible channels of energy. According to practitioners, the needles unblock and balance energy, or *qi*, easing health problems.)

Studies also show that regular exercise can regulate periods and strengthen the cardiovascular system in women with PCOS.

Now: A recent study by Dr. Stener-Victorin and her colleagues confirms the benefits of both these nondrug approaches—and shows how they might work.

The Mechanisms of Healing

The researchers studied 84 women with PCOS.

Thirty-three received acupuncture, with 14 treatments over four months. Thirty-four participated in an exercise program—brisk walking, cycling or another type of aerobic exercise, for 30 to 45 minutes, three days a week. And 17 didn't receive either treatment.

The researchers theorize that two factors fuel the disease…

1. Hyperactivity of the sympathetic nervous system, which is the part of the nervous system that responds to stress, speeding heart rate, spiking blood sugar and blood pressure and flooding the muscles with blood

2. High levels of testosterone

Result: Both acupuncture and regular exercise decreased the chronic hyperactivity of the sympathetic nervous system.

After four months, those receiving acupuncture had slimmer waists, better menstrual regularity and lower levels of testosterone.

Those who exercised lost weight.

The women who didn't receive either treatment had little or no changes in the activity of the sympathetic nervous system, and insignificant changes in their periods, testosterone levels and weight.

"The findings that acupuncture and exercise decrease sympathetic nerve activity in women with PCOS indicates a possible alternative nonpharmacological approach," says Dr. Stener-Victorin.

Acupuncture and Herbs

"The sympathetic nervous system is typically overstimulated in PCOS, and acupuncture can help normalize it," agrees Kathleen Albertson, LAc, PhD, an acupuncturist and nutritionist in Irvine, California, and author of *Acupuncture and Chinese Herbal Medicine for Women's Health* (CreateSpace).

How often should a woman receive treatment?

"It depends on her goals," says Dr. Albertson. "If infertility is the issue and she wants to get pregnant right way, I recommend acupuncture twice a week. If her goal is to reduce the symptoms of PCOS, I recommend once a week."

"Acupuncture combined with Chinese herbs is the best approach," she continues. "Chinese herbs can help promote circulation and normalize the menstrual cycle."

Although Chinese herbal formulas are customized for each person, two formulas that are often used for PCOS are...

1. Wen Jing Tang, also called "Warm the Menses." "It warms the meridians and helps with ovulation," says Dr. Albertson.

2. Liu Jun Zi Tang. "It tonifies the qi and also relieves the "stagnation" or sluggishness of internal fluids that characterizes PCOS," she says.

"Western medicine treats PCOS with prescription drugs—and their long-term use is more degenerating than regenerating," says Dr. Albertson. "Natural medicine treats the problem with modalities such as acupuncture, exercise and holistic nutrition—and they reduce stress and renew the body."

Exercise, Diet and Supplements

Humphrey used nondrug treatments to overcome her PCOS.

"I was diagnosed a few years ago with the condition," she says. "I was 30 pounds overweight, I had no menstrual cycle and I had other complications, such as hot flashes and mood swings—in fact, my doctor and friends thought I was premenopausal, even though I'm in my twenties."

Her doctor prescribed birth control pills for the problem. Her family had always embraced natural healing, so after a few months on the Pill, she decided to try a nondrug approach.

"I used exercise, diet and nutritional supplements to lose 30 pounds, restore regularity to my cycle and banish my other symptoms," she says. "I overcame PCOS naturally—without any medication."

Now, as a personal coach, she helps other women with PCOS do the same, as their doctors monitor symptoms. Her full program is outlined in her e-book, available at her Web site. *Some of her recommendations...*

●**Exercise.** "Women with PCOS have to follow a slightly different set of exercise guidelines—otherwise they'll further elevate testosterone, which can worsen menstrual irregularity, acne and other symptoms," says Humphrey.

She recommends three types of exercise...

1. Steady state aerobic exercise, such as brisk walking.

2. Interval training, involving one-minute bursts of intense exercise (such as a sprint), followed by two minutes of slow exercise (such as slow walking), followed by another one-minute burst, etc., for 20 to 30 minutes.

3. Weight training, lifting a lighter weight for 20 repetitions, rather than the standard recommendation of lifting the heaviest weight possible 10 to 12 repetitions.

She advises her clients to exercise aerobically three days a week, with interval training on at least one of those days, and to weight train two to three days a week. The other days are rest days.

● **Diet.** "I try to make a healthy, glucose-balancing diet as easy as possible—using the acronym EASY," Humphrey says.

E is for Eat every three to four hours.

A is for Always eat whole foods, combining protein and unrefined carbohydrates at every meal, such as a chicken sandwich on whole-wheat bread.

S is for Stay away from harmful foods, such as white sugar and refined carbohydrates.

Y is for You're allowed to have treats—but just eat a healthier version of the treat, such as a gluten-free cookie made with organic ingredients.

● **Nutritional supplements.** Humphrey herself uses the four nutritional supplements from the Insulite PCOS System, which are formulated to decrease testosterone, balance blood sugar and strengthen the cardiovascular system.

You can order the formulas at *www.pcos. insulitelabs.com* or call 888-986-4325.

Katie Humphrey, personal trainer in Palm Beach Garden, Florida and author of *Freedom from PCOS. www.freedom frompcos.com.*

Elisabet Stener-Victorin, PhD, associate professor, Department of Physiology, University of Gothenburg, Sweden.

Kathleen Albertson, LAc, PhD, acupuncturist and nutritionist in Irvine, California, and author of *Acupuncture and Chinese Herbal Medicine for Women's Health* (CreateSpace). *www.orangecountyacupuncture.com.*

A Female Secret to Better Sexual Health

Like a happy couple, sexual health and psychological well-being often go hand in hand.

New research: Australian researchers studied women aged 20 to 65 who had sexual intercourse at least two times a month, asking them if they were sexually satisfied or dissatisfied.

Those who said they were sexually satisfied also had a higher overall scores for "positive well-being" and "vitality," says study leader Sonia Davison, PhD, from the Women's Health Program at Monash University in Australia.

What characterized sexual dissatisfaction?

● Low levels of interest in and desire for sex

● Low levels of pleasure and satisfaction when they had sex

What might improve a woman's level of desire for and pleasure in sex?

The majority of American women might answer…*using a vibrator.*

The Silent (and Satisfied) Majority

"A vibrator is a handheld battery-powered device that produces pulses of varying intensity and frequency that enhance sexual arousal and time to orgasm," says Debby Herbenick, PhD, associate director of the Center for Sexual Health Promotion at Indiana University, and author of *Because It Feels Good: A Woman's Guide to Sexual Pleasure and Satisfaction* (Rodale).

Dr. Herbenick and her colleagues surveyed a nationally representative sample of more than 2,000 American women aged 18 to 60 and found that 53% of them had used a vibrator.

They also found that nearly one in four women had used a vibrator within the past month. And that those women had better sexual functioning—higher levels of desire, arousal, lubrication and easier orgasms.

And they found that vibrators are very safe—71% of users experienced zero side effects associated with vibrator use, and any side effects that were reported (such as numbness) were rare and of short duration.

"This study about women's vibrator use affirms what many doctors and therapists have know for decades—that vibrator use is common, it's linked to positive sexual function such as desire and ease of orgasm, and it's rarely associated with any side effects," says Dr. Herbenick.

Good Vibrations

"Women tend to say that they started using vibrators for fun, out of curiosity, to make it easier for themselves or their partners to have an orgasm or to otherwise spice up their sex lives," says Dr. Herbenick.

However: "Using a vibrator is a personal decision and is not for everyone," she adds.

For those who want to use and enjoy a vibrator, here are some of her recommendations...

●**Find a vibrator that feels good.** "Not all women like the same vibrator," she says. "More women prefer a vibrator for clitoral rather than vaginal stimulation, for example. Find one that feels good to you." And, she says, use it alone before using it with a partner, to develop comfort and ease with it.

●**Talk to your partner about using the vibrator.** "We've found that the vast majority of men feel comfortable with—or turned on by—the prospect of a partner using a vibrator or other sex toy," says Dr. Herbenick.

Her recommendations for acclimating your partner to the idea: Choose a time to talk when you're not having or about to have sex, asking him how he feels about using them and whether he'd be open to using one with you.

Share ideas about what would feel comfortable and pleasurable about using a vibrator together, as well as concerns you might have.

Focus on the pluses, and what it will bring to your sex life, such as making it easier for you to orgasm. Offer to show him how to use your vibrator.

●**Clean your vibrator.** "If you don't clean toys properly after each use, they can harbor bacteria, which increases your chances of a urinary tract infection, bacterial imbalance in the vagina or genital irritation," says Dr. Herbenick. "Most vibrators can be cleaned with warm water and soap, but they can't be safely held under water unless they are waterproof. If a vibrator is not waterproof, you can often take a damp cloth or cotton ball

soaked in soap and water or rubbing alcohol, and clean the toy by hand."

●**Resources.** You can stay up-to-date on the newest, most innovative and safest vibrators and other sex toys at Dr. Herbenick's Web site, *www.mysexprofessor.com.*

Dr. Herbenick recommends these "women-friendly" online sex-toy shops for purchasing a vibrator or other sex toys...

●A Woman's Touch (*www.a-womans-touch.com*)

●Babeland (*www.babeland.com*)

●Early to Bed (*www.early2bed.com*)

●MyPleasure (*www.mypleasure.com*)

●Pure Romance (*www.pureromance.com*)

●Tulip (*www.mytulip.com*)

Sonia Davison, PhD, Women's Health Program, Monash University, Australia.

Debby Herbenick, PhD, associate director of the Center for Sexual Health Promotion at Indiana University and author of *Because It Feels Good: A Woman's Guide to Sexual Pleasure and Satisfaction* (Rodale). *www.mysexprofessor.com.*

Natural Solutions for Female Incontinence

It's an embarrassing and distressing complaint among women, and also a common one. One minute you're laughing or coughing or sneezing or running, and the next you're mortified because you just leaked a little urine. Millions of women—twice as many women as men—suffer from urinary incontinence. A third of new mothers leak urine in the months after childbirth and a recent survey found that 16% of women—and up to 32% of older women—say they have some problems with incontinence.

For some women, urinary incontinence is merely a minor annoyance, but for others, it is so debilitating that they avoid social occasions or physical activities for fear of leakage. Andrew L. Rubman, ND, explains that there are many natural solutions for incontinence and most women who seek naturopathic treatment are able to avoid drastic measures like diapers, drugs (which may have multiple side effects) or surgery (which is never risk-free).

As in men, the *sacral plexus* exerts neurological control over urination, defecation and sexual function in women, but the female version of the story gets more complicated from there. A woman's urinary tract is structurally different from a man's, plus women undergo hormonal and physical changes related to pregnancy, childbirth and menopause.

What Causes Incontinence

Causes of female incontinence are very broad, ranging from structural issues, to hormonal issues, to bacterial and neurological challenges. *However, most of these problems can be helped with natural treatment...*

●**Pregnancy and childbirth can weaken the pelvic floor muscles and ligaments that support the bladder,** sometimes causing leakage. Forceps deliveries may raise risk, and the more times a woman has given birth, the greater her risk of pelvic weakness in the months and years to come.

●**Hysterectomy may cause shifts in how and where organs sit in the pelvis.**

●**Obesity stresses the bladder by putting additional pressure on it,** as well as on the pelvic floor.

●**Age and gravity.** Physiological changes in digestion that decrease the uptake of ingested calcium and magnesium can result in weakened muscle tone, says Dr. Rubman.

●**Misalignment in the sacroiliac joint.** The *sacroiliac joint*, which is located in the lower back between the spine and hip joint, sometimes gets moved out of alignment, often from childbirth. If it doesn't self-correct over time, this can lead to weakened pelvic muscles and ligaments.

●**Hormonal changes.** Lower estrogen levels following menopause may affect the muscles around the urethra, increasing the risk of leakage.

●**Urinary tract infections (UTIs).** Women are more apt to have urinary tract infections than men. Their shorter urethras make it easier for microbes to ascend into the urinary tract and embed in the lining of the bladder. Dr. Rubman notes that mold and yeast, which often underlie vulnerability to bacterial colonization, thrive in a moist environment, and the resulting inflammation and infection encourage leakage.

●**Antibiotic treatment or poor diet.** Antibiotics, which are often prescribed to women for UTIs, suppress the good bacteria right along with the bad. This can lead to fungal overgrowth and *Candida* infection at the urethral opening in the vulva. Eating too many processed foods and simple carbohydrates likewise can facilitate inflammation and microbial overgrowth.

●**Irritable bowel syndrome.** Inflammation in one area—for example, the bowel—can cause inflammation in another, Dr. Rubman explains. The physical proximity of these outlets also means that chronic microbial overgrowth in the bowel can potentially infiltrate the bladder.

●**Fibroids.** These benign uterine growths may press on the bladder and cause leakage.

●**Abnormal nerve signals.** Involuntary spasms of the bladder can be caused by damage to the nerves of the bladder, spinal cord or brain, typically the result of trauma or Parkinson's, stroke, MS or brain tumor.

Naturopathic Treatment of Incontinence

Just as there is no single reason for urinary incontinence, there is no single solution. *In his practice, Dr. Rubman prescribes a variety of strategies for his patients...*

●**Get tested for yeast and fungal infection.** Often doctors make the mistake of only testing for bacteria, then routinely prescribe antibiotics for UTIs, Dr. Rubman says, and might then miss an underlying problem with yeast, mold and fungi. Dr. Rubman typically orders a specific culture to check for the presence of yeast and fungus. Pending the results, he generally prescribes probiotics such as *lactobacillus* and *bifidobacterium* to bring microbial colonies back into balance.

• **Strengthen pelvic floor muscles.** Pelvic floor muscle training, both in late pregnancy and postpartum, may help prevent and/or treat incontinence related to childbirth.

To perform Kegel exercises: Locate your pelvic muscles by pretending to tighten your vagina around a tampon. Now alternately contract and relax your pelvic muscles, holding the relaxation phase for the same amount of time (about three seconds) as the contraction. Do three or four sets of 10 daily.

• **See a physical therapist.** There are physical therapists specially trained in women's health, who can teach women correct pelvic floor strengthening techniques. Ask your doctor for referral to someone in your area or go to the American Physical Therapy Association Web site at *www.apta.org.*

• **Maintain a proper weight.** A study in the *Journal of Urology* found that losing 5 to 10% of body weight can effectively treat urinary incontinence in women who are overweight or obese. Besides losing weight, other behavioral modifications that can help include quitting smoking, limiting alcohol and caffeine intake, and following an anti-inflammatory diet (high in lean protein such as fish and low in refined carbs and processed foods).

• **Get an adjustment.** If a misalignment in your sacroiliac joint is contributing to incontinence, see a chiropractic, osteopathic or naturopathic physician to properly align it.

• **Have a glass of cranberry juice...the unsweetened kind, that is.** Cranberry juice helps acidify urine, and contains a compound that makes the urinary tract more slippery. The resulting decrease in friction and reduced pH makes it harder for bacteria and other microorganisms to take hold. Supplements can help too. Dr. Rubman prescribes the freeze-dried extract produced by Eclectic Institute.

Note: Some women find cranberry juice irritating to the bladder.

• **Take vitamin C.** Like cranberry juice, vitamin C (ascorbic acid) helps acidify the urine. Dr. Rubman often prescribes vitamin C from Bronson Vitamins in doses varying with individual needs (*www.bronsonvita mins.com*).

The important thing to know is that incontinence is a largely treatable condition. See a naturopathic physician who will custom-design a treatment plan, and if necessary, coordinate care with your OB/GYN and urologist to bring the problem under control so you no longer have to be embarrassed by it.

Andrew L. Rubman, ND, medical director, Southbury Clinic for Traditional Medicines, Southbury, Connecticut.

The Dangers of Ill-Fitting Bras

Ladies, how does your bra fit? Chances are, not quite right. A British study that tested bra designs found that many women are unaware that they're wearing an ill-fitting bra. No big deal, you think? The truth is that when bras fit poorly, the bouncing that occurs can irreparably stretch the breast's connective tissues, causing sagging and pain, no matter what size your breasts are. "Breasts have little natural support," explains Joanna Scurr, PhD, author of the study and principal lecturer in the Department of Sport and Exercise Science at the University of Portsmouth, United Kingdom. Proper support is critical.

Best Bras Not Yet Available...

Dr. Scurr, a breast biomechanics expert, and her team are the first to conduct research in the 3D movement of breasts and how effective bras are at reducing it. They tested 50 or so bra designs on 200 women with a wide range of breast sizes. The women, who had sensors on their bodies, walked, jogged and ran on a treadmill while wearing different bra types. The researchers found that breasts bounce up to eight inches during exercise and that they move not only up and down, but also side to side and in and out. Slow jogging caused as much movement as did a full-out sprint. The problem is that most bras are designed to minimize only vertical motion, says Dr. Scurr, who is working with manufacturers to design a bra that can lessen movement in all three directions. Appropriate breast support is important even in the activities of daily life, she said.

Choose the Right Bra

Dr. Scurr advises shoppers to try on many different kinds of bras. Don't limit yourself to what you've always bought before or even what you think is most comfortable. The right bra may be different from the one you're accustomed to.

Specifically, she says, Get measured by a trained professional (usually employed at specialty/lingerie stores or high-end department stores) and use that measurement as a starting point, but try on lots of different-sized bras, constructed in different ways, since sizing varies among manufacturers.

Take a look and give a try to lots of different styles, too. Breasts come in different shapes and sizes, so not all styles will fit you well.

Make sure your chest band fits firmly, so you cannot easily fit your finger between the bra and your breastbone. The band provides the majority of support and a common mistake is having it fit too loose.

The underwire and shoulder straps should not dig into your flesh. The underwire should sit flat against your chest wall.

If you go down a band size (i.e., from a 36 to a 34) be aware that you then must go up a cup size.

The bra cup should not be baggy, nor should it press uncomfortably into breast tissue.

Always buy a bra that fits comfortably on the loosest setting—when you wash it, the material will stretch and you can then pull it in.

For the most support, buy an encapsulation bra, which has separate molded cups and limits motion in all directions. Avoid the compression bra (i.e., sports bras), which flattens the breasts, limiting only up and down movement.

Joanna Scurr, PhD, principal lecturer in the Department of Sport and Exercise Science at the University of Portsmouth, United Kingdom.

APPENDIX

NATURAL HEALING MODALITIES

Natural healing goes by many names. When natural healing techniques are used *instead* of conventional medicine, they are often called "alternative" healing. When they are used *with* conventional medicine, they are called "integrative" healing or "complementary medicine"—and dozens of top hospitals at major medical schools now feature "complementary and alternative medicine" or CAM. Regardless of the name, natural healing consists of *modalities*—the remedies and techniques that help the body heal itself, while avoiding or minimizing the troubling side effects of drugs. There are dozens of such modalities, from the energy-balancing needles of acupuncture to the healing postures of yoga therapy. In the following section, experts explain a number of time-tested natural healing modalities, many of them discussed in previous chapters. You'll discover why each specific modality works and how you can use it for better health and healing.

What Energy Healing Can Do for You

Many mainstream American doctors are taking a more open-minded look at so-called *energy healing*. In China, such forms of energy are known as *qi*...in India, the term is *prana*. The National Institutes of Health's National Center for Complementary and Alternative Medicine is actively involved in the scientific investigation of energy healing. And energy therapies are quietly gaining popularity among Western patients seeking alternatives to conventional medicine.

Gary E. Schwartz, PhD, one of the world's leading experts in the scientific study of energy healing, answers questions about how such therapies are being used in the US.

What exactly is energy healing?

To understand energy healing, it's useful to first discuss energy fields, which play a key role in our society. They support the radio-wave technology that allows us to use cell phones, satellite TV, garage-door openers and any number of other wireless technologies. These radio waves, which cannot be seen, are capable of transmitting data, conversations, music and visual images through the air, often over a distance of thousands of miles. Energy fields also are widely used in technology that diagnoses and treats disease. For example, electromagnetic fields are used in magnetic resonance imaging (MRI) scans and cardiac pacemakers.

Energy healing refers to the use of invisible frequencies of energy. Some of these frequencies have been measured via reproducible methods, while others are theorized. Practitioners of energy healing believe that disturbances in the energy fields that flow throughout the human body can result in illness.

There are studies suggesting that one person's energy fields can overlap and interact with another person's energy fields. For example, even when people are not touching each other, the electrical activity of one person's heart can be registered in the other person's *electroencephalogram* (EEG), a recorded image of the electrical activity in different parts of the brain.

How is energy healing now practiced in the US?

There are various forms. The most popular include Healing Touch (developed in the 1980s)...and Reiki (developed in 1922). With each of these therapies, the practitioner seeks to "manipulate" a patient's life force—or energy. The techniques can involve touching the patient or placing one's hands a few inches or feet from the patient's body. With Reiki, at least four 30- to 90-minute sessions are typically recommended. In a study of older adults receiving Healing Touch, pain reduction was reported after an average of 6.4 sessions.

How is energy healing believed to work?

I like to use the metaphor of a ladder, with each step providing a higher and wider view. On one step are electromagnetic fields generated by an energy healer's hands—fields that research shows can resonate with and change plant, animal and human cells. The energy of the healer's hands interacts with the energy of the patient and they respond to each other—something akin to two tuning forks resonating with each other.

Is there any scientific proof that energy healing is effective?

As a trained scientist, I started out as a skeptic, but after conducting research on energy healing for 10 years, I am certain that energy plays a role in health and healing.

One remarkable experiment that helped convince me that energy healing is real was conducted here at the University of Arizona and published in the *Journal of Alternative and Complementary Medicine*.

In the experiment, rats were subjected to daily stress from noise. One group of rats was treated with Reiki. Another group was "treated" by fake energy healers who stood in front of the animals' cages moving their arms in a way that mimicked the outward actions of the Reiki practitioners but with no intention to heal the rats.

At the end of the study, the rats treated with Reiki had significantly less stress-caused damage to small blood vessels. This study showed quite convincingly that energy healing is real—because with rats, there is no placebo effect.

Dozens of studies on humans have shown that energy healing, in the form of Reiki and Healing Touch, has improved such medical conditions as pain, wound healing and high blood pressure.

If the evidence is strong, why is there such widespread skepticism about energy healing?

There are several reasons. Many people tend to think of the world in material terms, as opposed to invisible, energetic terms. These individuals may not have grown up with cell phones and satellite TV or with the reality that there are unseen energies all around us that convey information. Also, the first energy healers tended to be "New Agers." Some were frauds and made outlandish claims—and people threw out the baby with the bathwater.

There are also powerful economic forces, such as those wielded by the pharmaceutical industry, that have a vested interest in not accepting a nondrug methodology that can reduce and, in some cases, eliminate the need for drugs.

New scientific ideas are always met with resistance, but I believe there will be a paradigm shift in which energy healing is accepted and becomes widely practiced by health professionals.

Why do critics of energy healing claim that the evidence is inconclusive?

Most of these critics have not reached their conclusions based on a thorough knowledge of the literature. Some applications of energy healing, such as its use in stress and pain reduction, are well documented, while other applications have not yet undergone rigorous scientific evaluation and are considered inconclusive.

Is energy healing particularly effective for certain health conditions?

Positive effects are uniformly reported in pain reduction, wound healing and stress relief. Energy healing also is effective in diseases caused or exacerbated by stress, such as high blood pressure.

Are there any risks associated with energy healing?

The risk for adverse effects is very low, particularly when compared with drugs and surgery. In rare cases, people who are particularly sensitive to energy may have an adverse response, such as a flare-up of allergies. But as a rule, energy healing is safe and can have profoundly powerful positive effects.

What's the best way to locate a competent energy healer?

Several organizations train and certify energy healers. To find lists of certified healers, go to the Healing Touch Program, 210-497-5529, *www.htpractitioner.com*…or the International Center for Reiki Training, 800-332-8112, *www.reiki.org*. You also can get a recommendation from a holistic physician or other health professional who is open to energy healing. Or talk to a friend who has had a positive experience with an energy healer.

Gary E. Schwartz, PhD, professor of psychology, medicine, neurology, psychiatry and surgery at the University of Arizona and director of the university's Laboratory for Advances in Consciousness and Health, both in Tucson. He is the author of The Energy Healing Experiments (Atria), www. drgaryschwartz.com.

Yoga Can Help You—But Which Kind Is Best?

Yoga is powerful medicine. It can improve balance, flexibility and posture… strengthen muscles and bones…lower blood pressure, ease pain and boost immune function…heighten sexual functioning…alleviate stress and depression…and bolster spiritual well-being.

Key: Finding a style that fits your abilities, temperament and goals. *With your doctor's okay, consider…*

●**Anusara.** This playful, warm-hearted and physically challenging style emphasizes body alignment (often with hands-on adjustments from the teacher) and a positive mindset that looks for the good in all people.

Best for: Physically fit people who want to be part of a like-minded community.

●**Ashtanga ("power" yoga).** A vigorous practice, it includes a fixed series of postures that flow rapidly and continuously, accompanied by energizing breathing techniques.

Best for: People who can handle an intense workout, want to build stamina and strength, and enjoy a set routine.

●**Bikram ("hot" yoga).** An invariable sequence of 26 poses is performed in a studio heated to at least 100°F to loosen muscles, tendons and ligaments.

Best for: People in good health who don't mind heat and want improved flexibility. Bikram, like other vigorous styles, may not be appropriate for frail or older students or those with serious illnesses.

●**Integral.** Beginning classes include gentle poses, breathing techniques, meditation and discussions of ancient yoga texts. The principle of selfless service (such as volunteer work) is emphasized. Some centers offer special classes for students with physical limitations or health problems (such as heart disease or cancer).

Best for: People interested in traditional Indian yoga that includes more than just poses.

●**Iyengar.** Emphasizing meticulous body alignment, this style makes use of blocks, straps and other props so students with limited flexibility can safely and comfortably assume poses. Teacher training requirements are among the strictest.

Best for: Anyone new to yoga or especially in need of better body alignment, such as people with arthritis or back pain.

●**Kripalu.** A blend of Western psychology and Eastern philosophy, this practice provides a safe place to explore emotional issues. Meditation and chanting accompany moderately vigorous and sometimes improvised movement.

Best for: People looking for stress relief and emotional release.

● **Kundalini.** This style includes a wide variety of breathing techniques, intense physical movements, chanting and meditation. The focus is on raising energy rather than on precise body alignment.

Best for: People who are seeking to build *prana* (life force) and who are open to yoga's spiritual dimensions.

● **Viniyoga.** Gentle flowing poses are held only briefly. Safety and breath work are emphasized. Teachers often focus on private one-on-one sessions rather than group classes.

Best for: People who are new to yoga or out of shape or who are looking to use yoga to help alleviate any of a variety of chronic ailments.

To find a class: Yoga Alliance (888-921-9642, *www.yogaalliance.org*) registers teachers who complete a certain number of hours of training in specific styles. If you have a medical condition, contact the teacher to see if a particular class is appropriate for you or to ask about private lessons. Yoga therapy has been shown in studies to be effective for a wide range of conditions, from diabetes and arthritis to cancer and chronic lung disease.

Timothy McCall, MD, board-certified internist, medical editor of *Yoga Journal* and author of *Yoga as Medicine: The Yogic Prescription for Health and Healing* (Bantam). *www.drmccall.com.*

So Much More Than a Foot Massage!

Reflexology has long been viewed by many Americans and medical professionals as little more than a relaxing foot massage.

Now: Recent scientific studies show that chronic pain, digestive disorders and other common health problems can be relieved through the use of this practice. Reflexology, which was developed by three medical professionals in the early 20th century, involves applying pressure to specific areas—known as "reflex points"—located on the feet, hands and ears.

How it works: When a body part is injured or stops functioning properly due to disease, irritating chemicals accumulate in distant but related nerve endings in the feet, hands and ears. Various studies have repeatedly shown that when certain parts of the feet, hands and ears are worked on with touch techniques, relief results in corresponding parts of the body.

Bonus: You can perform many basic forms of reflexology on yourself or a partner.*

For best results, work on all of the reflex points described in this article for at least five minutes twice a day, four or more times a week. Relief can be experienced within minutes, but it sometimes takes days or weeks of repeatedly working on the appropriate reflex areas to get results.

Caution: Do not work on bruises, cuts, sores, skin infections or directly on areas where you have damaged a bone or strained a joint during the preceding three to six months. If you've had surgery or suffered a bone fracture, ask your surgeon when it's safe to perform reflexology on these areas.

The main technique used on most parts of the feet and hands, including those points described below, is the "thumb roll."

What to do: Place gentle pressure with the pad of your thumb against the area on which you wish to work. Maintaining this pressure and moving slowly, bend the knuckle in the center of the thumb in an upward direction and roll your thumb from the pad toward the tip, moving it forward. Next, reverse the movement of the knuckle, so that once your thumb is flattened you can do another thumb

*To find a certified reflexologist in your area, contact the American Reflexology Certification Board, 303-933-6921, *www.arcb.net.*

roll, each time moving forward in the direction the thumb is pointing.

Reflex points that correspond to common complaints...

Heartburn

What to do: While sitting in a chair, place your left foot on your right knee. Use your left thumb to locate the "diaphragm line," which separates the ball of your foot and your instep, where the skin color changes between the pad and soft part of the sole. On this line, about an inch from the inner edge of the foot, press gently with the tip of your thumb while squeezing gently with your index finger on top of the foot for five to 10 minutes.

Next, place the tip of your right thumb on the soft part of your left palm at the point between the base of the knuckles below your index and middle fingers. With the fingers of your right hand gently squeezing the back of your left hand, apply gentle pressure with the tip of your right thumb for five to 10 minutes.

Headache

What to do: Start with the hand corresponding to the side of your head where the pain is most noticeable. On the back of that hand, locate a point about an inch below the base knuckle of your index finger in the fleshy web between your index finger and thumb. Place the tip of the thumb of your other hand on this point and the tip of your index finger of the other hand on the palm side of this point, squeezing to find a spot that's slightly thicker and more tender than the surrounding area. While maintaining steady pressure, gently move the tip of your thumb in small circles over this spot. (This movement is different from the thumb roll.) It usually takes about five minutes of work to alleviate a tension headache, and up to an hour to reduce or eliminate a migraine headache.

Caution: This point should not be worked on during the first trimester of pregnancy, as it could have an adverse effect on the fetus.

Instead, work only on the related point on the ear, as described in "neck pain" below.

After you have completed the hand reflexology, locate the small, hard flap of cartilage at the top of your earlobe, then feel where this flap and the earlobe meet. With the tip of your thumb on the front of the ear and the tip of your index finger behind the ear, gently squeeze this point between your index finger and thumb, feeling for a spot that's slightly thicker and more tender than the surrounding area. Squeeze both ears at once, holding for five to 10 minutes, while resting your elbows on a table or desk.

Irritable Bowel Syndrome

What to do: While sitting, place your left foot on your right knee. With your left hand, gently grasp the top of the foot. Using the thumb roll technique in repeated overlapping strips, work across from the inner edge to the outer edge of the foot, on all of the soft part of the sole and the entire heel, for 10 minutes. Repeat, using your right thumb on the bottom of your right foot.

After you have completed the foot reflexology, use your right thumb to perform the thumb roll technique on your left palm. Work from the outside to the inside of the palm, starting just below the base of the fingers and progressing toward the wrist. Repeat, using your left thumb to work on the right palm.

Neck Pain and Stiff Neck

What to do: Move your finger slightly above the cartilage flap described in the headache section, and find a ridge of cartilage running up and down the ear. Place the tips of your index fingers on the lower inch of this ridge on both ears while resting your elbows on a table or desk. Squeeze gently but firmly between your index fingers and thumbs, with your thumbs behind the ears. Continue for five to 10 minutes.

Bill Flocco, reflexology teacher and researcher, founder and director of the American Academy of Reflexology, based in Los Angeles and author of several books on reflexology, including *Reflexology Research: Anatomy of a Reflexology Research Study* (William Sanford).

Tai Chi Helps You Stay Young and Vital

I f you don't like to exercise, try *tai chi*—a Chinese martial art consisting of very slow controlled movements. It's great for stress reduction and for maintaining muscle tone and balance.

Tai chi expert Roger Jahnke, OMD, author of *The Healer Within* (HarperOne) and *The Healing Promise of Qi* (McGraw-Hill), trains teachers of tai chi at the Institute of Integral Qigong and Tai Chi (*www.IIQTC.org*). Here he describes easy-to-do beginner exercises that will help you find out immediately how great tai chi can make you feel.

Exercise 1 • Raise Hands

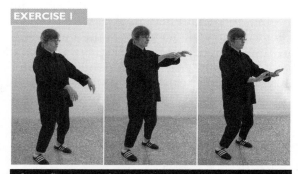

Arms float up to shoulder level, then float back down.

(This exercise also can be performed in a seated position with only the arm movements.)

Do 10 repetitions 1 to 2 times daily.

Helps: Develop a calm awareness of the body. Builds leg and arm strength.

1. Stand with feet shoulder-width apart or slightly wider (toes pointing forward). Bend your knees slightly. Don't let your knees extend past the front of your toes.

2. Rest your palms on the front of your thighs. Inhale as you straighten your legs (don't lock them). Keep your fingers slightly down (so that your wrists are bent) as you let your arms float up to shoulder level.

What Tai Chi Can Do

● **It can improve immune function.**

● **It can reduce pain** and safely increases movement in people with arthritis.

● **It reduces risk of falling by nearly 50%** in people age 65 and older by improving balance.

● **Its slow, gentle movements and the sensation of slowing down increase energy.** Some practitioners have said that it feels as though you are moving through water.

3. Bend your knees and let your arms float down—fingers pointed up—as you bend your elbows and sink further into the bent-knee position. Then slowly straighten your wrists so that your outstretched hands (palms facing down) are aligned with your arms.

4. Exhale as you slowly sink down, bending your knees as much as is comfortable. Keep your palms parallel to the ground as you come back to the starting position.

Exercise 2 • Swaying Bear

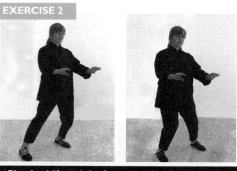

Slowly shift weight from one leg to the other.

(If this exercise is difficult, try it holding on to a chair. When you get stronger, you can try it without the chair.)

Do 10 repetitions on each side.

Helps: Develop a sense of balance and strengthen the leg muscles.

1. Stand with your feet a little wider than shoulder-width, toes facing forward. Bend your knees slightly.

2. Place your hands at your sides (at waist level) with your palms facing down and your elbows bent. Imagine your arms floating on top of water.

3. Very, very slowly shift your weight from side to side, keeping your knee over your foot and not bending your knee past your toes. Slowly shift to the right by bending and putting your weight onto your right leg—then slowly shift back and put more weight onto your left leg. Go to the point where the other leg is straight but not locked. As you advance, you can take a wider stance and bend your knees farther.

Roger Jahnke, OMD, tai chi expert and trainer, Institute of Integral Qigong and Tai Chi. *www.IIQTC.org.*

Mark A. Stengler, NMD, naturopathic medical doctor in private practice, La Jolla, California, and author of the *Bottom Line/Natural Healing* newsletter. *www.drstengler.com.*

Get Hypnotized, Get Healthier

Hear the word "hypnosis" and you may think of a stage show—a guy in a turban dangling a pocket watch and making you cluck like a chicken or behave in some other silly and uncharacteristic way.

This is not at all what modern hypnotherapy is like.

Reality: Ericksonian hypnosis (named after American psychiatrist Milton Erickson, who pioneered the techniques used today) is a collaboration between you and a trained health-care practitioner that can help you achieve specific health goals.

Hypnotherapy does not use commands, such as, "Now you will do what I say." Instead, the practitioner offers gentle, nonauthoritative suggestions when you are in a highly relaxed state. The idea behind hypnosis is that there is no separation between body and mind—so you can access the healing potential of the unconscious mind to move yourself in a healthful direction. Unlike classical hypnosis, which works on only a small subset of highly suggestible people, Ericksonian hypnosis can help almost anyone—though it is most effective for those who are motivated and accepting of treatment.

Help from Hypnosis

Research shows that hypnotherapy helps treat a variety of physical and psychological problems, including...

- Anxiety
- Chronic pain
- Insomnia
- Irritable bowel syndrome (recurring bouts of diarrhea and/or constipation)
- Menopausal
- Nausea
- Overeating
- Phobias, such as claustrophobia or fear of flying
- Sugar addiction
- Tobacco addiction

Examples: One study found that a single 15-minute hypnosis session significantly decreased pain and anxiety in women undergoing breast cancer surgery—and, for unknown reasons, also shortened the procedure time in the operating room. In another study, 68% of women with menopausal hot flashes showed reduced symptom severity and frequency, as well as decreased insomnia, after hypnosis.

How it works: Everybody has chatter in the conscious mind that can get in the way of healthful behaviors, such as controlling consumption of sweets or not panicking in an elevator. Hypnosis quiets the conscious mind so your unconscious can come in and say, "Wait a minute, we're trying to be healthier here"—making it easier to turn down that donut or stay calm in the elevator. Hypnosis relieves physical symptoms, such as pain or hot flashes, by reducing stress hormones that contribute to physical ailments.

Hypnosis by itself does not cure the problem—rather, it creates a heightened state of awareness that opens the way for your own willingness to bring about the desired changes. Hypnotherapy can focus on symptom reduction...strategies for coping with stress...resolution of personal problems...and/or personality development.

What to Expect in Treatment

Typically, the first session with a hypnotherapist lasts one hour. During this visit, the practitioner asks questions about your particular problem—when symptoms began, other treatments you have tried, how the issue affects your life and stress level. Because hypnotherapy is highly individualized, this information helps determine the most appropriate treatment for you. Hypnosis may or may not be done during this first session.

A course of hypnotherapy generally ranges from three to eight sessions, with each weekly hypnosis session lasting about 30 to 40 minutes. Sometimes patients return months or years later for a "booster" session.

During a session, you sit on a comfortable chair or couch in a quiet and softly lit room. Usually your eyes are closed, but you can hear everything around you.

Speaking in a soothing voice, the practitioner leads you into an *induction*, a trance-like state of deep relaxation. One common technique is the *body scan*. The practitioner asks you to focus on your feet, relaxing the muscles there. Next you focus on feeling the relaxed sensation in your ankles, your calves, your knees. Over five to 10 minutes, the practitioner guides you to relax your entire body.

While you are in a state of deep relaxation, the practitioner makes therapeutic suggestions, prompting your unconscious mind to deal more effectively with your health issue. The practitioner does not say something like, "You will not be afraid of the airplane," but rather, "You may find yourself feeling much more relaxed on the airplane than you have

in the past." Suggestions are tailored to the specific problem and person. The process generally is pleasant and completely safe. You do not reveal personal secrets or do anything that you don't want to do.

After the therapeutic suggestions, the practitioner typically brings you back to your normal state of consciousness by saying, "I'm going to be quiet now, and over the next few minutes, you can gradually bring yourself back to the room." You may or may not consciously remember what was said to you during hypnosis...you may come to the end of a session thinking that it lasted just a few minutes, when in reality it lasted half an hour.

Over the following few days or weeks, you may notice that your symptoms are improving—for instance, you sleep better, feel less nauseous or fearful, or find it easier to resist cravings for cigarettes.

Hypnotherapy Homework

The practitioner may assign you some simple self-hypnosis techniques to do on your own. For instance, if you are seeking to change a habit, such as compulsive overeating, self-hypnosis helps you handle cravings as they arise. These techniques typically include physical strategies, such as pressing two fingers together as a reminder of how to reach the relaxation state...or taking a series of deep breaths while focusing on a certain calming image or phrase.

For a physical problem, such as irritable bowel syndrome, the practitioner may tape-record an in-office hypnosis session and have you listen to it at home. As you reexperience the state of deep relaxation again and again, not only your mind but your entire body benefits—making your gut less susceptible to digestive upsets.

Finding a practitioner: In addition to being a licensed doctor, psychologist or social worker, a qualified practitioner should have about one year of hypnotherapy training. To ensure that your practitioner has met educational standards and training requirements in clinical hypnosis, you may want to verify that he/she is certified through the American

Society of Clinical Hypnosis (630-980-4740, *www.asch.net*).

Hypnotherapy costs about $125 to $300 per session. Although many insurance companies do not cover hypnosis per se, you may be able to collect under a mental-health benefit if your psychotherapist or integrative physician includes hypnosis among the treatments offered.

Benjamin Kligler, MD, MPH, vice chair of the department of integrative medicine at Beth Israel Medical Center and research director of the Continuum Center for Health and Healing, New York City. *www.healthandhealingny.org.*

Relief at Your Fingertips

You've probably heard of acupuncture, but there's something similar that you can do yourself—no needles involved—called *acupressure*. Acupressure can alleviate many physical, mental and emotional problems in only a few minutes—and it is free.

Acupressure involves stimulating acupoints on the body with fingertips or knuckles and is based on the principles of acupuncture, an ancient healing technique used by practitioners of Traditional Chinese Medicine (TCM). The acupoints often have ancient descriptive names, such as "Joining the Valley" and "Mind Clearing." Acupressure increases blood flow to the treated area and triggers the release of endorphins, pain-relieving brain chemicals.

Here are the acupressure techniques for various health problems. Unless otherwise noted, daily acupressure sessions, three times a day, are the best way to relieve a temporary or chronic problem. See the box on page 353 for specific advice.

Arthritis Pain

Joining the Valley is a truly amazing acupoint because it can relieve arthritis pain anywhere in the body.

Location: In the webbing between the thumb and index finger, at the highest spot of the muscle when the thumb and index finger are brought close together.

What to do: Rhythmically squeeze the acupoint. As you're squeezing, place the side of your hand that is closest to the little finger on your thigh or a tabletop. Apply pressure in the webbing as you press downward. This allows you to angle more deeply into the point, increasing the benefits.

Also good for: Headache, toothache, hangover, hay fever symptoms, constipation.

Caution: This point is forbidden for pregnant women because its stimulation can cause premature contraction in the uterus.

Memory Problems

The Mind Clearing acupoints are for improving recall instantly—for example, when you have forgotten a name or gone to the supermarket without your shopping list.

Location: One finger width (about one-half inch) directly above the center of each eyebrow.

What to do: Gently place your right thumb above your right eyebrow and your middle fingertip above the eyebrow on the left side. Hold very gently. You should feel a slight dip or indentation in the bone structure—the acupoints on both sides are in the dip. Press the indentation very lightly, hold and breathe deeply. After a minute or two, you'll experience more mental clarity and sharper memory.

Lower Back Pain

To help prevent and relieve lower back pain, practice this exercise for one minute three times a day. You can do it standing or sitting.

Location: Place the backs of your hands against your lower back, about one inch outside the spine.

What to do: Briskly rub your hands up and down—about three inches up and six inches down—using the friction to create heat in your lower back.

If you're doing the technique correctly, you'll need to breathe deeply to sustain the vigorous rubbing, and you'll break out in a slight sweat.

Also good for: Food cravings, especially sugar cravings, chronic fatigue, sexual problems, chills, phobias and fibromyalgia symptoms.

Emotional Upset

The Inner Gate acupoint can reduce emotional upset—such as anxiety, depression and irritability—in two to three minutes.

Location: On the inner side of the forearm, three finger widths up from the center of the wrist crease, in between two thick tendons.

What to do: Place your thumb on the point and your fingers directly behind the outside of the forearm between the two bones. Squeeze in slowly and firmly, hold for two to three minutes, breathing deeply. Repeat on the other arm for the same amount of time.

Also good for: Carpal tunnel syndrome, insomnia, indigestion and nausea.

Colds and Flu

If you think you're about to get a cold or flu, stimulating the Heavenly Rejuvenation acupoint may prevent infection.

Location: On the shoulders, midway between the base of the neck and the outside of the shoulders, one-half inch below the top of the shoulders, just above the tip of the shoulder blades.

What to do: There are two ways to stimulate this point...

Curving your fingers, hook your right hand on your right shoulder and your left hand on your left shoulder. You also can use your fingers on your opposite shoulder, which may be easier. With your fingertips, firmly press the point and take three slow, deep breaths.

If you don't have the flexibility to perform the first technique...lie down on your back, on a firm mattress or carpeted floor, with your knees bent and feet on the floor as close to your buttocks as possible. Bring your hands above your head, and rest the backs of your hands on the floor beside or above your head. Inhale and lift up your pelvis, pressing your feet against the floor to assist the lift. The higher your pelvis, the more weight will be transferred onto your shoulders, stimulating the acupoint. Hold this posture for one minute, taking long, slow, deep breaths, with your eyes closed. Lower your pelvis, and rest for three minutes.

Also good for: Nervous tension, stiff neck, high fever, chills, shoulder aches and irritability.

Insomnia

The acupoints Calm Sleep and Joyful Sleep—on the outer and inner ankles—can help relieve insomnia. Use these acupressure points whenever you want to deeply relax and sleep better.

Location: Calm Sleep is in the first indentation below the outer anklebone. Joyful Sleep is directly below the inside of the anklebone, in a slight indentation.

What to do: Place your thumb on one side of your ankle and your fingers on the other, and press firmly. If you're on the right spot, it will be slightly sore. Hold for two minutes, breathing deeply. Repeat on the other ankle. Do this again if you still are having trouble sleeping or if you wake up.

Headaches

The acupoints Gates of Consciousness relieve a tension headache or migraine.

Location: Underneath the base of your skull to either side of your spine, about three to four inches apart, depending on the size of your head.

What to do: Using your fingers, thumbs or knuckles, press the points under the base of your skull.

At the same time, slowly tilt your head back so that the angle of your head relaxes your neck muscles. Press forward (toward your throat), upward (underneath the base of your skull) and slightly inward, angling the pressure toward the center of your brain.

Continue to apply pressure for two minutes, breathing.

Also good for: Neck pain, insomnia, high blood pressure.

Michael Reed Gach, PhD, founder of the Acupressure Institute in Berkeley, California and author of self-healing instructional DVDs and CDs and many books, including *Acupressure's Potent Points* (Bantam), *Acupressure for Lovers* (Bantam) and *Arthritis Relief at Your Fingertips* (Warner). *www.Acupressure.com.*

Acupressure Basics

Unless otherwise noted, use your middle finger, with your index and ring fingers for support. Firmly and gradually, apply stationary pressure directly on the acupoint for three minutes.

● **Firmly means using an amount of pressure that causes a sensation between pleasure and pain—pressure that "hurts good."** If the pressure is applied too fast or too hard, the point will hurt. If the pressure is too soft, you won't get the full benefit.

● **Gradually means moving your finger into and out of the point in super-slow motion.** Applying and releasing finger pressure allow the tissue to respond and relax, promoting healing.

● **Stationary means you are not rubbing or massaging the area.**

● **Directly means at a 90-degree angle from the surface of the skin.** If you are pulling the skin, the angle of pressure is incorrect.

● **When you apply pressure, lean your weight toward the point.** If your hands are weak or it hurts your fingers when you apply pressure, try using your knuckles. You also can use a tool, such as a golf ball or pencil eraser.

● **Breathe slowly and deeply while you apply pressure.** This helps release pain and tension.

The Healing Powers Of Massage Therapy

Nearly 60% of doctors in the US recommend massage for some patients—almost twice as many as recommended it five years ago.

Why the dramatic increase?

For years, therapeutic massage was recommended primarily for musculoskeletal conditions, such as arthritis, low back pain and muscle tension. Now, credible research shows that massage has benefits that most doctors never expected. *What we now know...*

Why Massage Helps

Scientists now have evidence that massage affects virtually every major body function—from immunity to lung and brain function—and confers health benefits through a variety of mechanisms.

Even though massage therapists are usually trained in one or more massage techniques, such as Swedish, Shiatsu and deep tissue massage, there is no evidence that one technique is better than another for most conditions.

Studies indicate that the application of moderate pressure—firm enough to make an indentation in the skin—is the key to massage's health benefits. By stimulating pressure receptors under the skin, massage activates different branches of the vagus nerve, which regulates blood pressure, heart rate and many other physiological functions.

Massage also...

● **Reduces levels of stress hormones, such as cortisol.** This is important for pain relief, easing depression and increasing energy levels. Reductions in cortisol also enhance immune function, including the ability of natural killer cells to target viruses and cancer cells.

● **Enhances deeper sleep stages (known as *delta sleep*),** which helps reduce levels of a brain chemical, known as substance P, that is related to the sensation of pain.

Massage is now used to treat...

High Blood Pressure

Patients with elevated blood pressure often have high levels of stress hormones. Massage not only lowers levels of these hormones but also stimulates the branch of the *vagus nerve* that leads to the heart. Stimulating the nerve decreases heart rate and lowers blood pressure.

In one study, adults with hypertension were given 10 half-hour massages over five weeks. They showed a statistically significant decrease in diastolic (bottom number) blood pressure and reported less depression and anxiety—common problems in patients being treated for hypertension.

Carpal Tunnel Syndrome

The median nerve in the wrist passes through a narrow opening (the carpal tunnel) on the palm side of the wrist. Swelling or inflammation of the nerve, usually caused by repetitive movements such as typing or using a screwdriver, can result in chronic tingling, numbness and/or pain in the thumb as well as the index and middle fingers. Researchers at Baylor University Medical Center have recently reported that even gripping the steering wheel of a car for long hours may lead to carpal tunnel syndrome.

A daily self-massage can reduce pain and promote an increase in *nerve-conduction velocity*, a measure of nerve health.

15-minute self-massage: Using moderate pressure, stroke from the wrist to the elbow and back down on both sides of the forearm. Next, apply a wringing motion to the same area. Using the thumb and index finger, stroke the entire forearm and the hand in a circular or back-and-forth motion. Finish by rolling the skin with the thumb and index finger, moving across the hand and up both sides of the forearm.

Burns

Serious burns are among the most painful wounds. The standard treatments—including brushing away debris and cleaning the area—can be excruciatingly painful. Massage done before the skin is brushed appears to elevate the pain threshold of burn patients— perhaps by increasing levels of the brain chemical serotonin.

Example: If one hand is burned, another person can vigorously rub the patient's other hand. This activation of skin receptors, in effect, blocks the feeling of pain related to the burn.

Pain

Studies show that massage curbs back pain, migraine and cancer pain. It may do this by reducing the pain-promoting chemical *substance P* as well as the stress hormone *cortisol.*

Key findings: In three separate studies, patients with back pain were treated either with massage or a sham treatment (a massage with insufficient pressure to provide any benefit). Patients in both groups were treated twice weekly for 20 minutes. Those in the massage group consistently had less pain and better range of motion than patients in the sham group.

Massage also seems to help postsurgical pain. In a pilot study, researchers at Cedars-Sinai Medical Center in Los Angeles found that patients who received massages after heart-bypass surgery had less pain and fewer muscle spasms than those who didn't get massages.

To find a massage therapist, consult the American Massage Therapy Association, 877-905-2700, *www.amtamassage.org.*

Tiffany M. Field, PhD, author of *Touch* (MIT Press) and director of the Touch Research Institute at the University of Miami School of Medicine. *www.miami.edu/touch-research.*

The Essential Guide To Acupuncture

Acupuncture has been practiced in Asia for more than 5,000 years, but only recently has Western medicine begun to acknowledge this ancient healing therapy. Just over a decade ago, the FDA reclassified acupuncture needles from "experimental" status to "medical device." Around the same time, a consensus panel of the National Institutes of Health (NIH) found acupuncture to be an effective treatment for postoperative dental pain, chemotherapy-induced nausea and several other conditions.

Since then, people in the US have increasingly embraced acupuncture as an alternative or complementary therapy for numerous common ailments—and many health insurance companies now cover it. *What acupuncture can do for you...*

How It Works

The human body has 12 major energy *meridians* (pathways), each corresponding to a different organ system. Flowing through this network is the body's *qi* (pronounced chee), or life force. Health problems result when there is too much or too little qi in specific places.

Example: If qi flow is excessive, a woman may be congested, feverish or unable to sleep. If qi flow is insufficient, she may lack energy, feel chilly or catch a cold.

Acupuncture often eases arthritis, asthma, migraine and many other conditions (see the list on page 356). The practitioner inserts very fine needles into the skin at one or more of about 1,000 specific points. This either calms the flow of excessive energy or stimulates the point if the qi is blocked.

Among Western researchers, the most widely accepted theories are that acupuncture triggers the release of pain-relieving brain chemicals called endorphins...helps release substances that transmit nerve impulses to the brain...and/or stimulates the immune system.

To date, one of the largest and most rigorous trials on acupuncture in the US was an NIH study in 2004 involving 570 participants. The study evaluated acupuncture's usefulness in treating osteoarthritis of the knee.

Results: After receiving 23 acupuncture sessions over 26 weeks, participants showed, on average, 40% more improvement in pain plus significantly more improvement in movement and function compared with a control group that received sham acupuncture. (In sham treatments, fine needles are inserted but not in the appropriate points.)

What to Expect

Before seeing an acupuncturist for a health condition, it is best to have a diagnosis from a medical doctor or naturopathic doctor. This helps the acupuncturist provide appropriate complementary treatment. However, even if a doctor has not been able to diagnose your problem, acupuncture still may correct the underlying cause or causes of your symptoms.

Example: Effie Poy Yew Chow, PhD, RN, California-licensed acupuncturist, had a patient with severe asthma plus unexplained joint pain and digestive problems. Within two weeks of her first acupuncture session, the patient's symptoms were gone and she was able to discontinue her many medications.

Your acupuncturist also will want as complete a picture of you as possible—including your health history and medications...diet and supplement use...exercise and sleep patterns...relationships, emotional state and stress level. Healing is most complete when a patient takes responsibility for his/her own health—so getting stuck with needles is only

Should Acupuncture Ever Be Painful?

With acupuncture, fine needles inserted into the skin at specific points eliminate blockage of *qi*—the energy life force flowing through the body. Qi blockage leads to illness. Ideally, the needle precisely hits the blocked point, creating an "energy grabbing" of the needle called *dur-qi*. This feels like a slight electric shock or pinprick, but it may hurt if qi blockage is severe. Dur-qi activates the body's meridian system (network of energy channels), promoting healing.

part of the process. You may be advised to adjust your diet and lifestyle, keep a journal of your feelings and/or take steps to reduce stress.

At the start of every session, the acupuncturist checks the pulse points that correspond with the various meridians and examines your tongue color and coating, which provide clues to imbalances in qi flow. Then, depending on where the needles need to go, you'll lie face down, face up or on your side during treatment.

Does It Hurt?

Many people hesitate to try acupuncture for fear that it will hurt. In fact, the needles are so fine that they cause little pain. You may feel a brief uncomfortable sensation—like a pinprick or small electric shock—from the electromagnetic force or "energy grabbing" of the needle. This subsides within seconds, and then you may feel a wave of calmness. If you do feel a strong reaction when a needle goes in, it may mean that you have a lot of qi blockage. The needle disperses that blockage, so with each treatment, discomfort lessens.

Note: The needle should not cause prolonged discomfort. If it does, tell the practitioner so he/she can make adjustments.

The number of needles varies with the condition being treated, your individual needs and the practitioner's training. Needles may be inserted just a tiny fraction of an inch or as deep as an inch or more. They may be left in place for a few minutes, a few hours or even a few days.

A session usually lasts 20 to 60 minutes and costs from $60 to $100 or more, depending on the practitioner and location. Patients generally have a total of six to 10 sessions, going once or twice weekly at first and then gradually increasing the time between appointments as their symptoms improve. Patients may notice improvement during a session, hours after a session or sometimes only after a number of sessions.

Safety: When done by a qualified practitioner, acupuncture is safe for most people. The practitioner should swab treatment sites

Problems Often Treated with Acupuncture

Acupuncture may ease many conditions, including...

- Anxiety
- Arthritis
- Asthma
- Back pain
- Bladder infections
- Blood sugar imbalances
- Bursitis
- Carpal tunnel syndrome
- Dental pain
- Depression
- Fibromyalgia (widespread muscle and joint pain)
- Headache and migraine
- Insomnia
- Menopausal hot flashes
- Menstrual cramps
- Postoperative nausea
- Sciatica
- Seizures
- Sinus problems
- Stress
- Tendinitis

with disinfectant, then use sterile, single-use, disposable needles. Occasionally, patients experience very slight bleeding or bruising at a needle site.

Warning: Extra caution must be used when acupuncture is done on patients who have a bleeding disorder or who take a blood thinner. Acupuncture should not be used during pregnancy because there is a slight risk of miscarriage.

356

Best: Verify that your acupuncturist is certified by the National Certification Commission for Acupuncture and Oriental Medicine (904-598-1005, *www.nccaom.org*)...or by your state's licensing authority. For state-by-state information, visit *www.acupuncture.com/state laws/statelaw.htm.*

Effie Poy Yew Chow, PhD, RN, founder and president of East West Academy of Healing Arts in San Francisco (*www. eastwestqi.com*) and California-licensed acupuncturist.

Qigong for Beginners

The Chinese wellness system qigong (chee-GONG) combines four ancient practices, all meant to harness the body's self-healing powers. The basics are easy to learn and easy on the body, and they can be done at home. Here are samples of qigong movements and methods. Practice each daily to generate vitality and promote healing.

Body Movement

Slow, gentle exercises build awareness of posture...increase strength, endurance and flexibility...and unlike vigorous exercises, do not cause injury or consume internal resources (such as energy) to fuel muscles.

●**Gentle bending of the spine.** Stand with feet shoulder-width apart, knees slightly bent. Inhaling, raise arms above head, elbows slightly bent and palms facing skyward ...tip head back and tilt the pelvis, arching back slightly. On the exhalation, bend elbows and bring arms down in front of you, hands fisted and pressed together...tuck chin to chest, tilt the pelvis under and round your back. Repeat five to 10 times.

Breath Practice

Deep breathing sends more oxygen-rich blood toward tissues...and "pumps" lymph fluid through the lymphatic system, a major part of the immune system.

●**Gathering breath.** Sit with hands in your lap. Inhaling through the nose, move hands outward and upward, scooping up healing energy, until hands are just above face level, palms toward you and elbows slightly bent. Exhaling slowly, bring hands toward you, then downward past the chest and navel. Repeat five to 10 times.

Massage

Reflexes refer to areas of the body that are separated physically, yet linked via acupuncture and energy channels. Self-massage of points on the hands, ears and feet has a healing effect on the organs, joints or tissues to which these reflexes connect.

●**Healing hand massage.** Grasp your left hand with your right hand, thumb against the palm and fingers on the back of the hand. Starting gently and gradually increasing the pressure, knead your left hand, including fingers and wrist. Spend extra time on any sore points— these areas are linked to body functions and organs that are not operating optimally. Continue for three to five minutes, then switch hands.

Meditation

Stress overstimulates the nervous system and exhausts the adrenal glands (which secrete stress hormones). Meditation counteracts stress, enhancing healing brain chemicals and hormones.

●**Qigong meditation.** Stand, sit or lie comfortably. Inhale fully, imagining you are drawing in *qi* (vitality) from the universe through hundreds of energy gates (acupuncture points) all over your body's surface. Exhale slowly, visualizing healing resources circulating inside you. Continue for five to 15 minutes, mentally directing the healing flow to wherever your body needs it most.

Illustrations by Shawn Banner.

Roger Jahnke, OMD, board-certified doctor of oriental medicine, author of *The Healer Within* (HarperSanFrancisco), and director of the Institute of Integral Qigong and Tai Chi and CEO of Health Action Synergies, both in Santa Barbara, California. *www.instituteofintegralqigongandtaichi.org*.

Surprising Benefits of Biofeedback

The 1970s was an era of bizarre fads and funky ideas like the Pet Rock. Those disappeared quickly—but at least one idea that seemed weird then not only had staying power, but also proved visionary.

Mood rings, made with liquid crystal that changes color based on body temperature, were marketed as a tool to gauge state of mind. These novelties were an early form of biofeedback. Biofeedback was being studied in the 1970s, with research continuing even now, and it has become a highly sophisticated therapy for a host of different health challenges. In fact, even the American Cancer Society acknowledges that biofeedback can help improve cancer patients' quality of life and certain associated health conditions.

Celeste De Bease, PhD, the former chair of the Biofeedback Certification Institute of America, has taught biofeedback therapy for many years and practices it in Bala Cynwyd, Pennsylvania.

Are You "Over-reactive?"

Dr. De Bease explains that ideally the alarm or arousal levels people experience should be appropriate to the situations they encounter, but that's often not what happens. Many people chronically over-respond to stress and others go through daily life on "high alert" even when nothing particularly stressful is happening. Dr. De Bease calls this having a "hyperactive idling speed." Though they may have no clue that this is happening, they pay a high price in stress-related fatigue and illnesses. Through biofeedback, says Dr.

De Bease, such people can learn to "uncouple the primitive and physically taxing survival response of fight or flight from situations that do not call for it."

Biofeedback is used for a wide swath of disorders, many associated with some degree of stress, including Raynaud's disease, urinary incontinence, ADHD, fibromyalgia, anxiety, epilepsy, high blood pressure, migraine and other headaches, sleep disorders, IBS and tinnitus. Treatment usually starts with a psycho-physiological stress test in which people are exposed to stress-inducing situations, such as recounting a stressful experience or hearing a sudden loud noise. They are hooked up to equipment that measures the physical responses to determine their individual levels of reactivity and how long it takes them to recover afterward. Machines used in biofeedback therapy measure muscle tension, blood flow, heart rate and skin temperature, as well as sweat gland activity—all are extremely sensitive to thoughts and feelings. Additional equipment identifies brain activity (neurofeedback), which includes alpha waves (calm relaxation), beta (alert), theta (meditation and light sleep) and delta waves (deep sleep).

Learning a Better Way Through Biofeedback

Once problems are identified, the therapist uses various techniques to retrain clients to improve their physiological responses. One area of change centers on releasing muscle tension. This is the easiest biofeedback goal to achieve, says Dr. De Bease, because we control many of our muscles voluntarily. Then the work moves on to learning control of the autonomic nervous system, which affects vasoconstriction. For example, people who have Raynaud's disease often have cold hands, caused by constriction in the blood vessels leading to them. Biofeedback teaches them to focus on learning how to uncouple this subconscious response and pay attention to what triggered it.

Another key diagnostic area centers on heart rate. Normally the heart beats faster on inhalation and slows with exhalation (variability), but that pattern can be disrupted in people who are chronically stressed and whose hearts remain at a fast-paced "ready" rate. People can learn to normalize this heartbeat with breathing exercises, which Dr. De Bease explains is "a great bridge for helping people to balance the influences from the two components of autonomic nervous system function—sympathetic (preparing for attack) and parasympathetic (calm and relaxation)." Eventually people learn to consciously make changes that can affect their autonomic responses, including heart rate and perspiration. Rather than becoming inappropriately stressed yet again, you can learn to modify your response to fit the situation.

The Body-Mind Link

Dr. De Bease observes that using the body to calm the mind is exactly the opposite of the usual path in the Western world, where many believe that if you "think it, you can make it so." Biofeedback works in reverse, she says: "Change your body and it will change your mind." It's a tactic that reminds me of being told to smile when upset or angry—however silly you feel with a grin on your angry face, it does seem impossible to stay mad.

Much of the stress in our culture comes from time constraints and attempts to multitask, thinking about several things at once, says Dr. De Bease. When you find yourself overstressing because of commitments or distractions or fear of not getting everything done, slow down and regulate your breathing. Breathing slowly in and out will help balance the function of the parasympathetic and sympathetic nervous system, allowing for a more appropriate autonomic response to external stressful stimuli.

Biofeedback can help all sorts of health problems—and is generally considered safe. You can find a practitioner near you by going to the Web site of the Biofeedback Certification Institute of America (*www.bcia.org*). Most biofeedback sessions run about 45 minutes and cost in the same range as psychotherapy. Insurance generally pays at least part of the cost—sometimes all, depending on your health condition. Don't expect to solve your problems in one visit, however. Most people require a session a week for 20 weeks or so and some may continue even longer.

Celeste De Bease, PhD, former chair of the Biofeedback Certification Institute of America, biofeedback therapy teacher and therapist, Bala Cynwyd, Pennsylvania. *www.bioneurofeedback.com.*

INDEX

ABOUT THE AUTHOR

Bill Gottlieb is a health educator and author of seven books, including *Alternative Cures* (Ballantine), *Speed Healing* (Bottom Line Books), *Breakthroughs in Drug-Free Healing* (Bottom Line Books) and *The Natural Fat-Loss Pharmacy* (Broadway). His articles on health and healing have appeared in *Bottom Line Personal*, *Bottom Line Health*, *Reader's Digest*, *Prevention*, *Men's Health*, *Self* and many other national publications. He is the former editor-in-chief of Rodale Books and Prevention Magazine Books. He lives in northern California.